Cartilage and Osteoarthritis

METHODS IN MOLECULAR MEDICINE™

John M. Walker, SERIES EDITOR

111. **Chemosensitivity:** *Volume 2, In Vivo Models, Imaging, and Molecular Regulators,* edited by *Rosalyn D. Blumethal, 2005*
110. **Chemosensitivity:** *Volume 1, In Vitro Assays,* edited by *Rosalyn D. Blumethal, 2005*
109. **Adoptive Immunotherapy,** *Methods and Protocols,* edited by *Burkhard Ludewig and Matthias W. Hoffman, 2005*
108. **Hypertension,** *Methods and Protocols,* edited by *Jérôme P. Fennell and Andrew H. Baker, 2005*
107. **Human Cell Culture Protocols,** *Second Edition,* edited by *Joanna Picot, 2005*
106. **Antisense Therapeutics,** *Second Edition,* edited by *M. Ian Phillips, 2005*
105. **Developmental Hematopoiesis:** *Methods and Protocols,* edited by *Margaret H. Baron, 2005*
104. **Stroke Genomics:** *Methods and Reviews,* edited by *Simon J. Read and David Virley, 2004*
103. **Pancreatic Cancer:** *Methods and Protocols,* edited by *Gloria H. Su, 2004*
102. **Autoimmunity:** *Methods and Protocols,* edited by *Andras Perl, 2004*
101. **Cartilage and Osteoarthritis:** *Volume 2, Structure and In Vivo Analysis,* edited by *Frédéric De Ceuninck, Massimo Sabatini, and Philippe Pastoureau, 2004*
100. **Cartilage and Osteoarthritis:** *Volume 1, Cellular and Molecular Tools,* edited by *Massimo Sabatini, Philippe Pastoureau, and Frédéric De Ceuninck, 2004*
99. **Pain Research:** *Methods and Protocols,* edited by *David Z. Luo, 2004*
98. **Tumor Necrosis Factor:** *Methods and Protocols,* edited by *Angelo Corti and Pietro Ghezzi, 2004*
97. **Molecular Diagnosis of Cancer:** *Methods and Protocols, Second Edition,* edited by *Joseph E. Roulston and John M. S. Bartlett, 2004*
96. **Hepatitis B and D Protocols:** *Volume 2, Immunology, Model Systems, and Clinical Studies,* edited by *Robert K. Hamatake and Johnson Y. N. Lau, 2004*
95. **Hepatitis B and D Protocols:** *Volume 1, Detection, Genotypes, and Characterization,* edited by *Robert K. Hamatake and Johnson Y. N. Lau, 2004*
94. **Molecular Diagnosis of Infectious Diseases,** *Second Edition,* edited by *Jochen Decker and Udo Reischl, 2004*
93. **Anticoagulants, Antiplatelets, and Thrombolytics,** edited by *Shaker A. Mousa, 2004*
92. **Molecular Diagnosis of Genetic Diseases,** *Second Edition,* edited by *Rob Elles and Roger Mountford, 2004*
91. **Pediatric Hematology:** *Methods and Protocols,* edited by *Nicholas J. Goulden and Colin G. Steward, 2003*
90. **Suicide Gene Therapy:** *Methods and Reviews,* edited by *Caroline J. Springer, 2004*
89. **The Blood–Brain Barrier:** *Biology and Research Protocols,* edited by *Sukriti Nag, 2003*
88. **Cancer Cell Culture:** *Methods and Protocols,* edited by *Simon P. Langdon, 2003*
87. **Vaccine Protocols,** *Second Edition,* edited by *Andrew Robinson, Michael J. Hudson, and Martin P. Cranage, 2003*
86. **Renal Disease:** *Techniques and Protocols,* edited by *Michael S. Goligorsky, 2003*
85. **Novel Anticancer Drug Protocols,** edited by *John K. Buolamwini and Alex A. Adjei, 2003*
84. **Opioid Research:** *Methods and Protocols,* edited by *Zhizhong Z. Pan, 2003*
83. **Diabetes Mellitus:** *Methods and Protocols,* edited by *Sabire Özcan, 2003*
82. **Hemoglobin Disorders:** *Molecular Methods and Protocols,* edited by *Ronald L. Nagel, 2003*
81. **Prostate Cancer Methods and Protocols,** edited by *Pamela J. Russell, Paul Jackson, and Elizabeth A. Kingsley, 2003*
80. **Bone Research Protocols,** edited by *Miep H. Helfrich and Stuart H. Ralston, 2003*
79. **Drugs of Abuse:** *Neurological Reviews and Protocols,* edited by *John Q. Wang, 2003*
78. **Wound Healing:** *Methods and Protocols,* edited by *Luisa A. DiPietro and Aime L. Burns, 2003*
77. **Psychiatric Genetics:** *Methods and Reviews,* edited by *Marion Leboyer and Frank Bellivier, 2003*
76. **Viral Vectors for Gene Therapy:** *Methods and Protocols,* edited by *Curtis A. Machida, 2003*

METHODS IN MOLECULAR MEDICINE™

Cartilage and Osteoarthritis

VOLUME 2

Structure and In Vivo Analysis

Edited by

Frédéric De Ceuninck

Massimo Sabatini

Philippe Pastoureau

Division de Rhumatologie
Institut de Recherches Servier
Suresnes, France

HUMANA PRESS ✻ TOTOWA, NEW JERSEY

Softcover reprint of the hardcover 1st edition 2004
999 Riverview Drive, Suite 208
Totowa, New Jersey 07512

www.humanapress.com

This publication is printed on acid-free paper. ∞
ANSI Z39.48-1984 (American Standards Institute)

Permanence of Paper for Printed Library Materials.

Cover design by Patricia F. Cleary.
Cover illustrations: Stained sections of normal (background) and osteoarthritic cartilage (foreground). Artwork courtesy of Massimo Sabatini, Philippe Pastoureau, and Frédéric De Ceuninck.

For additional copies, pricing for bulk purchases, and/or information about other Humana titles, contact Humana at the above address or at any of the following numbers: Tel.: 973-256-1699; Fax: 973-256-8341; E-mail: humana@humanapr.com; or visit our Website: www.humanapress.com

10 9 8 7 6 5 4 3 2 1

eISBN 1-59259-821-8

ISSN 1543-1894

Library of Congress Cataloging-in-Publication Data

Cartilage and osteoarthritis.
p. ; cm. — (Methods in molecular medicine ; 100, etc.)
Contents: v. 1. Cellular and molecular tools / edited by Massimo Sabatini, Philippe Pastoureau, Frédéric De Ceuninck.
Includes bibliographical references and index.
ISBN 978-1-61737-606-1 e-ISBN 978-1-59259-821-2
1. Cartilage cells—Laboratory manuals. 2. Osteoarthritis—Laboratory manuals. I. Sabatini, Massimo. II. Pastoureau, Philippe. III. De Ceuninck, Frédéric. IV. Series.
[DNLM: 1. Chondrocytes—pathology. 2. Osteoarthritis. 3. Chondrocytes—metabolism. WE 348 C3268 2004]
QP88.23.C36 2004
616.7'223—dc22

200302809

Preface

Osteoarthritis (OA), the most common form of arthritis, is generally characterized by a slowly progressive degeneration of articular cartilage, particularly in the weight-bearing joints. It has a stronger prevalence in women, and its incidence increases with age. OA is a major and growing health concern in developed countries, owing to steadily increasing life expectancy and the demand for better quality of life. Because of its chronic nature and nonfatal outcome, OA affects the growing population of the elderly over an increasing time span. Moreover, despite its relatively benign character, OA is one of the most disabling diseases; it is responsible for increasing financial and social burdens in terms of medical treatments, forced inactivity, loss of mobility, and dependence.

Despite a growing awareness of OA as a medical problem that has yet to reach its maximum impact on society, there is a surprising absence of effective medical treatments beyond pain control and surgery. So far, only symptom-modifying drugs are available, while a major demand remains for disease-modifying treatments of proven clinical efficacy. This demand will hopefully be met in the future by some of the drugs that have been pressed into development and are now at different stages of clinical investigation. Nevertheless, the current lack of effective treatments reflects a still insufficient knowledge of cartilage with respect to its metabolism, interactions with other joint tissues, and causes and mechanisms (possibly of very different nature) that lead to failure of its turnover. As is seen in other therapeutic fields, the future availability of better drugs will depend on a deeper knowledge of OA physiopathology, allowing rational definition of new molecular targets for pharmacological intervention. This new interest in OA is fostering an intense research effort both in academic institutions and in the pharmaceutical industry.

In this context, two volumes of the *Methods in Molecular Medicine*™ series are dedicated to research protocols on cartilage and osteoarthritis. *Cartilage and Osteoarthritis*, Volume 1: *Cellular and Molecular Tools* combines classical but still evolving techniques with emerging methods that promise to add critical knowledge to cartilage metabolism in health and disease. Authors with hands-on expertise have described protocols for the in vitro study of normal and osteoarthritic cartilage through biochemical, biomolecular, immunological, and physical approaches. Volume 2: *Structure and In Vivo Analysis* is dedicated to procedures for study at the tissue level of turnover, structure, and functioning of normal and diseased articular cartilage, through invasive and noninvasive means.

We hope and expect that these two volumes constitute a welcome addition to the literature of research protocols, as well as a helpful and trusted laboratory companion.

Frédéric De Ceuninck
Massimo Sabatini
Philippe Pastoureau

Acknowledgments

We would like to thank Corinne Morlat, Research Assistant, Institut de Recherches Servier, for her invaluable secretarial help in editing this book.

Contents of Volume 2

Structure and In Vivo Analysis

Contents of Companion Volume

Volume 1: *Cellular and Molecular Tools*

Contributors

Thomas Aigner • *Cartilage Research, Department of Pathology, University of Erlangen-Nürnberg, Erlangen, Germany*
Klaus Arnold • *Institute of Medical Physics and Biophysics, Medical Department, University of Leipzig, Leipzig, Germany*
Won C. Bae • *Department of Bioengineering and Whitaker Institute of Biomedical Engineering, University of California, San Diego, La Jolla, CA*
Olivier Beuf • *Laboratoire de RMN, CNRS UMR 5012 et Plate-forme Animage, Université Claude Bernard Lyon I –ESCPE, Lyons, France*
Albert C. Chen • *Department of Bioengineering and Whitaker Institute of Biomedical Engineering, University of California, San Diego, La Jolla, CA*
Agnès Chomel • *Division de Rhumatologie, Institut de Recherches Servier, Suresnes, France*
Frédéric De Ceuninck • *Division de Rhumatologie, Institut de Recherches Servier, Suresnes, France*
Pierre D. Delmas • *INSERM Unit 403, Pavillon F, Hôpital E. Herriot, Lyon, France*
Felix Eckstein • *Institute of Anatomy, Paracelsus Medical Private University, Salzburg, Austria*
Klaus Engelke • *Institute of Medical Physics, University of Erlangen, Erlangen, Germany*
Beate Fuchs • *Institute of Medical Physics and Biophysics, Medical Department, University of Leipzig, Leipzig, Germany*
Patrick Garnero • *INSERM Unit 403 and SYNARC, Lyon, France*
Steffen Gay • *Center for Experimental Rheumatology, Department of Rheumatology, University Hospital Zürich, Zürich, Switzerland*
Peter Ghosh • *The Institute of Bone and Joint Research, The University of Sydney (Department of Surgery) at the Royal North Shore Hospital, St. Leonards, Australia*
Kenneth R. Gratz • *Department of Bioengineering and Whitaker Institute of Biomedical Engineering, University of California, San Diego, La Jolla, CA*
Caroline D. Hoemann • *Department of Chemical Engineering, École Polytechnique de Montréal, Montréal, Quebec, Canada*
Daniel Huster • *Junior Research Group "Solid-state NMR Studies of the Structure of Membrane-Associated Proteins," Biotechnological Biomedical Center/Institute of Medical Physics and Biophysics, Medical Department, University of Leipzig, Leipzig, Germany*

MARTIN JUDEX • *Department of Internal Medicine I, University of Regensburg, Germany; Sidney Kimmel Cancer Center, San Diego, CA*
JÖRN KAUFMANN • *Clinics of Neurology II, Medical Department, University of Magdeburg, Germany*
STEPHEN M. KLISCH • *Department of Mechanical Engineering, California State University, San Luis Obispo, San Luis Obispo, CA*
ROBERT KNAUSS • *Institute of Medical Physics and Biophysics, Medical Faculty, University of Leipzig, Leipzig, Germany*
ALEXANDER KUHLMANN • *Cartilage Research, Department of Pathology, University of Erlangen-Nürnberg, Erlangen, Germany*
PASCAL LAUGIER • *Laboratoire d'Imagerie Paramétrique, Université Paris VI–CNRS UMR 7623, Faculté de Médecine Broussais, Hôtel-Dieu, Paris, France*
SANDRA MARTELLI • *Istituti Ortopedici Rizzoli, Laboratorio di Biomeccanica, Italian Ministry of Healthcare, Bologna, Italy*
KEVIN B. MCGOWAN • *Department of Bioengineering and Whitaker Institute of Biomedical Engineering, University of California, San Diego, La Jolla, CA*
JAMES MELROSE • *The Institute of Bone and Joint Research, The University of Sydney (Department of Surgery) at the Royal North Shore Hospital, St. Leonards, Australia*
ULF MÜLLER-LADNER • *Department of Internal Medicine I, University of Regensburg, Germany*
LAMA NAJI • *Department of Natural Sciences, Institute of Experimental Physics, Magdeburg, Germany*
ELENA NEUMANN • *Department of Internal Medicine I, University of Regensburg, Germany*
WILFRED NGWA • *Institute of Medical Physics and Biophysics, Medical Faculty, University of Leipzig, Leipzig, Germany*
PHILIPPE PASTOUREAU • *Division de Rhumatologie, Institut de Recherches Servier, Suresnes, France*
JEAN-CHARLES ROUSSEAU • *INSERM Unit 403, Pavillon F, Hôpital E. Herriot, Lyon, France*
ANNA-MARJA SÄÄMÄNEN • *Department of Medical Biochemistry and Molecular Biology, University of Turku, Turku, Finland*
MASSIMO SABATINI • *Division de Rhumatologie, Institut de Recherches Servier, Suresnes, France*
ROBERT L. SAH • *Department of Bioengineering and Whitaker Institute of Biomedical Engineering, University of California, San Diego, La Jolla, CA*
AMENA SAÏED • *Laboratoire d'Imagerie Paramétrique, Université Paris VI–CNRS UMR 7623, Faculté de Médecine Broussais, Hôtel-Dieu, Paris, France*

LINDA J. SANDELL • *Department of Orthopaedic Surgery, Washington University School of Medicine at Barnes-Jewish Hospital, St Louis, MO*

JÜRGEN SCHILLER • *Institute of Medical Physics and Biophysics, Medical Faculty, University of Leipzig, Leipzig, Germany*

BARBARA L. SCHUMACHER • *Department of Bioengineering and Whitaker Institute of Biomedical Engineering, University of California, San Diego, La Jolla, CA*

SUSAN SMITH • *The Institute of Bone and Joint Research, The University of Sydney (Department of Surgery) at the Royal North Shore Hospital, St. Leonards, Australia*

STEPHAN SOEDER • *Cartilage Research, Department of Pathology, University of Erlangen-Nürnberg, Erlangen, Germany*

MICHELE M. TEMPLE • *Department of Bioengineering and Whitaker Institute of Biomedical Engineering, University of California, San Diego, La Jolla, CA*

ROBERT TRAMPEL • *Max Planck Institute for Human Cognitive and Brain Sciences, Germany*

EERO VUORIO • *Department of Medical Biochemistry and Molecular Biology, University of Turku, Turku, Finland*

LYDIA WACHSMUTH • *Institute of Medical Physics, University of Erlangen, Erlangen, Germany*

STEFANO ZAFFAGNINI • *Istituti Ortopedici Rizzoli, Laboratorio di Biomeccanica, Italian Ministry of Healthcare, Bologna, Italy*

1

Generation and Use of Transgenic Mice As Models of Osteoarthritis

Anna-Marja Säämänen and Eero Vuorio

Summary

The term osteoarthritis (OA) represents a group of diseases characterized by gradual degradation of articular cartilage and a number of associated degenerative processes within the joint. Consequently, no single animal model is likely to fulfil all the criteria of OA. The present chapter discusses the possibilities of using transgenic technologies for modification of the mouse genome to generate animal models of OA. After discussing the different approaches available, we provide an example of the generation of a traditional transgenic mouse strain and describe techniques and practical aspects of genotyping as well as the preparation of skeletal samples for radiological, histological, immunohistological, and molecular biologic analyses for phenotype characterization. We also present a histological grading system to evaluate the progression of OA lesions, with examples of other degenerative alterations in the knee joint structures.

Key Words: Transgenic mouse; osteoarthritis; cartilage; bone; collagen; proteoglycan; mRNA; safranin O; polarized light microscopy; joint loading; knee joint degeneration; animal model.

1. Introduction

It is now commonly agreed that osteoarthritis (OA) is not a single disease but a group of diseases with a similar final outcome, a gradual degradation of articular cartilage with a number of associated symptoms *(1)*. A logical corollary of this viewpoint is that there cannot exist any single animal model that would fulfill all the criteria of OA. Against this background, it is striking how few well-characterized animal models for OA exist *(2)*. Currently, several techniques are available for manipulation of the mouse genome, either by generating transgenic mice harboring a variety of gene constructs or by inactivating specific genes *(3)*. Despite these possibilities, only a few genetically manipu-

From: *Methods in Molecular Medicine, Vol. 101: Cartilage and Osteoarthritis, Volume 2: Structure and In Vivo Analysis*
Edited by: F. De Ceuninck, M. Sabatini, and P. Pastoureau © Humana Press Inc., Totowa, NJ

lated mouse models for OA have been reported, and even fewer have been characterized in detail *(2)*. There are probably several reasons for this. First, despite considerable research efforts, only a few candidate genes have been identified in familial human OA *(4–6)*. Consequently, only a small number of gene-protein systems are available for proof-of-concept testing through production of transgenic mice. Most of the information available concerns mutations in the proα1(II) collagen gene coding for the constituent chains of the homotrimeric type II collagen and in the proα1(IX) and proα2(IX) collagen genes coding for two of the three constituent chains of the heterotrimeric type IX collagen *(2,7)*.

Doubt about the usefulness of a small rodent is likely to be another reason for the limited number of transgenic mouse models for OA. Although remarkable differences in the size, life span, and weight distribution in articular cartilages have been presented to justify these claims, it is interesting to note that mutations affecting type II, IX, and XI collagens in the mouse result in osteoarthritic cartilage degeneration in much the same way as in humans *(2,4)*. In both species the degeneration is often associated with mild chondrodysplasia of the epi/metaphyseal type, or with arthro-ophthalmopathies of the Stickler/Wagner type *(8–12)*.

In humans, the development of OA is usually a slow and inconspicuous process. Consequently, an "ideal" mouse model should also exhibit slow progression of articular cartilage degeneration. This invariably means that large numbers of mice must be kept in animal facilities for extended periods with regular monitoring for OA symptoms. Compared with surgical models of OA, which exhibit rapid progression, experiments on transgenic mouse models are quite time-consuming and expensive, which may also contribute to the small number of transgenic models available.

The purpose of this chapter is to discuss and describe the generation and use of genetically modified mice for models of human OA. As the techniques for genetic manipulation differ depending on the gene-protein system selected, our presentation focuses on three main themes:

1. General strategies for designing genetic manipulations in mice.
2. Techniques used for monitoring and grading of OA lesions in the mouse.
3. Practical aspects of performing detailed radiographic, histological, and molecular biological analyses on OA mice.

We first consider the gene manipulative techniques in the mouse—particularly those intended for generation of a slowly progressing degenerative diseases such as OA—which are expensive and time-consuming. Thus it is imperative to pay special attention to the design of experiments involving genetic manipulation. At least three important considerations must be kept in mind:

1. Generation of animal models for OA can be based on information on human gene–protein systems known to be affected in human OA. Transgenic and targeting techniques can be used to reproduce mutations that are similar (or equivalent to) those described in human OA ***(13)***. The dominant-negative nature of most mutations affecting the triple-helical domain of collagen molecules has made it possible to use conventional transgenic techniques successfully to generate mouse models for cartilage disorders using the genes for proα1(II), α1(IX), and α2(IX) collagens. A characteristic feature of the mouse lines produced is dose-dependent severity of the mouse phenotypes: when produced at high levels, mutant α-chains result in severe, even perinatally lethal chondrodysplasias, whereas at lower expression levels the only consequence appears to be early-onset OA ***(2,14)***. The Del1 mice presented below serve as an example of the transgenic approach toward producing a mouse model for OA ***(15–19)***.
2. It is possibile to disturb normal cartilage metabolism by interfering with the expression of known or putative cartilage genes under a cartilage-specific or -inducible promoter. Such mice are generated by the transgenic approach. An example is tetracycline-regulated transcription of human collagenase-3 in transgenic mice ***(20)***. This type of approach helps to elucidate the role of specific regulatory factors, e.g., growth factors, cytokines, and signal pathway components, for the integrity of cartilage.
3. The function of a gene–protein system may be interrupted by inactivation of a specific gene (or several genes) known or expected to be normally active in articular cartilage. This approach helps us to understand the role of specific gene–protein systems for cartilage structure and metabolism. In some cases, an OA phenotype has been observed either in mice heterozygous (*Col2a1*) or homozygous (*Col9a1* and *Col11a2*) for the inactivated allele ***(21–23)***. Inactivation of noncollagenous genes expressed in cartilage, such as fibromodulin and α1-integrin, have also resulted in development of knee OA ***(24,25)***.

Yet another alternative for obtaining an animal model for OA is to characterize one of the many mouse lines harboring natural mutations predisposing them to OA ***(2)***. Some of the natural mutations have been characterized at the genomic level, making them equivalent to targeted mutations in endogenous genes. The best known examples are the heterozygous Dmm mice harboring a *Col2a1* mutation and heterozygous cho mice harboring a *Col11a1* mutation, both of which develop mild OA ***(26)***.

After the gene–protein system to be mutated and the strategy to be employed have been selected, generation of transgenic mice continues by isolation (or purchasing) of a genomic clone for the gene to be manipulated. The example presented below of transgenic Del1 mice is one of the many available for producing transgenic mice ***(15)***.

2. Materials

2.1. Generation of Transgenic Mice

2.1.1. Gene Constructs

1. Genomic clones covering the gene of interest, either isolated from phage or cosmid libraries or purchased (e.g., BAC clones, Genome Systems, St. Louis, MO).
2. Appropriate cloning tools to manipulate the gene ***(3,27)***.

2.1.2. Microinjection

1. Quick-Pick Electroelution Capsule Kit (Qiagen, Valencia, CA).
2. Elutip DEAE columns (Schleicher & Schüell, Dassel, Germany).
3. Ultrapure toxin-free water.

2.1.3. Genotyping

2.1.3.1. Isolation of Tail DNA

1. Tail solution: add 5 mL of 1 *M* Tris-HCl, pH 8.0, 20 mL of 0.5 *M* Na_2 ethylenediaminetetraacetic acid (EDTA), pH 8.0, 2 mL of 5 *M* NaCl, and 5 mL of 20% sodium dodecyl sulfate (SDS), and fill to 100 mL with dH_2O.
2. TE buffer: 10 m*M* Tris-HCl, 1 m*M* Na_2EDTA, pH 8.0. Prepare by adding 1 mL of 1 *M* Tris-HCl, pH 8.0, 0.2 mL of 0.5 *M* Na_2EDTA, pH 8.0, and fill to 100 mL with dH_2O. Autoclave.
3. Proteinase K (Promega, Madison, WI cat. no. 3021), 20 mg/mL. Dissolve in dH_2O and store at –20°C in small aliquots.
4. Phenol (Sigma Aldrich, Steinheim, Germany cat. no. P-4557) and buffer for saturated phenol, pH 10.5 (Sigma Aldrich cat. no. P-5658).
5. Chloroform, technical grade.
6. Polyethylene glycol (PEG) 6000 (Baker grade, Baker, Deventer, Holland).

2.1.3.2. Southern Hybridization

1. Appropriate restriction enzymes, preferably at high concentration (Promega).
2. TAE buffer: 40 m*M* Tris acetate, pH 8.0, 1 m*M* Na_2EDTA. Prepare 50X stock: weigh 242 g of Tris base, add 57.1 mL of glacial acetic acid and 100 mL of 0.5 *M* Na_2EDTA, pH 8.0, and fill to 1000 mL with water. Autoclave. Dilute 50-fold in dH_2O for running buffer in agarose gel electrophoresis.
3. Ethidium bromide. Prepare a 10 mg/mL stock solution in dH_2O and store the bottle in the dark. (Wrap in aluminum foil; *see* **Note 1**.)
4. 0.9% Agarose gel (SeaKem LE agarose, BMA Products, Rockland, ME) prepared in TAE. Add ethidium bromide to a final concentration of 0.5 μg/mL for visualization of DNA in ultraviolet (UV) light.
5. Hybond N+ nylon membrane (Amersham Biosciences, Piscataway, NJ).
6. Whatman 3MM filter paper.
7. 20X SSC: 0.3 *M* sodium citrate, 3 *M* NaCl. To prepare the solution, weigh 175.3 g of NaCl and 88.2 g of sodium citrate × 2 H_2O, and fill with dH_2O to 1000 mL.

8. Stop solution: to prepare BPB-Ficoll, dissolve 12.5 mg of bromphenol blue and 1 g of Ficoll 400 (Pharmacia Biotech, Uppsala, Sweden) in 5 mL of dH_2O. Store in aliquots at room temperature.

2.1.3.3. POLYMERASE CHAIN REACTION

1. Primers to amplify the region across the deletion of exon 7 and intron 7 of the mouse *Col2a1* gene:
   Ex6 primer: 5'-AAC TTC GCG GCT CAG ATG GCT G-3'.
   Ex8 primer: 5'-AGA CAC CAG GCT CGC CAG GTT C-3'.
2. Deoxynucleotides dATP, dCTP, dGTP, and dTTP. Prepare a dNTP mix of 2.5 m*M* each in RNase-free sterile distilled MilliQ water and store at –20°C.
3. *Taq* DNA polymerase (Roche Diagnostics, Mannheim, Germany).

2.2. Characterization of Osteoarthritic Phenotype in Transgenic Mice

2.2.1. Radiographic Analysis

1. Diagnostic film designed for mammography imaging (Min-RL, Kodak, Windsor, CO).
2. Faxitron X-ray cabinet system (Faxitron X-ray Corporation, Wheeling, IL).

2.2.2. Histologic Analysis

1. Phosphate-buffered saline (PBS): to prepare 10X PBS stock solution, weigh 80 g of NaCl, 21.6 g $Na_2HPO_4 \cdot 7H_2O$, 2.0 g KH_2PO_4, and 2.0 g KCl, fill to 1000 mL with dH_2O and autoclave.
2. Fixation solution: freshly prepared 4% paraformaldehyde in 1X PBS. To make 100 mL, heat 90 mL of distilled water to 60°C on a heating platform in a hood, and add 4 g of paraformaldehyde and a drop of 2 *N* NaOH (*see* **Note 2**). Close the container with aluminum foil. Turn off the heating, but keep the container on the heating platform with constant stirring to dissolve the paraformaldehyde. *Do not allow the temperature to rise above 65°C.* Add 10 mL of 10X PBS. Cool the paraformaldehyde solution on ice, and filter through a filter paper.
3. Biopsy cassettes: Uni-Cassette 4088 (Tissue-Tek, Miles, Elkhart, IN).
4. Decalcification solution: 0.1 *M* phosphate buffer, pH 7.0, 10% Na_2EDTA (*see* **Note 3**). Prepare stock solutions: 1 *M* NaH_2PO_4, 0.5 *M* Na_2HPO_4, and 20% Na_2EDTA. To dissolve Na_2EDTA, adjust the pH to 7.4–7.6 by adding solid NaOH with constant stirring. Autoclave all stock solutions for longer storage. Store at room temperature. To prepare decalcification solution, add 30.5 mL of 1 *M* NaH_2PO_4, 218.5 mL of 0.5 *M* Na_2HPO_4, 500 mL of 20% Na_2EDTA, and fill to 1000 mL with dH_2O. Autoclave for longer storage.
5. Dehydration solutions: 40, 50, and 70% ethanol (technical grade) and xylene.
6. Paraffin: Histowax, melting point 56–58°C (Histolab Products, Göteborg, Sweden).
7. Dehydration automat (Pathcenter, Shandon, Pittsburg, PA).
8. Embedding unit and stainless steel molds soaked in 5% glycerol in 70% ethanol.
9. Rotating microtome (Leica Microsystems, Heidelberg, Germany cat. no. RM 2155).

10. Disposable microtome blades, e.g., Tissue-Tek Accu-Edge Disposable Microtome Blades (Sakura Finetek, Torrance, CA).
11. Cardboard boxes, e.g., 1.0 × 20 × 30 cm.
12. SuperFrost® Plus Microscope Slides (Menzel Gläser, Göttingen, Germany).
13. Delafield's hematoxylin: mix 16 g of hematoxylin (Fluka Riedel de Haën, Buchs, Germany cat. no. 51260) and 100 mL of 94 % ethanol. Dissolve hematoxylin in ethanol by heating slightly and slowly. Add 1600 mL of saturated ammonium sulfate into solution. Leave in an open container for 3–5 d. Filter, and add 400 mL of glycerol (87%, Merck, Whitehouse Station, NJ cat. no. 4094) and 400 mL of 94% ethanol. Leave in daylight for 1–2 mo. Store in the dark after the solution is ready. Filter just before every use (*see* **Note 4**).
14. 1% eosin solution in ethanol: mix 25 g of eosin Y (BDH, Poole, UK cat. no. 34197) and 500 mL of dH_2O and add 2000 mL of 94% ethanol. Just before use for staining, add 0.5 mL glacial acetic acid per 100 mL of dye solution and filter.
15. 1% HCl, 70% ethanol: mix 1400 mL of 94% ethanol and 600 mL of dH_2O. Then pour 20 mL of strong HCl slowly into ethanol solution. Remember to do it in this order to prevent excess heating of the solution.
16. 0.5% Safranin O (Fisher, Fair Lawn, NJ), in 0.1 *M* NaAc, pH 4.6. Dissolve 2.5 g of safranin O in 500 mL of sodium acetate buffer, allow to dissolve overnight, and filter before use. Store in the dark.
17. 1000 U/mL Testicular hyaluronidase (EC 3.2.1.35, type IV-S from bovine testes, Sigma Aldrich): prepare freshly in 0.1 *M* Na-phosphate, pH 6.9.
18. DPX mounting medium (Difco, West Molesey, UK).
19. Cover slips (Knittel-Gläser, Germany).

2.2.3. Isolation of Total RNA From Skeletal Tissues

1. Liquid nitrogen.
2. Tissue pulverization unit (*see* **Note 5**).
3. Diethyl pyrocarbonate (DEPC; Sigma Aldrich).
4. GIT solution: 4 *M* guanidinium isothiocyanate (GIT), 25 m*M* sodium citrate, pH 7.0, 0.5% SDS, 0.7% β-mercaptoethanol, 0.1% antifoam A (Sigma Aldrich cat. no. A-5758). To prepare the solution, add 50 g of GIT (Fluka BioChemica, Buchs, Germany), 0.5 g of SDS, 2.5 mL of 1 *M* sodium citrate, pH 7.0, 0.7 mL of β-mercaptoethanol, 0.33 mL of 30% antifoam A and fill with dH_2O to 100 mL. Stir overnight at room temperature, filter through glass fiber paper and a 0.45-μm filter (Nalgene, Nalge Nunc International, Rochester, NY). Adjust pH to 7.0 with 1 *N* NaOH.
5. 5.7 *M* CsCl, 25 m*M* sodium citrate, pH 5.0, DEPC-treated: to prepare the solution, add 95.8 g of CsCl (technical grade, molecular biology certified, IBI Shelton Scientific, Shelton, CT), 2.5 mL of 1 *M* sodium citrate, pH 5 (25 m*M*), 0.2 mL of DEPC, fill with dH_2O to 100 mL, leave in a hood overnight, and autoclave.
6. Ultracentrifuge (Beckman Optima cat. no. LE-80K) equipped with a swing-out rotor (Beckman cat. no. SW 55TI) and ultracentrifuge tubes (Polyallomer, 13 × 51 mm, Beckman Instruments, Palo Alto, CA).

7. DEPC-treated dH_2O: add 0.2 mL of DEPC to 100 mL of dH_2O, leave in hood overnight, and autoclave.
8. 3 *M* NaAc, pH 5.5: prepare 100 mL of buffer, add 0.2 mL of DEPC, leave in a hood overnight, and autoclave.
9. SET buffer, 10 m*M* Tris-HCl, pH 7.5, 4 m*M* Na_2EDTA, 1% SDS, DEPC-treated: add 5 mL of 20% SDS (1%) prepared in DEPC-treated water, 0.8 mL of 0.5 *M* DEPC-treated Na_2EDTA, pH 7.5, and 1 mL of 1 *M* DEPC-treated Tris-HCl, pH 7.5 (10 m*M*). Fill with dH_2O to 100 mL and autoclave.
10. 20 mg/mL Proteinase K, RNase-free (Promega cat. no. V 3021). Dissolve in DEPC-treated dH_2O and store at –20°C in small aliquots.
11. RNase-free Eppendorf tubes, pipet tips, and glass Pasteur pipets.
12. Disposable scalpels.

3. Methods

3.1. Generation of Transgenic Mice

3.1.1. The Gene Construct

After isolation of the complete gene for mouse *Col2a1* gene coding for the proα1(II) collagen chain ***(28)***, the detailed planning for a dominant-negative mutation was based on the nucleotide sequence and the restriction map of the gene. **Figure 1** summarizes the cloning steps used to generate the construct for microinjection. To remove exon 7 and intron 7 sequences, a genomic subclone was digested with *Apa*I, which released a 150-bp fragment containing both the exon and the intron ***(15)***. Ligation recreated a splice signal followed by an exon 8 sequence. As exon 7 contained 45 bp, the deletion resulted in an in-frame deletion and shortening of the resultant proα1(II) chain by 15 amino acids (five complete Gly-X-Y triplets). Reassembly of the complete mutant *Col2a1* gene was produced by subsequent cloning steps, as illustrated in **Fig. 1**. The final construct for microinjection thus carried 3 kb of (endogenous) promoter sequence, the entire 5'-untranslated sequence, all exons and introns (excluding exon 7 and intron 7), the entire 3'-untranslated sequence and 7 kb of the 3'-flanking sequence. With this and other similar constructs, good tissue specificity and copy number-dependent expression have been obtained in transgenic mice ***(15,29,30)***.

3.1.2. Microinjection

For successful microinjection, the DNA construct has to be exhaustively purified using any of the existing protocols ***(3)***. One of the recent protocols we have used for construct purification involves cleavage of the construct from the vector by appropriate restriction enzymes and purification by a Quick-Pick Electroelution Capsule Kit and Elutip DEAE columns. For microinjection, the DNA is diluted to a final concentration of 2 ng/L in embryo-tested (toxin-free)

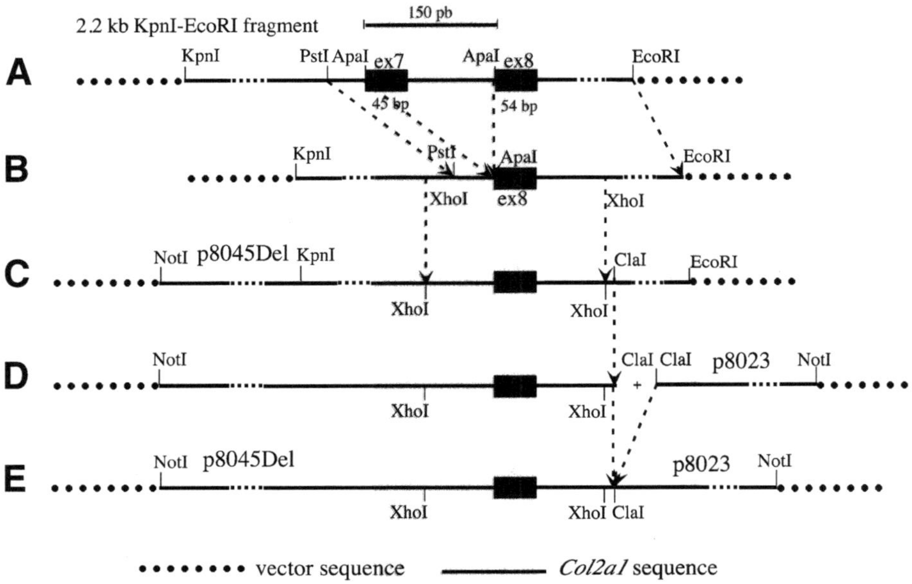

Fig. 1. Generation of the Del1 contruct. A 0.8-kb *Pst*I-*Eco*RI fragment was removed from a 2.2-kb *Kpn*I-*Eco*RI genomic clone, and subcloned. **(A)** Deletion was generated by removal of a 150-bp *Apa*I fragment from a *Pst*I-*Eco*RI clone. A shortened *Pst*I-*Eco*RI fragment was subcloned back to a 2.2-kb *Kpn*I-*Eco*RI clone (**B**), followed by subcloning of an *Xho*I-*Xho*I fragment into genomic clone p8045, containing the 5' half of the gene (**C**). **(D)** The gene was reconstituted by addition of a 26-kb *Cla*I fragment from clone p8023, which contained the 3' half of the gene. **(E)** The reconstituted gene was liberated from the cosmid vector by *Not*I digestion and subjected to microinjection after exhaustive purification.

Ultrapure water. Transgenic founder mice can then be generated in the desired genetic background by microinjecting the DNA into pronuclei of fertilized oocytes using standard techniques *(3)*. It is advisable to have the next steps (purification of fertilized oocytes, the actual microinjection step, and reintroduction of the oocytes into recipient mice) be performed by a transgenic core facility, as the techniques employed require considerable experience. A detailed laboratory manual of the techniques is available for those interested *(3)*.

3.1.3. Genotyping

The next step the investigator is likely to be involved in is genotyping the offspring of recipient female mice. For this purpose DNA will have to be extracted from the pups (usually from the tails) for analysis by both Southern

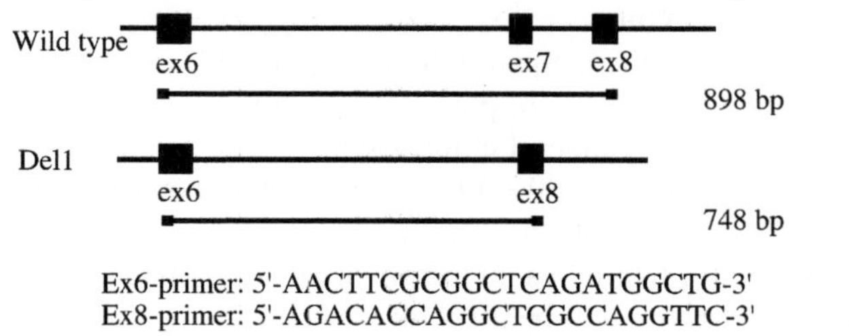

Fig. 2. Genotyping by polymerase chain reaction (PCR). Transgenic and wild-type mice were identified by amplification of a genomic DNA fragment defined by primers from the beginning of exon 6 (Ex6-primer) and the end of exon 8 (Ex8-primer). Since transgenic mice contain both the transgene and the wild-type *Col2a1* gene, two PCR products are observed on the agarose gel, a 748-bp transgene fragment and a 898-bp wild-type fragment. The amplified fragments are shown as lines, with the black boxes at each end denoting the primers.

hybridization and polymerase chain reaction (PCR). In most cases it is important to know the number of transgene copies integrated into the genome of the transgenic mice produced. This can be estimated by Southern hybridization using the two endogenous genes and a dilution series of transgenes for reference. The transgene-positive mice (referred to as founder mice) will then be subjected to a mating program to produce animals for the actual experiments. Southern analysis is also needed later to identify heterozygous and homozygous embryos of heterozygote × heterozygote breedings.

It is advisable to plan the transgene construct in a way that allows for easy identification of the transgene in the genome of the recipient mice. In case of the Del1 mice this could be conveniently accomplished by PCR across the site of deletion (**Fig. 2**). Since the Del1 mice homozygous for the mutation die prenatally, the transgenic strain is maintained by breeding the heterozygotes with nontransgenic mice sharing the same genetic background. Therefore the genotype of all the offspring mice has to be determined to identify the transgenics.

3.1.3.1. Isolation of DNA From Mouse Tails

1. Cut a 3–5-mm-long piece of tail and place it in an 1.5-mL Eppendorf tube.
2. Add 350 µL of tail solution (50 m*M* Tris-HCl, pH 8.0, 100 m*M* EDTA, 100 m*M* NaCl, 1% SDS) or 700 µL if the tail piece is big.
3. Add 10 µL proteinase K or 20 µL if you have used 700 µL of tail solution.
4. Incubate overnight at 55°C, and vortex during incubation, if possible.

5. Vortex and spin at full speed for 1 min in an Eppendorf microcentrifuge. Remove supernatant to a fresh tube.
6. Extract supernatant with an equal volume of phenol.
7. Extract with an equal volume of phenol/chloroform (1:1).
8. Extract with an equal volume of chloroform.
9. Add 0.4 vol (about 160 µL) 30% PEG 6000 prepared in 1.8 *M* NaCl. Mix well.
10. Incubate on ice for 2 h or at 4°C overnight.
11. Spin at full speed for 6 min in a microcentrifuge at room temperature, and decant immediately. The pellet will be difficult to see.
12. Wash by adding 1 mL of 70% ethanol at room temperature and vortex.
13. Spin at full speed for 10 min at room temperature and decant immediately; be careful not to touch the pellet. The pellet will now be clearly visible.
14. Repeat **steps 12** and **13**.
15. Dry in a speed vac and resuspend in 50–100 µL of TE buffer. Leave at 4°C for overnight to dissolve DNA properly.
16. Measure the OD of a 1:100 dilution at 280 nm. Calculate the DNA concentration.

3.1.3.2. Southern Hybridization

Digest genomic DNA overnight with appropriate restriction enzyme(s) (*Pst*I in Del1 mice) cleaving at both sides of the transgene mutation, and run on agarose gel along with copy number standards and a DNA size marker. Transfer the DNA on nitrocellulose or nylon membrane and perform Southern hybridization. Use a ^{32}P-dCTP–labeled cDNA probe covering the transgene mutation ***(15)*** to detect the wild-type and transgene fragments. Measure the relative ratios of wild-type and transgene bands visualized by autoradiography or phosphor imaging to identify the homozygous and heterozygous mice. Compare the intensities with the lanes containing different dilutions of transgene to estimate the number of integrated transgenes in the genome.

1. Digest the genomic DNA overnight with *Pst*I at 37°C:
   a. enzyme (0.8 µL of 60 U/µL).
   b. 2 µL 10X H buffer (Promega).
   c. dH_2O ad 20 µL.
2. Prepare the dilutions of transgenes for reference, if you wish to measure the copy number of transgenes in the genome. Linearize the transgene vector with appropriate restriction enzyme(s) (*Pst*I).
3. Stop the reactions by adding 2 µL of BPB-Ficoll into the tubes. Heat the tubes at 65°C for 10 min.
4. Run the samples, copy number standards, and DNA size marker on 0.9% agarose gel prepared in TAE, until BPB has migrated about 10 cm.
5. Take a digital image in 1:1 scale or a photograph with a UV-visible ruler alongside.
6. Prepare the gel for transfer, performing the treatments on a rocking or rotating platform (gently):

a. Depurinate the gel in 0.25 *M* HCl for 20 min.
b. Rinse in distilled water.
c. Denaturate in 1.5 *M* NaCl, 0.5 *M* NaOH for 30 min.
d. Rinse in distilled water.
e. Neutralize in 1.5 *M* NaCl, 0.5 *M* Tris-HCl, pH 7.2, 1 m*M* EDTA for 20 min.

7. Transfer the DNA on a Hybond N+ filter membrane by using the capillary flow of 20X SSC through the gel. Assemble the transfer tower with Whatman 3MM paper and a 5–10-cm-high stack of paper towels and weight ***(27)***. Transfer overnight.
8. After transfer, place the membrane on two Whatman 3MM paper sheets moistened in 0.4 *M* NaOH for 30 min, with the DNA side facing up. Then rinse briefly in 5X SSC and dry for 1 h on a filter paper (DNA side upward) at 80°C. Store the filter between filter papers in a dry place at room temperature until used for hybridization.
9. Prepare the probe: liberate the insert from plasmid E5.1/Pst0.8 plasmid (contains the *Pst*I-*Eco*RI fragment, as shown in **Fig. 1A**) by double digestion with *Eco*RI and *Pst*I. Use a random labeling kit (e.g., Roche or Promega) for radioactive labeling of the probe with ^{32}P-dCTP, and perform standard Southern hybridization, as suggested by the filter supplier.

3.1.3.3. Genotyping by PCR

1. Prepare the reactions: 0.5 µg genomic DNA; 4 µL dNTP mix; 75 pmol Ex6 primer; 75 pmol Ex8 primer; and 5 µL 10X Buffer.
2. 0.25 µL (1.25 U) Taq DNA polymerase.
3. Fill to 50 µL with sterile dH_2O.
4. Run the PCR program: 30 cycles of 94°C for 1 min, 57°C for 2 min, and 72°C for 2 min, with a 72°C 7-min extension, and a 4°C soak.
5. Take a 16-µL aliquot of PCR product, add 3 µL of PBP, and run on a 1% agarose gel. A 898-bp band—originating from the wild-type gene—should be observed in all samples, as well as one additional 748-bp band in samples containing the transgene (**Fig. 2**).

3.2. Characterization of Osteoarthritic Phenotype in Transgenic Mice

The phenotypic changes and development of knee OA in mice are usually first studied by means of radiography, histology, immunohistochemistry, and mRNA expression analyses (Northern hybridization, quantitative reverse transcriptase [RT]-PCR, RNase protection assay). This chapter describes the sample preparation for these studies and the OA grading analysis used to estimate the degree of joint degeneration ***(16–19)***. Sample preparation protocols for analysis of proteoglycans by safranin O staining and collagen fibril orientation by polarized light microscopy of unstained tissue sections are also described.

3.2.1. Radiography of Hind Limbs

1. Dissect the hindlimbs free of skin. Remove the fat and most of the muscle, but leave a little to protect the bone and joint structures. Wrap the hindlimbs in a piece of paper towel moistened in PBS, and place them on ice until the radiography has been performed. Then process the limbs for histology.
2. Take the X-rays in both the anterior-posterior and lateral projections. This is advisable, as possible varus deformity can be observed only in the anterior-posterior projection, whereas possible ectopic ossification (ossicles) deep to the tendon can be observed in the lateral projection. Fix the limbs on the plastic sheet in the proper orientation using tape at the peripheral sites, and place the sheet on a light-tight envelope containing the X-ray film. Take the radiographs with a Faxitron X-ray cabinet or equivalent X-ray device suitable for small-specimen radiography.
3. To analyze the radiographs, either examine them by loop or scan the films and analyze the enlarged images by using image analysis software, e.g., Adobe PhotoShop 5.0 (Adobe Systems, San Jose, CA).

3.2.2. Histological Analysis

1. Bend the knee into a 90° angle, and place it into a biopsy cassette with the patella of the bent knee facing the corner of the cassette to maintain the proper angle during fixation. If you do not wish to study the histology of the tarsal or hip joints, cut the tibial and femoral bones at the level of the middle diaphysis. This will help considerably in processing the tissue sections in later steps.
2. Fix the samples for 24 h in freshly prepared 4% paraformaldehyde in PBS on a rocking platform at 4°C.
3. Rinse in tap water: first rinse briefly, and then three times for 10 min on a rocking platform (*see* **Note 6**).
4. Decalcify the samples in 10% Na_2EDTA in PBS, pH 7.4, at room temperature on a rocking platform until they are soft. Change the solution once or twice a week. Decalcification time depends on the age of the animal. The status can be tested with a thin needle (e.g., 22 gage) at peripheral parts of the bone, or by X-ray. This is a rough estimate for the decalcification times that we have used:

Age (mouse)	Decalcification time
5 d	1 d
10 d	2–3 d
1 mo	1–2 wk
>3 mo	2–4 wk

5. When the decalcification is complete, rinse the samples thoroughly in tap water on a rocking platform, 4 × 10 min.
6. Dehydrate the samples in increasing concentrations of ethanol on a rocking platform at room temperature before embedding in paraffin: 40% ethanol for 1 h, 50% ethanol for 1 h, and 70% ethanol for 1 h. Tissue samples can be stored for a

short period (a few d or wk) in 70% ethanol at +4°C if necessary before embedding in paraffin. From this step onward, it is advisable to carry out dehydration under vacuum in an automat (Pathcenter, Shandon): 70% ethanol 1 × 1 h, 97% ethanol 5 × 1 h, xylene 2 × 50 min, paraffin 4 × 60 min (60°C).

7. Embed the tissues in paraffin either in the sagittal plane, with the lateral side facing down and taking care that the longitudinal plane of the patella is horizontal, or in the anterior–posterior plane, with the longitudinal plane of the tibial bone adjusted horizontally and the femur pointing upward. The embedding plane depends on what you wish to analyze: soft tissue calcification can best be analyzed in sagittal sections, whereas simultaneous analysis of erosions on both medial and lateral condyles and osteophytes can best be analyzed in anterior-posterior sections.
8. Using a rotating microtome, cut 5-μm serial sections through the entire block, or at least through the tibial condyles, if you have the tissue in the anterior-posterior orientation. Collect the sections into cardboard boxes and store at 4°C.
9. Pick every 20th section on the microscope slide, and dry overnight at 37°C or for 1 h at 50°C to fix the sections on slides.
10. Stain the sections with H&E:
    a. Xylene, 2 × 5 min.
    b. Absolute ethanol, 2 × 2 min.
    c. 96% Ethanol, 2 × 2 min.
    d. Distilled water, 30 s.
    e. Delafield's hematoxylin, 9 min.
    f. Running tap water, 5 min.
    g. Removal of excess dye: 1% HCl, 70% ethanol, 4–5 s.
    h. Running tap water, 10 min.
    i. 1% Eosin in ethanol, 30 s.
    j. 96% Ethanol, 2 × 2 min.
    k. Absolute ethanol, 2 × 2 min.
    l. Xylene, 3 × 5 min
    m. Mount the sections with DPX and allow to dry in a hood.
11. Examine the sections by light microscopy for characterization of the knee joint degeneration.

For characterization of glycosaminoglycan distribution, stain the sections with safranin O. If you wish to do a semiquantitative analysis of proteoglycans in tissue sections, include 0.5% safranin O in the fixation solution and in the following decalcification solution to inhibit proteglycan extraction from the tissue (**steps 2** and **4**). To cut down the dye consumption (expensive!), reduce the sample size to a minimum. Embed tissue blocks in paraffin manually (**step 6**), as the dye will partially dissolve in xylene and paraffin, and hence also stain other blocks. Cut blocks into 3-μm sections to keep absorbance values in a linear region. Safranin O stains sulfated glycosaminoglycans deep purple red.

12. Safranin O staining:
    a. Xylene, 2 × 5 min.
    b. Absolute ethanol, 2 × 2 min.
    c. 96% Ethanol, 2 × 2 min.
    d. Distilled water, 30 s.
    e. Safranin O staining solution, 10 min.
    f. Running tap water, 10 min.
    g. 96% Ethanol, 2 × 2 min.
    h. Absolute ethanol, 2 x 2 min.
    i. Xylene, 3 × 5 min
    j. Mount the sections with DPX and allow to dry in a hood.

For semiquantitative analysis of glycosaminoglycans, perform analysis with scanning microspectrophotometry of 3-μm sections ***(31)***.

13. Preparation of unstained tissue sections for polarized light microscopy ***(16,32)***. To analyze the orientation/content of collagen fibrils, prepare the paraffin sections from **step 10** as follows:
    a. Xylene, 4 × 10 min.
    b. Absolute ethanol, 2 × 2 min.
    c. 96% Ethanol, 2 × 2 min.
    d. Distilled water, 2 × 2 min.
    e. Digestion with hyaluronidase, 1000 U/mL in 0.1 *M* sodium phosphate, pH 6.9, for 18 h at 37°C in a moist chamber. Perform the following treatments gently as the sections may detach from the glass:
    f. Distilled water, 3 × 3 min; perform in horizontal plane.
    g. 96% Ethanol, 2 × 2 min.
    h. Absolute ethanol, 2 × 2 min.
    i. Xylene, 3 × 5 min.
    j. Mount the sections with DPX and allow to dry in a hood.

A sophisticated method of analyzing collagen-induced birefringency of unstained tissue sections has been developed by using a computer-assisted quantitative polarized light microscopy ***(32)***.

3.2.2.1. Grading of Degenerative Lesions

Grading of cartilage erosion in knee joints of Del1 mice is based on the classification method modified from Wilhelmi and Faust ***(16,33,34)***. Every 20th section of each tissue block (*see* **Subheading 3.2.2., step 9**) is stained with H&E, microscopically examined for the articular cartilage erosion, and graded according to the depth of erosion penetrating from the articular surface (**Fig. 3**). If more than one grade is observed within the section, the greatest score value is given to the sample (*see* **Note 7**).

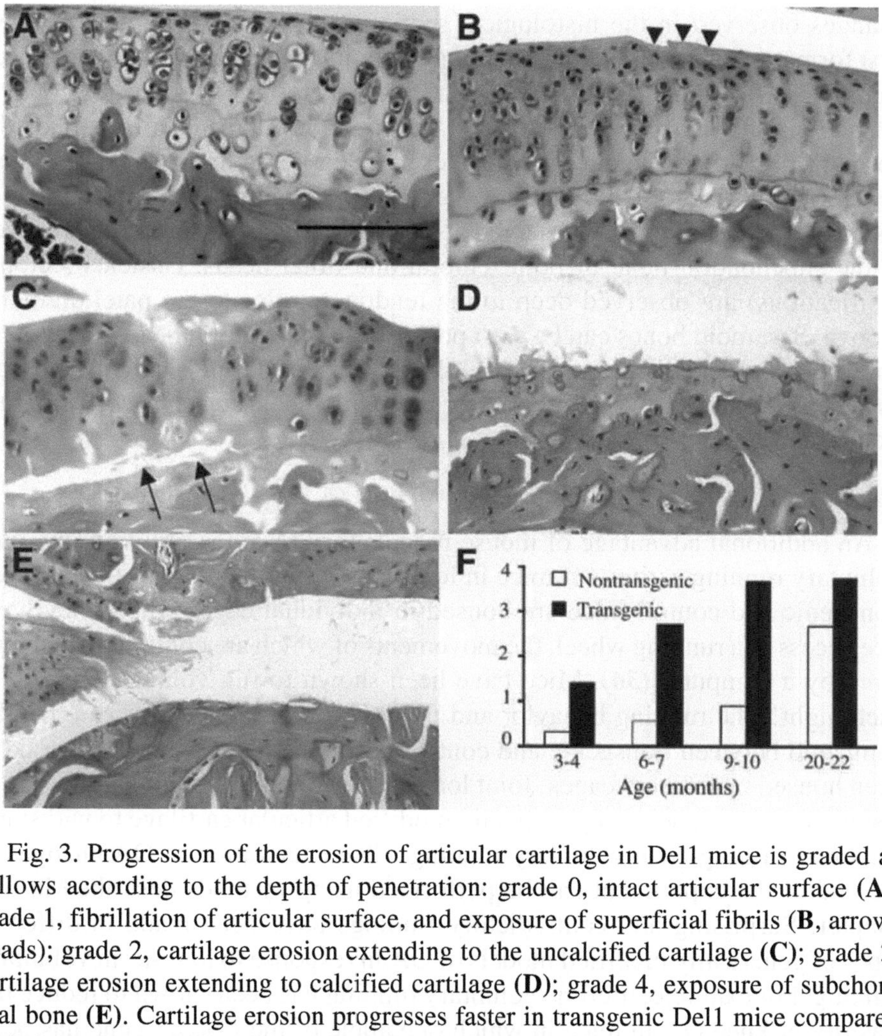

Fig. 3. Progression of the erosion of articular cartilage in Del1 mice is graded as follows according to the depth of penetration: grade 0, intact articular surface (**A**), grade 1, fibrillation of articular surface, and exposure of superficial fibrils (**B**, arrowheads); grade 2, cartilage erosion extending to the uncalcified cartilage (**C**); grade 3, cartilage erosion extending to calcified cartilage (**D**); grade 4, exposure of subchondral bone (**E**). Cartilage erosion progresses faster in transgenic Del1 mice compared with the nontransgenic controls (**F**). Columns represent the average grade values within each age group. The number of animals per group is between 3 (age 20–22 mo) and 36 (age 3–4 mo). Note also detachment of articular cartilage at the tide mark (C, arrows) and subchondral bone sclerosis in (**D**) and (**E**). Scale bar, 100 μm in (A) (also applies to B–E).

Knee joint degeneration of Del1 mice is characterized by a number of other alterations that are observed in radiographical and histological analysis of the knee joints. Radiography provides a noninvasive method to follow up the progression of knee joint degeneration but is less sensitive, and observation of the early changes requires a radiologist's trained eye. The late degenerative changes observed in the histological sections and/or in radiographs involve cyst formation in subchondral bone, fragmentation and calcification of menisci, ectopic ossifications in soft tissues, tendons, and sesamoid bones, osteophyte formation, and subchondral sclerosis. Ossification of menisci is part of the normal aging process in mice, but it takes place earlier in transgenic Del1 mice. In Del1 mice the menisci are severely fragmented and disorganized. Osteophytes are commonly observed at the age of 15 mo. Cysts can be observed in the subchondral bone of both femoral and tibial heads. Ossicles (ectopic ossifications) are observed deep to the tendon anterior to the patellofemoral groove. Sesamoid bones can be seen posterior to the femoral head. From these criteria, subchondral sclerosis, osteophytes, meniscal calcification, and soft tissue calcification, have been used for radiographical scoring of OA progression ***(24,35)***.

3.2.2.2. Effect of Loading on the Development of OA

An additional advantage of mouse models for OA is the ability to monitor voluntary running activity of mice in long-term experiments. For this purpose transgenic and control mice are housed in individual cages where they have free access to a running wheel, the movements of which are continuously monitored by a computer ***(36)***. Mice have been shown to run voluntarily 4–6 km each night! The running behavior and progression of OA defects can then be compared between transgenic and control mice, and also with mice that have been housed in ordinary cages. Joint loading by voluntary running allows us to test in vivo the capacity of genetically modified articular cartilage to withstand the stress of long-term voluntary running. Characterization of OA changes at the end of the experiment can be performed using methods described in this chapter. Surprising and contradictory findings have been made in different types of genetically modified models of OA in response to long-term voluntary running. For example, lifetime voluntary running has been shown to reduce the severity of knee OA in mice in which one allele of the *Col2a1* gene has been inactivated ***(22)***. In contrast, a similar running program increased the severity of knee OA in the lateral compartment of Del1 transgenic mice ***(37)***. The differences between these two types of mutations in response to running probably reflect distinct mechanisms by which OA develops in these mice.

3.2.3. Isolation of Total RNA From Skeletal Tissues

RNA isolation from tissues rich in fibrillar collagen and proteoglycans and of low cell density is a difficult task. Another problem in the isolation of RNA from mouse knee joints is a small sample size. The sampling method presented here was adopted as a result of compromise since dissecting of articular cartilage from the knee epiphyses was too time-consuming and the RNA yield too

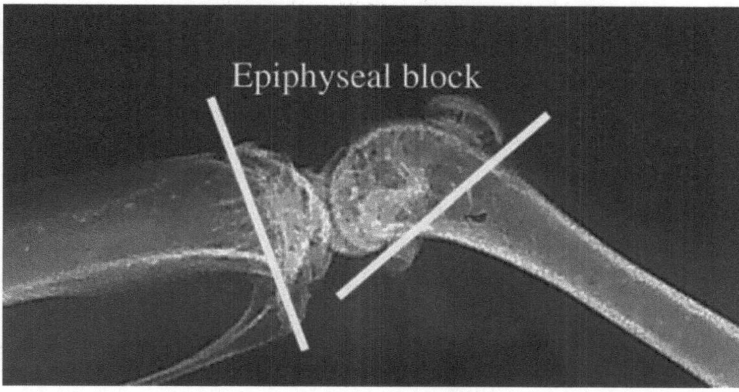

Fig. 4. Tissue sampling for RNA isolation. Knee epiphyses are cleared from soft tissue, and the knee joint is cut with a scalpel at standardized sites on tibial and femoral heads, as indicated by the white lines in the sagittal radiograph of a hindlimb. The epiphyseal block thus contains patella, ligaments, menisci, subchondral bone, and growth plates in addition to articular cartilage.

low to allow Northern hybridizations of individual samples. The total RNA yield isolated from articular cartilage samples is generally less than 10 μg/joint, in contrast to the 100–150 μg isolated from epiphyseal block. The results obtained with these samples represent the average changes taking place in the articular cartilage, subchondral bone, growth plate, menisci, synovium, and ligaments. Hence the changes observed between nontransgenic and transgenic groups must be verified and localized by immunohistochemistry. An alternative for epiphyseal blocks is to collect tibial condyles dissected just above the growth plate, which better represents the articular cartilage compartment and has a smaller influence from the subchondral bone and other joint tissues (yield, 20–30 μg/joint). For screening of mRNA expression levels in the knee epiphyses, quickly and carefully dissect the hindlimb free of muscle, and cut with a scalpel at the level of the growth plates of the tibia and femur (**Fig. 4**). Punch a small hole with an injection needle in the cap of the microcentrifuge tube to keep the tube from exploding when moving it from the liquid nitrogen container to the freezer. Place the sample in a microcentrifuge tube, freeze the sample in liquid nitrogen, and store it at –70°C until processing for RNA isolation. Isolate total RNA using GIT and CsCl buoyant density gradient centrifugation using a modification of a method presented by Chirgwin et al. ***(38)*** (*see* **Notes 8** and **9**):

1. Pulverize the sample in liquid nitrogen (*see* **Note 5**).
2. In a hood, soak the dispersing tool for 30 min in active DEPC-treated dH_2O (2.0 mL of DEPC in 100 mL of dH_2O) before homogenization. Transfer the powder

with spatula (cooled in liquid nitrogen) into a 10 mL tube containing 2 mL of GIT solution on ice; homogenize with Ulra Turrax. Lift the tool up from the sample and rinse foam with 1 mL of GIT to the sample tube to fill the volume to 3 mL.

3. Remove the tissue debris by centrifugation (tabletop centrifuge, 3000*g*, 15 min).
4. During this centrifugation, prepare the ultracentrifuge tubes: pipet 2 mL of 5.7 *M* CsCl solution to the bottom of the tubes.
5. Layer the supernatant from **step 3** on top of CsCl solution in the ultracentrifuge tube. Fill and balance the tubes with GIT, leaving less than 2 mm empty space on top of the tube, and with less than 0.01 g difference in the weights of the opposite tubes.
6. Centrifuge for 18–21 h at 175,000*g* at 20°C (Beckman Optima LE-80K Ultracentrifuge and SW 55 TI swing-out rotor).
7. Remove the supernatant by suction halfway down with a glass capillary pipet.
8. Switch to a clean aspiration pipet and remove the remaining supernatant by suction. Be careful not to touch the inner surface of the tube to avoid any contamination with RNases that migrate to the top fraction of the gradient during centrifugation and may be bound to the inner surface.
9. After suction, invert the tubes to drain with a quick turn on a soft tissue or a paper towel.
10. Keep the tubes inverted, and cut off the bottom of tube containing the RNA pellet with a scalpel. Invert and transfer the tube bottoms on ice. Dissolve one sample at a time on ice with ice-cold solutions (**steps 11** and **12**).
11. Rinse the pellet once with 200 µL of 95% DEPC-treated ethanol.
12. Add 200 µL of DEPC-treated dH_2O to dissolve the pellet. This takes a while: pipet up and down. The pellet looks like cellophane. Remove the solution into an Eppendorf tube on ice. Repeat, dissolving with 100 µL of DEPC-treated dH_2O. The RNA sample is now in 300 µL of DEPC-treated dH_2O on an ice bath.
13. Since proteoglycans also migrate to the same fraction as RNA, remove them by digestion with proteinase K: add 500 µL of SET buffer + 20 µL of RNase-free proteinase K (20 mg/mL). Incubate for 1–3 h at 37°C.
14. Divide the sample into two Eppendorf tubes, 400 µL in each, add 400 µL of phenol/chloroform (1:1) into each tube and vortex for 30 s at room temperature.
15. Separate the phases by centrifugation for 2–3 min in a microcentrifuge at full speed and transfer the water phase into a new tube. Carefully avoid taking any of the lower phase.
16. Add 1:10 vol 3 *M* NaAc, pH 5.5, and vortex.
17. Add 1 µL of 95% ethanol, vortex carefully, and keep overnight at –20°C (or 1 h at –70°C).
18. Centrifuge at full speed for 15 min at +4°C; decant the supernatant and dry the precipitate in a SpeedVac.
19. Dissolve in DEPC-treated dH_2O (100 µL).
20. Take a 1-µL aliquot for determination of RNA amount (1 + 99 µL dH_2O) by UV absorption at 260/280 nm.
21. Store RNA at –70°C.

4. Notes

1. **Caution:** Ethidium bromide is a strongly mutagenic agent. Always wear protective gloves when handling the solutions and gels containing ethidium bromide.
2. **Caution:** paraformaldehyde is an irritating and allergenic compound; during weighing, always wear a protective face mask to prevent inhalation, and work with the solution in the hood.
3. DEPC treatment: when performing *in situ* hybridizations, add 2 mL of DEPC for 1000 mL of decalcification solution and distilled water to be used for rinsing. Mix the solutions, and let stand in a hood overnight. Autoclave the next day. Also prepare ethanol dilutions in DEPC-treated dH_2O, (2 mL/L). **Caution:** DEPC is an irritant; avoid eye and skin contact and inhalation, wear protective cloves, and work in a hood when handling active DEPC. DEPC degrades to ethanol and CO_2 in water solution.
4. Ready-to-use Instant hematoxylin (Shandon cat. no. 9990107) can be used to replace Delafield's hematoxylin.
5. To pulverize the tissue, we use a stainless steel unit composed of a cylinder, a bottom piece, and a piston, which are cooled by soaking in liquid nitrogen. Soak the sample in liquid nitrogen, place between the bottom piece and the piston, and pulverize by hitting the piston with a shot hammer two to three times.
6. Fix the samples in paraformaldehyde at 4°C for 24 h on a rocking platform. Do not prolong the fixation time, as it will decrease the signal in immunohistochemistry and *in situ* hybridization.
7. Simultaneously with the screening for cartilage erosion of the tissue sections, it is advisable to make notes about the different tissue compartments that are observed within each section, e.g., in which sagittal section the tibial or femoral condyles are seen, whether the section is from the lateral or medial condyle (if it is a sagittal section), or if the patella, patellar tendon, or cross ligaments are present in the sections. This helps in later selection of tissue sections for the immunohistochemical analysis to be made of certain tissue compartments. It is also possible to estimate from these notes whether the tissue had been embedded in the proper orientation. In samples embedded properly in horizontal plane, the patella, patellofemoral groove, and cross ligaments appear in the same sections.
8. For RNA isolation, all plastic and glass material needs to be RNase-free. Incubate the glassware at 180°C for at least 2 h, and gas-sterilize the plastic pipet tips and Eppendorf tubes. Treat all the solutions with DEPC, add 2 mL of DEPC to 1 L of solution, allow to stand overnight at room temperature, and autoclave. GIT solution does not need to be DEPC-treated, as the reagent itself inhibits RNase activity.
9. Advantages of GIT-CsCl buoyant density gradient centrifucation method: RNA isolated with this method is stable and tolerates several freeze-thaw cycles. We have succesfully used such RNA for RT-PCR, Northern hybridization, and RNase protection analyses even after 5–10 yr of storage in DEPC-treated dH_2O solution at –70°C. The method suits particularly for isolation of total RNA from tissues rich in fibrillar collagen and/or low in cell density, such as cartilage, bone, cor-

nea, and skin. mRNA isolated by this method has proved to give excellent results in different cDNA array analyses, e.g., Affymetrix chips, even when RNA samples have been stored for several years at –70°C. Our attempts to purify RNA from skeletal tissues have failed with all silica-based microspin column kits we have tested. They are ineffective at removing all DNA. Another problem is that these tissues are rich in collagen fibers and proteoglycans and have relatively low cell density, which all together result in low quality and quantity of RNA. Single-step isolation methods have given better results ***(39)***, but the RNA often needs further purification steps if it is used as a template for quantitative RT-PCR or cDNA chip arrays. Also the RNA purified by single-step procedure is less resistant for repeated freezing-melting cycles than the RNA purified through CsCl buoyant density gradient centrifugation.

Disadvantages: The method is time-consuming and requires expensive equipment such as ultracentrifuge and titanium rotors. Only four to six samples can be processed at a time, depending on the rotor. Also, CsCl is rather expensive.

References

1. Felson, D. T. and Zhang, Y. (1998) An update on the epidemiology of knee and hip osteoarthritis with a view to prevention. *Arthritis Rheum.* **41,** 1343–5135.
2. Helminen, H. J., Säämänen, A.-M., Salminen, H., and Hyttinen, M. M. (2002) Transgenic mouse models for studying the role of cartilage macromolecules in osteoarthritis. *Rheumatology* **41,** 848–856.
3. Hogan, B., Beddington, F., Costantini, F., and Lacy, E. (eds.) (1994) *Manipulating the Mouse Embryo. A Laboratory Manual.* Cold Spring Harbor Laboratory Press, Cold Spring Harbor, NY.
4. Jimenez, S. A., Williams, C. J., and Karasik, D. (1998) Hereditary osteoarthritis, in *Osteoarthritis* (Brandt, K. D., Doherty, M., and Lohmander L. S., eds.), Oxford University Press, New York, pp. 31–49.
5. Prockop, D. J. and Kivirikko, K. I. (1995) Collagens: molecular biology, diseases, and potentials for therapy. *Annu. Rev. Biochem.* **64,** 403–434.
6. Myllyharju, J. and Kivirikko, K. I. (2001) Collagens and collagen-related diseases. *Ann. Med.* **33,** 7–21.
7. Mundlos, S. and Olsen, B. R. (1997) Heritable diseases of the skeleton. Part II: Molecular insights into skeletal development-matrix components and their homeostasis. *FASEB J.* **11,** 227–233.
8. Jacenko, O. and Olsen, B. R. (1995) Transgenic mouse models in studies of skeletal disorders. *J. Rheumatol.* **43 (suppl),** 39–41.
9. Olsen, B. R. (1995) Mutations in collagen genes resulting in metaphyseal and epiphyseal dysplasias. *Bone* **17 (suppl 2)**, 45S–49S.
10. Vikkula, M., Mariman, E. C., Lui, V. C., et al. (1995) Autosomal dominant and recessive osteochondrodysplasias associated with the COL11A2 locus. *Cell* **80,** 431–437.
11. Snead, M. P. and Yates, J. R. (1999) Clinical and molecular genetics of Stickler syndrome. *J. Med. Genet.* **36,** 353–359.

12. Ihanamäki, T., Salminen, H., Säämänen, A. M., Sandberg-Lall, M., Vuorio, E., and Pelliniemi, L. J. (2002) Ultrastructural characterization of developmental and degenerative vitreo-retinal changes in the eyes of transgenic mice with a deletion mutation in type II collagen gene. *Curr. Eye Res.* **24,** 439–450.
13. Vandenberg, P., Khillan, J. S., Prockop, D. J., Helminen, H., Kontusaari, S., and Ala-Kokko, L. (1991) Expression of a partially deleted gene of human type II procollagen (COL2A1) in transgenic mice produces a chondrodysplacia. *Proc. Natl. Acad. Sci. USA* **88,** 7640–7644.
14. Vuorio, E., Elima, K., Perälä, M., and Säämänen, A.-M. (1998) Transgenic mice as models for cartilage and eye diseases, in *Wenner-Grenn Foundation Symposium: Connective Tissue Biology: Integration and Reductionism* (Reed, R. and Rubin, C., eds.), Portland Press, London, pp. 135–145.
15. Metsäranta, M., Garofalo, S., Decker, G., Rintala, M., de Crombrugghe, B., and Vuorio, E. (1992) Chondrodysplasia in transgenic mice harboring a 15-amino acid deletion in the triple helical domain of proα1(II) collagen chain. *J. Cell Biol.* **118,** 203–212.
16. Säämänen, A.-M. K., Salminen, H. J., de Crombrugghe, B., Dean, P. B., Vuorio, E. I., and Metsäranta, M. P. H. (2000) Osteoarthritis-like lesions in transgenic mice harboring a small deletion mutation in type II collagen gene. *Osteoarthritis Cartilage* **8,** 248–257.
17. Salminen, H., Perälä, M., Lorenzo, P., et al. (2000) Up-regulation of cartilage oligomeric matrix protein at the onset of articular cartilage degeneration in a transgenic mouse model for osteoarthritis. *Arthritis Rheum.* **43,** 1742–1748.
18. Salminen, H., Vuorio, E., and Säämänen, A.-M. (2001) Expression of Sox9 and type IIA collagen during attempted repair of articular cartilage damage in a transgenic mouse model for osteoarthritis. *Arthritis Rheum.* **44,** 947–955.
19. Salminen, H. J., Säämänen, A.-M. K., Vankemmelbeke M. N., Auho, P. K., Perälä, M. P., and Vuorio, E. I. (2002) Differential expression patterns of matrix metalloproteinases and their inhibitors during development of osteoarthrosis in a transgenic mouse model. *Ann. Rheum. Dis.* **61,** 591–597.
20. Neuhold, L. A., Killar, L., Zhao, W., et al. (2001) Postnatal expression in hyaline cartilage of constitutively active human collagenase-3 (MMP-13) induces osteoarthritis in mice. *J. Clin. Invest.* **107,** 35–44.
21. Li, S. W., Takanosu, M., Arita, M., et al. (2001) Targeted disruption of Col11a2 produces a mild cartilage phenotype in transgenic mice: comparison with the human disorder otospondylomegaepiphyseal dysplasia (OSMED). *Dev. Dyn.* **222,** 141–152.
22. Lapveteläinen, T., Hyttinen, M., Lindblom, J., et al. (2001) More knee joint osteoarthritis (OA) in mice after inactivation of one allele of type II procollagen gene but less OA after lifelong voluntary wheel running exercise. *Osteoarthritis Cartilage* **9,** 152–160.
23. Fässler R., Schnegelsberg, P. N., Dausman, J., et al. (1994) Mice lacking alpha 1 (IX) collagen develop noninflammatory degenerative joint disease. *Proc. Natl. Acad. Sci. USA* **91,** 5070–5074.

24. Ameye, L., Aria, D., Jepsen, K., Oldberg, Å., Xu, T., and Young, M. (2002) Abnormal collagen fibrils in tendon of biglycan/fibromodulin-deficient mice lead to gait imparment, ectopic ossification, and osteoarthritis. *FASEB J.* **16,** 673–680.
25. Zemmyo, M., Meharra, E. J., Kuhn, K., Creighton-Achermann, L., and Lotz, M. (2003) Accelerated, aging-dependant development of osteoarthritis in α-1 integrin-deficient mice. *Arthritis Rheum.* **48,** 2873–2880.
26. Seegmiller, R. E., Ryder, V., Jackson R., et al. (2001) Comparison of two collagen mutant mouse lines that serve as models of early-onset osteoarthritis in human chondrodysplasia. *Osteoarthritis Cartilage* **9 (suppl. B),** S15.
27. Sambrook, J. and Russell, D.W., eds. (2001) *Molecular Cloning. A Laboratory Manual.* Cold Spring Harbor Laboratory Press, Cold Spring Harbor, NY, pp. 6.33–6.35.
28. Metsäranta, M., Toman, D., de Crombrugghe, B., and Vuorio, E. (1991) Mouse type II collagen gene. Complete nucleotide sequence, exon structure, and alternative splicing. *J. Biol. Chem.* **266,** 16862–16869.
29. Garofalo, S., Vuorio, E., Metsäranta, M., et al. (1991) Reduced amounts of cartilage collagen fibrils and growth plate anomalies in transgenic mice harboring a glycine-to-cysteine mutation in the mouse type II procollagen alpha 1-chain gene. *Proc. Natl. Acad. Sci. USA* **88,** 9648–9652.
30. Garofalo, S., Metsäranta, M., Ellard, J., et al. (1993) Assembly of cartilage collagen fibrils is disrupted by overexpression of normal type II collagen in transgenic mice. *Proc. Natl. Acad. Sci. USA* **90,** 3825–3829.
31. Kiviranta, I., Jurvelin, J., Tammi, M., Säämänen, A.-M., and Helminen, H. J. (1985) Microspectrophotometric quantitation of glycosaminoglycans in articular cartilage sections stained with safranin O. *Histochemistry* **82,** 249–255.
32. Kiraly, K., Hyttinen, M. M., Lapveteläinen, T., et al. (1997) Specimen preparation and quantification of collagen birefringence in unstained sections of articular cartilage using image analysis and polarizing light microscopy. *Histochem. J.* **29,** 317–327.
33. Wilhelmi, G. and Faust, R. (1976) Suitability of the C57 black mouse as an experimental animal for the study of skeletal changes due to ageing, with special reference to osteo-arthrosis and its response to tribenoside. *Pharmacology* **14,** 289–296.
34. Helminen, H. J., Kiraly, K., Pelttari, A., et al. (1993) An inbred line of transgenic mice expressing an internally deleted gene for type II procollagen (COL2A1). *J. Clin. Invest.* **92,** 582–595.
35. Evans, R. G., Collins, C., Miller, P., Ponsford, F. M., and Elson, C. J. (1994) Radiological scoring of osteoarthritis progression in STR/ORT mice. *Osteoarthritis Cartilage* **2,** 103–109.
36. Lapveteläinen, T., Tiihonen, A., Koskela, P., et al. (1997) Training a large number of laboratory mice using running wheels and analyzing running behavior by use of a computer-assisted system. *Lab. Anim. Sci.* **47,** 172–179.
37. Lapveteläinen, T., Hyttinen, M. M., Säämänen, A.-M., et al. (2002) Lifelong voluntary joint loading increass osteoarthritis in mice housing a deletion mutation in

type II procollagen gene, and slightly also in non-trangenic mice. *Ann. Rheum. Dis.* **61,** 810–817.

38. Chirgwin, I. M., Przybyla, A. E., MacDonald, R. J., and Rutter, W. J. (1989) Isolation of biologically active ribonucleic acid from sources enriched in ribonuclease. *Biochemistry* **18,** 5294–5299.
39. Chomczynski, P. and Sacchi, N. (1987) Single-step method of RNA isolation by acid guanidinium thiocyanate-phenol-chloroform extraction. *Anal. Biochem.* **162,** 156–159.

2

Development and Clinical Application in Arthritis of a New Immunoassay for Serum Type IIA Procollagen NH2 Propeptide

Jean-Charles Rousseau, Linda J. Sandell, Pierre D. Delmas, and Patrick Garnero

Summary

Type II collagen, the most abundant protein of cartilage matrix, is synthesized as a procollagen molecule including the N-(PIINP) and C-(PIICP) propeptides at each end. Type II procollagen is produced in two forms as the result of alternative RNA splicing. One form (IIA) includes and the other form (IIB) excludes a 69-amino acid cysteine-rich globular domain encoded by exon 2 in PIINP. During the process of synthesis, these N-propeptides are removed by specific proteases and released in the circulation, and their levels are believed to reflect type II collagen synthesis. In this chapter we describe the development of a specific enzyme-linked immunosorbent assay (ELISA) for the measurement of the IIA form of PIINP (PIIANP) in serum based on a polyclonal antibody raised against recombinant human exon 2 fusion protein of type II procollagen. We show that this ELISA is highly specific for circulating PIIANP and has adequate technical precision. In patients with knee osteoarthritis and rheumatoid arthritis, serum PIIANP was decreased by 53% ($p < 0.0001$) and 35% ($p < 0.001$), respectively, suggesting that type IIA collagen synthesis is altered in these arthritic diseases. The measurement of serum PIIANP may be useful for the clinical investigation of patients with joint diseases.

Key Words: Type II collagen; N-propeptide; joint disease; osteoarthritis; rheumatoid arthritis; cartilage; biological marker; ELISA.

1. Introduction

The hallmark of osteoarthritis (OA), the most common joint disease, is cartilage loss leading to joint destruction. Molecular markers are molecules or fragments thereof of connective tissue matrices that are released into biological fluids during the process of tissue biosynthesis and turnover and that can be measured by immunoassays. Several molecular markers of bone, cartilage, and synovium have been described, and their changes have been investigated in

From: *Methods in Molecular Medicine, Vol. 101: Cartilage and Osteoarthritis, Volume 2: Structure and In Vivo Analysis*
Edited by: F. De Ceuninck, M. Sabatini, and P. Pastoureau © Humana Press Inc., Totowa, NJ

patients with OA, mainly in cross-sectional studies (for a review, *see* **ref. *1***). Because the loss of cartilage is believed to result from the combination of a decreased reparative process coupled with an increased degradative phenomenon, thereby limiting the capacity of cartilage repair, and because type II collagen is the most abundant protein of cartilage matrix, the assessment of type II collagen synthesis and degradation is an attractive approach for the investigation of OA. After many years of unsuccessful research, the recent development of assays specific for type II collagen breakdown is probably a breakthrough in the field of biological markers for OA, given that degradation of collagen fibers is associated with irreversible cartilage destruction ***(2–5)***. Conversely, there is still a lack of a specific and sensitive biological marker reflecting the rate of type II collagen synthesis.

Type II collagen is synthesized as a procollagen molecule including the N-(PIINP) and C-(PIICP) propeptides at each end. Type II procollagen is produced in two forms as the result of alternative RNA splicing. One form (IIA) includes and the other form (IIB) excludes a 69-amino acid cysteine-rich globular domain encoded by exon 2 in the PIINP (**Fig. 1**). During the process of synthesis, these N-propeptides are removed by specific proteases before the mature molecules are incorporated into fibrils ***(6)***. Theoretically, serum levels of these propeptides can be used as specific markers of collagen synthesis. This IIA form is known to be expressed in skeletal progenitor cells and noncartilaginous tissues in embryos but to be absent from mature and normal cartilage, in which IIB is known to be expressed ***(7–10)***. Aigner et al. ***(11)*** showed the re-expression of type IIA collagen by adult articular chondrocytes in OA disease. This re-expression may contribute to the reported increase of mRNA and protein expression of type II collagen during OA disease ***(12–16)*** but also implies a significant modulation of chondrocyte phenotype. Together, these results suggest that the N-propeptide IIA could be a specific marker of OA disease, reflecting the synthesis of IIA collagen. Currently, no immunoassays have been developed allowing the measurement of N-propeptide IIA. This chapter describes the development of an immunoassay for serum N-propeptide IIA, the characterization of circulating immunoreactive forms detected by this assay, and preliminary clinical evaluation in arthritis.

2. Materials

2.1. Materials for Immunoassay

1. Maxisorp microtiter plates (Nunc, Roskilde, Denmark).
2. Bovine serum albumin (BSA), radioimmunoassay (RIA) grade (Sigma, St Louis, MO).
3. Tween-20 (Sigma).

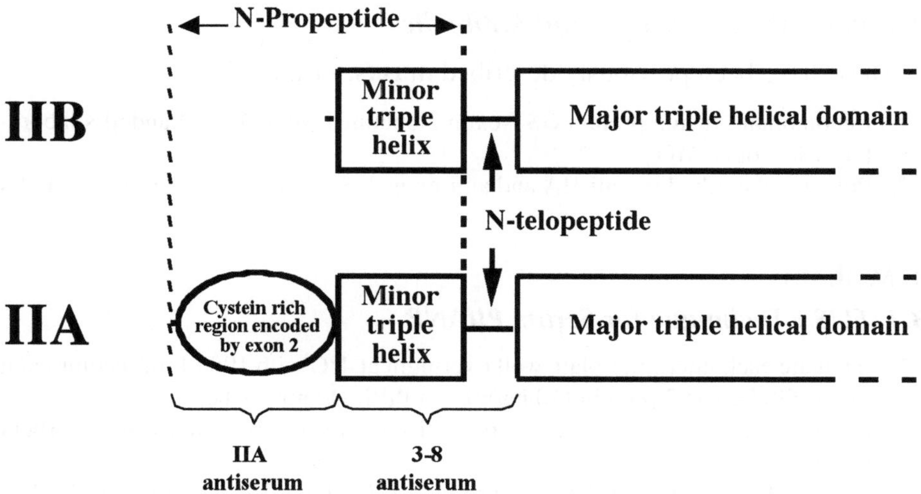

Fig. 1. Schematic reprensentation of type IIA/IIB procollagen. Type II collagen is expressed in two forms of IIA and IIB, as the result of alternative splicing of exon 2 in the NH2-propeptide region. IIA polyclonal antibodies specifically recognize IIA N-propeptide, and exon 3–8 polyclonal antibodies recognize the two forms (IIA and IIB) of the N-propeptide.

4. Phosphate-buffered saline (PBS), pH 7.4.
5. Anti-rabbit IgG peroxidase conjugate (Sigma).
6. H_2O_2 and tetramethylbenzidine substrate indicator solution (Sigma).
7. H_2SO_4 (VWR, Gibbstown, NJ).
8. Dynatech microtiter plate reader MR 7000 (Labsystems, Vantaa, Finland).

2.2. Materials for Specificity Characterization

1. 5% Tris/tricine gel electrophoresis and Western blot equipment.
2. Nitrocellulose membrane (Hybond ECL, Amersham, Buckinghamshire, England).
3. Polyclonal anti-von Willebrand factor (Dako, Carpinteria, CA).
4. Polyclonal antithrombospondin (NeoMarkers, Fremont, CA).
5. Polyclonal anti-GST–exon 2 recombinant protein (IIA antiserum).
6. Polyclonal anti-GST–exon 3–8 recombinant protein (3–8 antiserum, developed in chicken).
7. Rabbit nonimmune serum.
8. Goat antirabbit horseradish peroxidase (HRP) conjugate (Jackson ImmunoResearch, West Grove, PA).
9. Antichicken IgG (whole molecule) peroxidase conjugate (Sigma).
10. Western Lightning Chemiluminescence reagent (Perkin Elmer, Boston, MA).
11. BioMax MS-1, Kodak film (Sigma).

2.3. Recombinant Protein and Antibodies

These have been previously described in **refs. *11*** and ***17***.

1. Recombinant fusion protein GST-exon 2 obtained from Dr. L. Sandell's laboratory (St. Louis, MO).
2. Polyclonal antibodies anti-IIA and anti-exon 3–8 obtained from Dr. L. Sandell's laboratory.

3. Methods

3.1. ELISA Technique for Serum PIIANP

1. Incubate each microtiter plate well overnight at 4°C with 100 µL of recombinant fusion GST-exon 2 protein (10 ng/mL) in PBS. Do not shake.
2. Empty well contents and tap the plate firmly two to three times on absorbent paper.
3. Saturate for 2 h at room temperature with PBS, BSA 1% on a microwell plate rotation apparatus (gentle agitation).
4. Wash microwells with 200 µL of PBS, 1% BSA, 0.05% Tween-20.
5. Repeat three times and check that there is no residual washing solution in wells after each washing cycle. Repeat washes after each step of the protocol.
6. Dispense 100 µL/well of standards (recombinant fusion protein GST-exon 2; 0 [PBS/BSA/Tween], 2.5, 5, 7.5, 10, 15, 20, 30, 40 ng/mL) or serum (samples and controls). Serum must be centrifuged for 15 min at 4°C (14,000*g*) before use.
7. Add 100 µL/well of IIA antiserum (1:1650 final) and incubate for 4 h at room temperature on a microwell plate rotation apparatus (40 rpm).
8. Add the peroxidase-conjugated antirabbit antibodies (diluted 1:8000; 100 µL/well) and incubate at room temperature for 1 h on a microwell plate rotation apparatus (40 rpm).
9. Incubate at room temperature with 100 µL/well H_2O_2/tetramethylbenzidine substrate indicator solution (one tablet in 10 mL of 0.05 *M* phosphate citrate buffer, pH 5.0 with 2 µL H_2O_2) on a microwell plate rotation apparatus (40 rpm).
10. After 30 min, stop the color reaction by addition of 100 µL 2 *M* H_2SO_4/well.
11. Read the optical density at 450 nm with a Dynatech Reader.

3.2. Characterization of Antigens Recognized by Antiserum IIA

1. Select a pool of sera from healthy donors and dilute this pool 10 times in PBS buffer.
2. Boil the samples for 5 min and resolve them (15 µL/well) in a 5% Tris/tricine gel under reducing conditions.
3. Transfer overnight (50 V) in 100 m*M* CAPS (3-[cyclohexylamino]-1-propanesulfonic acid), 5% methanol on a nitrocellulose membrane (Hybond ECL, Amersham Pharmacia Biotech).
4. Saturate the membranes for 1 h with 5% nonfat milk in PBS with shaking.
5. Wash the membranes 4 × 10 min in PBS, 0.05% Tween-20.

6. Incubate with primary antibodies overnight at 4°C with shaking (IIA antiserum, 1:400; 3–8 antiserum, 1:500; nonimmune serum, 1:400; anti-von Willebrand factor, 1:400; antithrombospondin, 1:400).
7. Wash the membranes 4 × 10 min in PBS, 0.05% Tween-20.
8. Incubate with the specific secondary antibodies (anti-rabbit 1:3000 or anti-chicken 1:20,000) for 1 h at room temperature with shaking.
9. Wash the membranes 4 × 10 min in PBS, 0.05% Tween-20.
10. Use the Perkin Elmer kit for the revelation of the membranes.

3.3. Populations Used in the Study

1. Healthy subjects. Reference values were obtained from 67 women ranging in age from 31 yr to 75 yr (mean age: 53 ± 13 yr) and 21 men ranging in age from 53 yr to 77 yr (mean age: 63.4 ± 6.9 yr). All belonged to large population-based cohorts involved in prospective studies on the determinants of bone loss in women (OFELY [Os des Femmes de Lyon] study) ***(18)*** and men (MINOS study) ***(19)***. The cohort of the OFELY study comprises 1039 healthy white female volunteers (31–89 yr of age), and the cohort of the MINOS study comprises 842 healthy white male volunteers (50–85 yr of age). All healthy subjects came from the same region of France as the patients with knee OA and rheumatoid arthritis (RA). None of the control subjects had evidence of OA as assessed by clinical examination, questionnaire, and X-ray films of the thoracic and lumbar spine, and all subjects were without disease or treatment that could interfere with bone or joint metabolism including hormone replacement therapy in postmenopausal women.
2. Osteoarthritis patients. The study group included 43 outpatients suffering from knee OA ranging in age from 41 yr to 83 yr (23 women and 20 men; median age: 62.6 ± 9.6 yr). They consulted at the Department of Rheumatology of the Centre Hospitalier Lyon Sud (Lyon, France). All patients fulfilled the American College of Rheumatology criteria for primary knee OA ***(20)***. All patients had had chronic daily pain of the knee for at least 3 mo (median: 10 yr) and also had radiographical evidence of OA with joint space narrowing when using the posteroanterior view of the knees flexed at 30° (Schuss view). Patients presenting with an advanced stage of OA with a minimum joint space width of less than 1 mm were excluded. All women were postmenopausal and all patients were without treatment that could interfere with bone metabolism including estrogen replacement therapy, dilantin, thyroid replacement therapy, and diuretics. Pain and physical function were assessed by the Western Ontario and McMasters Universities multifunctional (WOMAC) index ***(21)***, using a visual analog scale as a grading system. A subset of 53 healthy age and sex-matched subjects (32 women and 21 men, mean age: 62.4 ± 7.7 yr) was used as a control for patients with knee OA.
3. Rheumatoid arthritis patients. We investigated 66 women who met the American College of Rheumatology criteria for RA disease revised in 1987 ***(22)*** ranging in age from 15 to 84 yr (median age: 54 ± 16 yr; median disease duration: 6 yr). Twenty-four were on low-dose corticosteroids (<10 mg/d prednisone). Patients

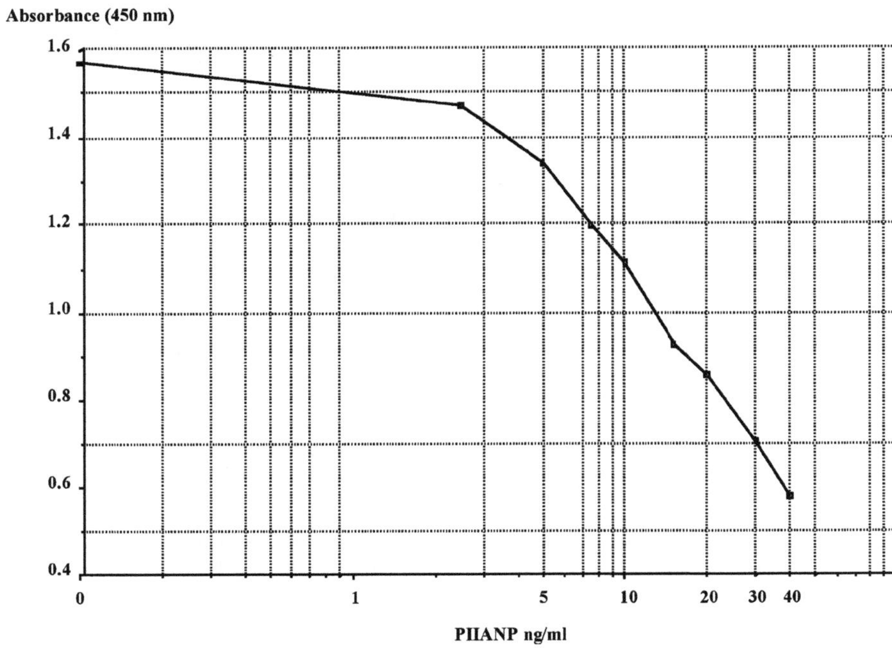

Fig. 2. Standard curve produced by duplicate measurements of the mean optical density at 450 nm of nine PIIANP standards.

with renal insufficiency were excluded. A subset of 67 healthy age-matched women (mean age: 53 ± 13 yr) was used as controls for patients with RA.

3.4. Statistical Analysis

Comparison of serum PIIANP levels between healthy controls and patients with OA or RA was assessed by the nonparametric Mann-Whitney U test.

3.5. Analytical Performances of PIIANP ELISA

A typical standard curve using the recombinant fusion protein GST-exon 2 as a standard is shown on **Fig. 2**. The competitive polyclonal antibody-based enzyme-linked immunosorbent assay (ELISA) demonstrated adequate intra- and interassay precisions (coefficient of variation [CV] <10%) and dilution recovery (**Tables 1–3**). The detection limit, defined as the concentration 2 SDs above that of the lowest calibrator, was 1.13 ng/mL.

3.6. Characterization of Serum Antigens Recognized by Antiserum IIA

1. The major part of PIIANP is encoded by exon 2 (**Fig. 1**), which has the highest sequence homology with the interstitial collagen chain $\alpha 1(I)$. It also has signifi-

Table 1
Intraassay Precision of the PIIANP Assay[a]

Serum PIIANP (ng/mL)	CV (%)
9.6	7.4
12.8	8.5
25.4	9.0

[a]Intraassay variability was assessed by measuring three serum samples 10 times in the same run.

Table 2
Interassay Precision on the PIIANP Assay[a]

Serum PIIANP (ng/mL)	CV (%)
9.0	8.6
27.0	6.0
36.3	1.5

[a]Interassay variability was assessed by measuring three serum samples in duplicate in five runs.

Table 3
Dilution Recovery

Sample	Dilution (%)	Serum PIIANP (ng/mL) Expected	Serum PIIANP (ng/mL) Measured	Recovery (%)
A	Net	—	259	—
	80	20.7	21.1	102
	60	15.5	13.3	86
	40	10.3	9.5	92
B	Net	—	24.2	—
	80	19.3	14.0	72
	60	14.5	13.9	96
	40	9.7	12.4	128
C	Net	—	30.4	—
	80	24.3	23.2	95
	60	18.2	17.8	98
	40	12.2	12.1	99

cant sequence homology with thrombospondins 1 and 2 and the von Willebrand factor C domain *(10)*. Consequently we analyzed the specificity of IIA antiserum with these circulating proteins.

2. Western blot analysis showed that antiserum IIA recognizes two immunoreactive forms with molecular weights of 90 kDa (band a) and 120 kDa (band b) respectively (**Fig. 3A**, lane 1 and **Fig. 3B**, lane 1). These two bands were also recognized by an antiserum raised against the protein part encoded by exon 3–8 in the collagen II N-propeptide, which is present in both PIIANP and PIIBNP (**Fig. 3B,** lane 2). Thus circulating PIIANP appears to be present in at least two different immunoreactive forms (*see* **Note 1**). The antibody raised against exon

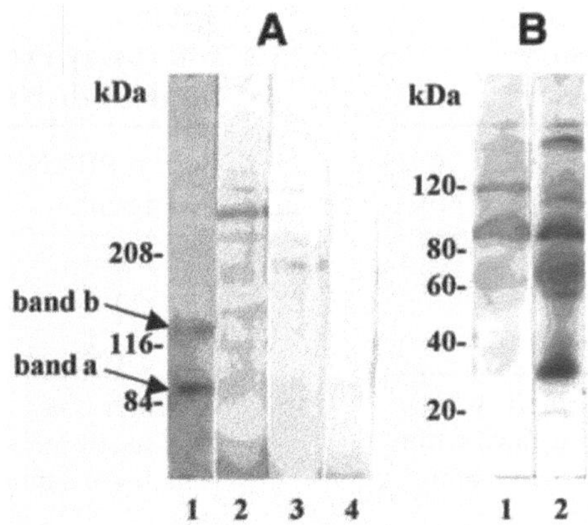

Fig. 3. Western blot analysis of the serum pool from healthy patients. The membranes were probed with **(A)** anti-IIA (lane 1), anti-von Willebrand factor (lane 2), antithrombospondin (lane 3), or nonimmune serum (lane 4) and **(B)** with anti-IIA (lane 1) or anti-exon 3–8 (lane 2).

3–8 recognized additional immunoreactive forms that are not detected by anti-IIA antibody and that probably correspond to circulating PIIBNP forms (*see* **Note 2**).

3. We then verified that bands a and b were not recognized by antithrombospondin and anti-von Willebrand factor antibodies (**Fig. 3A**, lanes 2 and 3) and additionally that antiserum IIA did not recognize bands corresponding to thrombospondin and von Willebrand factor (**Fig. 3A**, lanes 1 and 2). As negative control, a nonimmune serum showed no crossreactivity with bands a and b (**Fig. 3A**, lane 4).
4. The specificity of ELISA for PIIANP was also confirmed by the lack of significant crossreactivity of the PIIANP antiserum with purified intact human N-propeptide of type I collagen (PINP) composed of two $\alpha1$(I) chains and one $\alpha2$(I) chain, in agreement with previously reported findings ***(10)*** (data not shown).
5. The mol wt of bands a and b were higher than the estimated weight of monomeric N-propeptide IIA, approx 20–30 kDa. It is unlikely that these bands correspond to aggregates with binding serum protein because Tris/tricine gels were performed under reducing conditions after samples were boiled. We can hypothesize that bands a and b are composed of multiple propeptides with triple-helical regions bound to each other by the crosslinking molecules such as pyridinoline in the N-telopeptide region, located upstream to the cleavage site of matrix metalloproteinases (MMPs)-3, -7, -9, -13, and -14 ***(17)***.

3.7. Concentration of Serum PIIANP in Patients With Knee OA and Rheumatoid Arthritis

The mean serum concentration of PIIANP was significantly decreased ($p <$ 0.0001) in patients with knee OA (12.0 ± 3.2 ng/mL vs 25.8 ± 7.5 ng/mL; **Fig. 4A**)

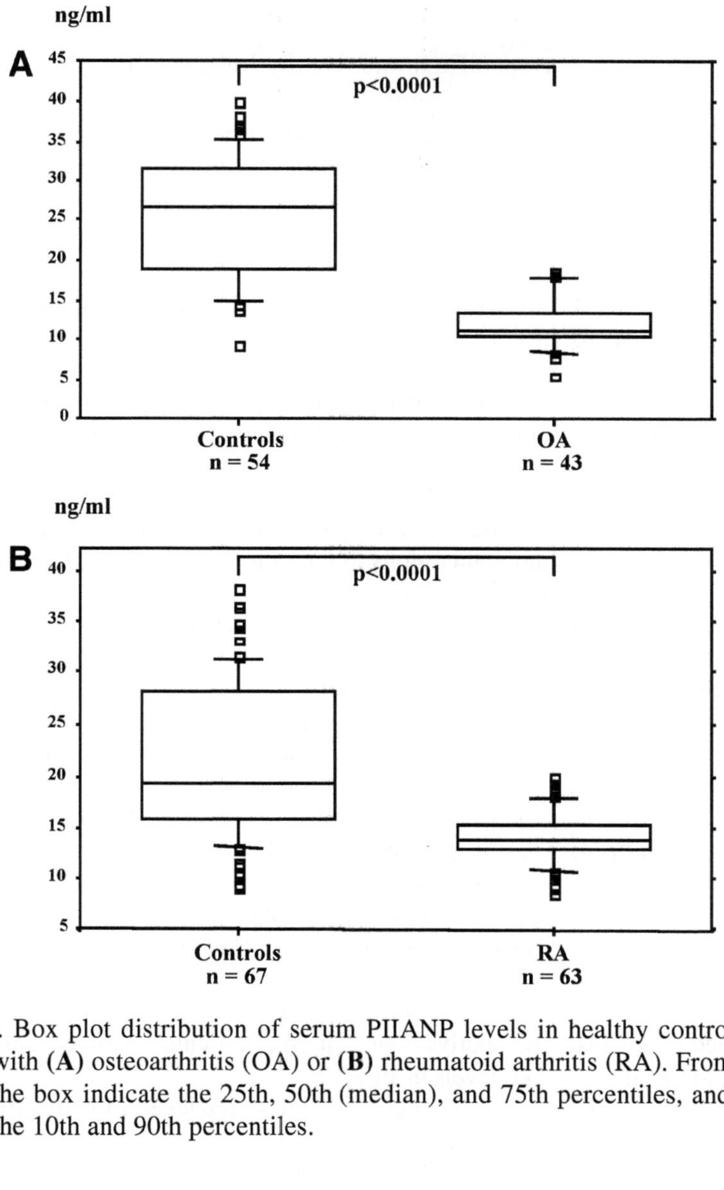

Fig. 4. Box plot distribution of serum PIIANP levels in healthy controls and in patients with **(A)** osteoarthritis (OA) or **(B)** rheumatoid arthritis (RA). From the bottom up, the box indicate the 25th, 50th (median), and 75th percentiles, and the bars indicate the 10th and 90th percentiles.

and RA (14.1 ± 2.5 ng/mL vs 21.7 ± 7.6 ng/mL; **Fig. 4B**) compared with sex- and age-matched healthy controls (*see* **Notes 3–5**). When using the mean –1 SD of the controls as the lower limit of the normal range, 97 and 57% of patients with knee OA and RA, respectively, had serum levels below that limit. The distribution of PIIANP serum levels was narrower in patients with OA or RA than in healthy controls (**Figs. 4A** and **4B**).

3.8. Concluding Remarks

We have developed a specific immunoassay for serum PIIANP. This assay has adequate technical performance and should be useful to predict the progression of OA—probably in combination with markers of type II collagen degradation, as recently reported *(33)*—and also to monitor the efficacy of disease-modifying OA therapy, especially anabolic treatments.

4. Notes

1. We showed that IIA antiserum recognizes two forms of circulating PIIANP without significant crossreactivity with other proteins in the serum of healthy people. Additionally, the sequence encoded by exon 2 is highly conserved between human and mouse (85%) or human and rabbit (92%), suggesting that this immunoassay could be useful in the evaluation of preclinical studies using these animal models.
2. The development of an assay specific for the PIIBNP form would be an alternative complementary approach to assay for PIIANP. Indeed, this would allow the investigation of potential alterations in the ratio between type IIA and type IIB collagen synthesis in arthritic diseases.
3. The tissue origin of N-propeptide IIA in healthy controls is still a matter of discussion. Although immunohistochemistry studies were unable to detect type IIA procollagen in mature cartilage of healthy controls even after extensive protease treatments *(11)*, animal studies showed mRNA expression of type IIA procollagen in culture of adult bovine chondrocytes *(23)* and in articular cartilage of healthy dogs *(24)* and mice *(25)*. In addition, detectable concentrations of type IIA procollagen protein were shown in the pellets of adult bovine chondrocytes *(26)*. Thus, it may be possible that part of the circulating PIIANP arises from adult cartilage. Besides articular cartilage, type IIA collagen may also arise in part from other tissues such as adult vitreous humor or intervertebral disc tissues *(27–29)*. Nevertheless, it remains unclear whether or not these tissues synthesize type IIA in adults, and their contributions to the serum concentration are likely to be low compared with articular cartilage. Additional studies are needed to elucidate the relative contribution of articular cartilage and other tissues to the global serum levels of PIIANP.
4. In patients with knee OA, we found decreased serum levels of PIIANP compared with controls. The clinical significance of decreased serum PIIANP levels in patients with knee OA should, however, be interpreted with caution. Nelson et al. *(30)* showed that the content of PIICP—another index of type II collagen synthesis—in cartilage tissue extract was increased in patients with knee OA. Measurements of PIICP in synovial fluid and serum have yielded conflicting results. Increased levels of PIICP in the synovial fluid of the signal joint were found in patients with knee OA compared with healthy controls *(31)*. These increased levels are, however, mainly found in early and mid-stage OA, whereas levels decrease in end-stage disease, possibly because of decreased cartilage mass and

chondrocytes end-stage failure. Contrasting with increased PIICP levels in synovial fluid, Nelson et al. ***(30)*** reported in another population depressed levels of that marker in the serum of patients with knee OA compared with healthy controls. Thus, it could be speculated that decreased serum PIICP levels in OA may reflect systemic alterations of type II collagen metabolism, which may not be related to the signal joint ***(30)***. In our study, we only analyzed serum, and thus it remains to be determined whether the conflicting data between synovial fluid and serum PIICP levels will also apply to PIIANP. Clearly further studies comparing serum and synovial fluid levels of both PIICP and PIINP in well-characterized populations of patients with OA and controls are required to delineate the clinical significance of the serum levels of these markers. The PIIANP decrease was larger (58% vs 19%) than that of PIICP, suggesting that serum PIIANP may be more sensitive than serum PIICP in detecting alteration of type II collagen metabolism in OA. However, because no direct comparison of these two markers was performed in the same subjects, an increased sensitivity of PIIANP over PIICP needs to be confirmed in other studies.

5. Our study showed that serum PIIANP levels are markedly decreased in RA patients compared with controls. Conversely, levels of serum PIICP were found to be increased in serum ***(30)*** without significant differences between aggressive and nonaggressive disease ***(32)***. The reasons for this discrepancy between serum levels of PIIANP and PIICP in patients with RA is unclear, but it may result from differences in population characteristics, our patients being characterized by long-standing disease. It seems unlikely that this decrease was the result of increased proteinase degradation of PIIANP at the tissue level. Indeed, Fukui et al. ***(17)*** showed recently that the antibody raised against IIA that was used in the ELISA still recognizes recombinant N-propeptide IIA even after cleavage by the differents MMPs known to be involved in the destruction of articular cartilage.

References

1. Garnero, P., Rousseau, J.-C., and Delmas, P. D. (2000) Molecular basis and clinical use of biochemical markers of bone, cartilage and synovium in joint diseases. *Arthritis Rheum.* **43,** 953–968.
2. Dean, D. D., Martel-Pelletier, J., Pelletier, J. P., Howell, D. S., Woessner, J. F., Jr. (1989) Evidence for metalloproteinase inhibitor imbalance in human osteoarthritis cartilage. *J. Clin. Invest.* **84,** 678–685.
3. Poole, A. R. (1997) Cartilage in health and disease, in *Arthritis and Allied Conditions: A Textbook of Rheumatology*, 13th ed. (Koopman, W. J., ed.) Lippincott Williams and Wilkins, Baltimore, MD, pp. 255–308.
4. Campbell, C. J. (1969) The healing of cartilage defects. *Clin. Orthop.* **64,** 45–63.
5. Kim, H. K., Moran, M. E., and Salter, R. B. (1991) The potential for regeneration of articular cartilage in defects created by chondral shaving and subchondral abrasion: an experimental investigation in rabbits. *J. Bone Joint Surg. Am.* **73,** 1304–1345.
6. van der Rest, M. and Garrone, R. (1991) Collagen family of proteins. *FASEB J.* **5,** 2814–2823.

7. Sandell, L. J., Morris, N., Robbins, J. R., and Goldring, M. R. (1991) Alternatively spliced type II procollagen mRNAs define distinct populations of cells during vertebral development: differential expression of the amino-propeptide. *J. Cell Biol.* **114,** 1307–1319.
8. Ng, L. J., Tam, P. P., and Cheah, K. S. E. (1993) Preferential expression of alternatively spliced mRNAs encoding type II procollagen with a cystein-rich amino-propeptide in differentiating cartilage and nonchondrogenic tissues during early mouse development. *Dev. Biol.* **159,** 403–417.
9. Sandell, L. J., Nalin, A., and Reife, R. (1994) Alternative splice form of type II procollagen mRNA (IIA) is predominant in skeletal precursors and non-cartilaginous tissues during early mouse development. *Dev. Dyn.* **199,** 129–140.
10. Oganesian, A., Zhu, Y., and Sandell, L. J. (1997) Type IIA procollagen aminopropeptide is localized in human embryonic tissues. *J. Histochem. Cytochem.* **45,** 1469–1480.
11. Aigner, T., Zhu, Y., Chansky, H. H., Martsen, F. A., Maloney, W., and Sandell, L. J. (1999) Reexpression of type IIA procollagen by adult articular chondrocytes in osteoarthritic cartilage. *Arthritis Rheum.* **42,** 1443–1450.
12. Eyre, D., McDewitt, C. A., Billingham, M. E., and Muir, H. (1980) Biosynthesis of collagen and other matrix proteins by articular cartilage in experimental osteoarthritis. *Biochem. J.* **188,** 823–837.
13. Carney, S. L., Billingham, M. E. J., Muir, H., and Sandy, J. D. (1984) Demonstration of increased proteoglycan turnover in cartilage explants from dogs with experimental osteoarthritis. *J. Orthop. Res.* **2,** 201–216.
14. Sandy, J. D., Adams, M. E., Billingham, M. E., Plaas, A., and Muir, H. (1984) *In vivo* and *in vitro* stimulation of chondrocyte biosynthetic activity in early experimental osteoarthritis. *Arthritis Rheum.* **27,** 388–397.
15. Matyas, J. R., Adams, M. E., Huang, D. Q., and Sandell, L. J. (1995) Discoordinate gene expression of aggrecan and type II collagen in experimental osteoarthritis. *Arthritis Rheum.* **38,** 420–425.
16. Aigner, T., Gluckert, K., and von der mark, K. (1997) Activation of fibrillar collagen synthesis and phenotypic modulation of chondrocytes in early human osteoarthritis cartilage lesions. *Osteoarthritis Cartilage* **5,** 183–189.
17. Fukui, N., McAliden, A., Zhu, Y., et al. (2002) Processing of type II procollagen aminopropeptide by matrix metalloproteinases. *J. Biol. Chem.* **277,** 2193–2201.
18. Garnero, P., Sornay-Rendu, E., Chapuy, M. C., and Delmas P. D. (1996) Increased bone turnover in late postmenopausal women is a major determinant of osteoporosis. *J. Bone Miner. Res.* **11,** 827–834.
19. Szulc, P., Marchand, F., Duboeuf, F., and Delmas, P. D. (2000) Cross-sectional assessment of age-related bone loss in men: the MINOS study. *Bone* **26,** 123–129.
20. Altman, R., Asch, E., Bloch, D., et al. (1986) Development of criteria for the classification and reporting of osteoarthritis: classification of osteoarthritis of the knee. *Arthritis Rheum.* **29,** 1039–1049.
21. Bellamy, N., Buchanan, W. W., Goldsmith, C. H., and Campbell, S. L. W. (1988) Validation of the WOMAC: a health status instrument for measuring clinically

important patient relevant outcomes to antirheumatic drug therapy in patients with osteoarthritis of the hip or knee. *J. Rheumatol.* **15,** 1833–1840.
22. Arnett, F. C., Edworthy, S. M., Block, D. J., et al. (1988) The American Rheumatism Association 1987 revised criteria for the classification of rheumatoid arthritis. *Arthritis Rheum.* **31,** 315–324.
23. Ryan, M. C. and Sandell, L. J. (1990) Differential expression of a cystein-rich domain in the amino-terminal propeptide of type II (cartilage) procollagen by alternative splicing of mRNA. *J. Biol. Chem.* **265,** 10,334–10,339.
24. Matyas, J. R., Adams, M. E., Dinqqin, H., and Sandell, L. J. (1997) Major role of collagen IIB in the elevation of total type II procollagen messenger RNA in the hypertrophic phase of experimental osteoarthritis. *Arthritis Rheum.* **40,** 1046–1049.
25. van der Kraan, P. M., Vitters, E. L., Meijers, T. H., Poole, A. R., and van der Berg, W. B. (1998) Collagen type I antisense and collagen type IIA messenger RNA is expressed in adult murine articular cartilage. *Osteoarthritis Cartilage* **6,** 417–426.
26. Rebuck, N., Croucher, L. J., and Hollander, A. P. (1999) Distribution of two alternatively spliced variants of type II collagen N-propeptide compared with the C-propeptide in bovine chondrocyte pellet cultures. *J. Cell Biochem.* **71,** 313–327.
27. Reardon, A. J., Sandell, L. J., Jones, C. J., McLeod, D., and Bishop, P. N. (2000) Localisation of pN-type IIA procollagen on adult bovine vitreous collagen fibrils. *Matrix Biol.* **19,** 169–173.
28. Bishop, P. N., Reardon, A. J., McLeod, D., and Ayad, S. (1994) Identification of alternatively spliced variants of type II procollagen in vitreous. *Biochem. Biophys. Res. Commun.* **203,** 289–295.
29. Zhu, Y., McAliden, A., and Sandell, L. J. (2001) Type IIA procollagen in development of the human intervertebral disc: regulated expression of the NH_2-propeptide by enzymatic processing reveals a unique developmental pathway. *Dev. Dyn.* **220,** 350–362.
30. Nelson, F., Dahlberg, L., Laverty, S., et al. (1998) Evidence for altered synthesis of type II collagen patients with osteoarthritis. *J. Clin. Invest.* **102,** 2115–2125.
31. Lohmander, L. S., Yoshihara, Y., Roos, H., Kobayashi, T., Yamada, H., and Shinmei, M. (1996) Procollagen II-C propeptide in joint fluid: changes in concentration with age, time after injury and osteoarthritis. *J. Rheumatol.* **23,** 1765–1769.
32. Mansson, B., Carey, D., Alini, M., et al. (1995) Cartilage and bone metabolism in rheumatoid arthritis: differences between rapid and slow progression of disease identified by serum markers of cartilage metabolism. *J. Clin. Invest.* **95,** 1071–1077.
33. Garnero, P., Ayral, X., Rousseau, J.-C., et al. (2002) Uncoupling of type II collagen and degradation predicts progression of joint damage in patients with knee osteoarthritis. *Arthritis Rheum.* **46,** 2613–2624.

3

Histological and Immunohistological Studies on Cartilage

James Melrose, Susan Smith, and Peter Ghosh

Summary

The material properties of dense avascular connective tissues such as cartilage present unique challenges to the development of any prospective histological procedures. This chapter documents some of the protocols we have developed in our laboratories for the histological and immunohistochemical evaluation of extracellular-matrix components in normal and pathological articular cartilage. Illustrative examples are provided of specimens from an ovine meniscectomy model of osteoarthritis. A major strength of this experimental animal model is that spatial and temporal changes in joint matrix components can be followed longitudinally in an animal population of well-defined pedigree that minimizes biological variation. Furthermore, a systematic experimental approach can be adopted with this model using cartilage specimens from early predegenerative stages to later advanced stages of joint degeneration. Significantly, the histological changes observed in this model closely parallel changes evident in joint tissues during osteoarthritis in humans and have provided significant insights into these degenerative processes.

Key Words: Immunohistology; cartilage; osteoarthritis; toluidine blue; polarization microscopy; Masson's trichrome; picrosirius red; collagen; proteoglycan; aggrecan.

1. Introduction

Tissue sampling, fixation, staining, and microscopic assessment are the cornerstones of histochemistry. Many histological and histochemical textbooks are available that document these techniques. Such material, however, deals almost exclusively with soft connective tissues and bone *(1,2)*. To date only one definitive review on the histology of articular cartilage has appeared *(3)* and only a single textbook dealing with cartilage and bone histology *(4)*.

Articular cartilage has an extensive extracellular matrix but relatively few cells compared with softer connective tissues and subsequently displays quite different fixation characteristics and diffusive properties to the solvents and

From: *Methods in Molecular Medicine, Vol. 101: Cartilage and Osteoarthritis, Volume 2: Structure and In Vivo Analysis*
Edited by: F. De Ceuninck, M. Sabatini, and P. Pastoureau © Humana Press Inc., Totowa, NJ

dyes commonly used in histological processing. Existing histochemical protocols for soft connective tissues therefore cannot be applied directly to cartilage without extensive modification. Furthermore, cartilage is not uniform in composition: it displays spatial and temporal variations and may also vary focally with particular disease processes. Cartilage also abuts bone and thus requires decalcification to facilitate the histochemical processing of the cartilage tissue sections. Decalcification may, however, be detrimental to the subsequent histochemical or immunohistochemical staining of cartilage. Even so, it is important that the underlying bony tissues be preserved, since these keep the native shape of the cartilage and facilitate the correct spatial orientation of specimens. Because of the nonuniform composition of cartilage, a distortion in native tissue architecture can occur if precautions are not taken to prevent differential swelling artifacts during histological processing. Articular cartilage therefore presents considerable and unique technical challenges to the development of any prospective histology procedure. The present chapter documents some of the protocols we have so far developed in our laboratories for the histological assessment of extracellular matrix components in normal age-matched and pathological articular cartilage specimens from an ovine meniscectomy model of osteoarthritis (***5,6***; *see* **Fig. 1**).

2. Materials

2.1. Equipment

1. Rotary-type tissue processor Citadel 1000 (Shandon).
2. Embedding apparatus (Tissue Tek III, Bayer).
3. Rotary microtome (Reichert-Jung 2035, Leica).
4. Flotation bath (Medite TFB 35).
5. Decalcification apparatus (Bone Decalcifier, Lipshaw).
6. Bandsaw (190 mm, HBS 7600, Ryobi).
7. Vacuum pump and chamber for vacuum embedding of specimens.
8. Microscope (Leica DMLB) equipped for use with transmitted light in combination with polarization and interference contrast (Nomarski optics) modes.
9. Photomicroscope documentation system (Leica MPS 60, 35-mm camera) equipped with databack slide labeling accessory.
10. Microtek 35t plus 35-mm slide scanner, Adobe Photoshop software 5.0, and Power Macintosh personal computer for processing of digitized slide images and assembly of composite histology figures.
11. Stainless steel molds and plastic embedding cassettes (Bayer).
12. Disposable microtome blades (A3) and trimming and dissecting knives (F130 European, F60, 61 types, Feather Safety Razor, Osaka, Japan).
13. Racks for histochemical staining of microscope slides.
14. Sequenza vertical cover plate immunostaining chamber apparatus (Shandon).
15. Humidified trays for some immunohistology incubation steps.
16. SuperFrost® Plus microscope slides (Menzel-Glaser).

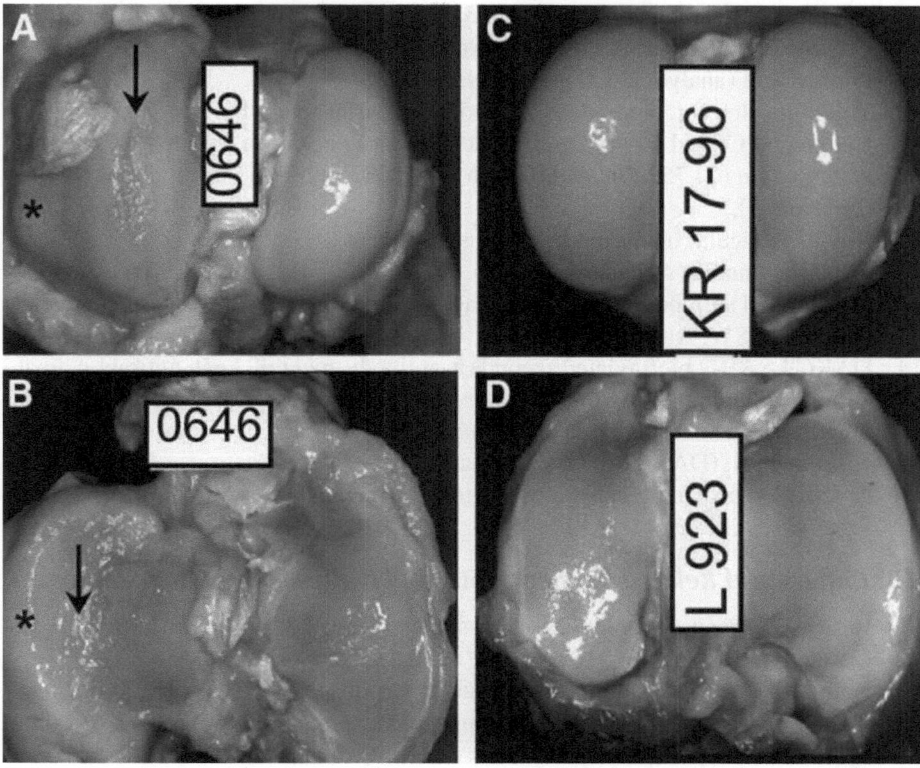

Fig. 1. Morphologies of the femoral condyle and tibial plateau cartilages of laterally meniscectomized ovine stifle joints 6 mo post meniscectomy (**A**, **B**) and a control sham operated joint for comparison (**C**, **D**). The arrows and asterisks in (A) and (B) depict areas of focal damage to the weight-bearing surfaces of the laterally meniscectomized joints and osteophyte formations in the joint margins, which frequently accompany these changes in the meniscectomized joints. The sham operated control stifle joint surfaces presented in (C) and (D) have smooth, shiny, well-lubricated articulating surfaces and no marginal osteophytes.

2.2. Chemicals

1. Paraplast wax for preparation of paraffin blocks (Paraplast, Oxford Labware, Sherwood Medical, St. Louis, MO).
2. Celloidin for double embedding of tissue specimens (NBS Biologicals via Lab Supply, Sydney, Australia).
3. Methyl benzoate (Ajax Chemical, Crown Scientific, Sydney, Australia) (*see* **Note 1**).
4. Tricresyl phosphate (Fluka) (*see* **Note 2**).
5. 10% Neutral buffered formalin fixative, pH 7.2.
6. Ethanol (absolute).

7. Xylene (analytical grade) (*see* **Note 3**).
8. Chloroform (analytical grade) (*see* **Note 3**).
9. Formic acid (analytical grade) (*see* **Note 4**).
10. Toluidine blue O (color index [CI] 0152040), sirius red F3BA (cat. no. 314492F), fast green FCF (CI 42053), picric acid (BDH); Ponceau de Xylidene (CI 16150), hematoxylin (CI 75290), acid fuchsin (CI 42685), phosphotungstic acid (Sigma) (*see* **Note 5**).
11. Bovine testicular hyaluronidase (Sigma).
12. Mounting media (Aquaperm, Eukitt).
13. Monoclonal antibodies to type II collagen (clone II-4CII) *(7)* (ICN Biochemicals, N. Ryde, NSW, Australia).
14. DAKO LSAB-2 biotinylated secondary antibody cocktail, goat–antirabbit, goat–antimouse immunoglobulins (cat. no. K0690); DAKO LSAB+ streptavidin-conjugated horseradish peroxidase (cat. no. K1015), immunohistology substrates and consumables, (DAKO Australia, Botany, NSW, Australia).
15. NovaRED peroxidase substrate (Vector, Burlingame, CA).
16. Proteinase K reagent (DAKO cat. no. S03020).

2.3. Buffers and Related Reagents, Stains, Fixatives, and Other Materials

1. Buffer A: testicular hyaluronidase digestion buffer, 0.1 *M* phosphate buffer, pH 5.0.
2. Decalcification solution: 10% formic acid, 5% formalin.
3. Neutral buffered formalin: 10% formalin in phosphate buffer pH 7.0–7.2. Dissolve 4.0 g sodium dihydrogen orthophosphate monohydrate and 6.5 g disodium hydrogen orthophosphate, anhydrous in MilliQ double-distilled water and combine with 100 mL 40% formaldehyde. Mix thoroughly and bring the mixture to a final volume of 1000 mL. Formalin is supplied as a solution of approx 37% formaldehyde gas in water. This solution is regarded by most histologists as 100% formalin when preparing fixative solutions.
4. Buffer B: toluidine blue O stain buffer, 0.1 *M* sodium acetate buffer, pH 4.0.
5. Bouin's fixative/mordant solution: combine 40% formalin (25 mL), saturated aqueous picric acid (75 mL), and glacial acetic acid (5 mL), and mix thoroughly (stable for 2 yr).
6. Weigert's hematoxylin solution: prepare a stock solutions of 1% w/v hematoxylin in ethyl alcohol and dissolve overnight (Weigert stock A, stable for 1 yr). Combine 4 mL of 30% w/v aqueous ferric chloride solution, concentrated HCl (1 mL), and distilled water (100 mL) with thorough mixing (Weigert stock B, stable for 1 yr). Combine equal parts of Weigert A and B stock solutions to prepare the working reagent. The working reagent is reported to be stable for 3–4 d; in this study it was used within 1 h.
7. Scott's tap water substitute: blueing solution. Dissolve 2.0 g potassium bicarbonate and 20.0 g magnesium sulfate in distilled water with thorough mixing and bring to a final volume of 1000 mL.
8. Ponceau de Xylidine/acid fuchsin staining solution: prepare 1% w/v Ponceau de Xylidene (ponceau 2R) and 1% w/v acid fuchsin solutions in 1% v/v acetic acid,

and combine two parts ponceau 2R reagent with one part acid fuchsin reagent to prepare the working stain. The working reagent should be made up freshly just before use.

9. Phosphotungstic acid solution: dissolve phosphotungstic acid (50.0 g) in 1000 mL distilled water (stable for 6 mo).
10. Tris-buffered saline-Tween (TBS-T): 50 m*M* Tris-HCl buffer, pH 7.6, containing 0.15 *M* NaCl and 0.05% Tween-20.

3. Methods

3.1. Introductory Comments

3.1.1. Safety Considerations

1. The microtome and knife should be treated with respect; these are precisely engineered instruments manufactured to very fine tolerances.
2. **Caution:** Many of the chemicals associated with histochemical processing are hazardous to health. Pregnant staff should take particular care, as many of the chemicals routinely used in histochemical processing can cause fetal damage or death.
3. Tissue processors should be kept in rooms with efficient fume extraction.
4. All transfers of chemicals from storage bottles to tissue processor containers should be performed in a spark-proof fume hood.
5. Protective clothing, long-sleeved laboratory coats, rubber gloves, safety glasses/goggles, or face masks should be worn during all histochemical procedures.

3.1.2. Specific Details of Some Hazardous Reagents Used in Histochemistry

The following information was obtained from Materials Safety Data Sheets (MSDS) provided by Ajax Chemicals Australia (Auburn, NSW, Australia), BDH Chemicals Australia (Kilsyth, Victoria, Australia), Fisher Chemical, (Queensland, Australia), and the web site MSDS.online.com. This is a particularly convenient and up to date web-based source of information. Numerous other web-based sites can also be consulted for MSDS information. MSDS data should be routinely obtained when any new histology reagents are purchased and kept on file for subsequent reference purposes. *Laboratory Histopathology: A Complete Reference* *(8)* was also a useful source of safety information.

Caution is required for all the reagents listed:

1. *Alcian blue 8GX* is a water-soluble, copper phthalocyanin dye, it is an irritant combustible powder that should never be handled close to heat or a naked flame, skin contact should be avoided.
2. *Sirius red* is a disazo dye. Little is known about the hazards associated with its use, but other disazo dyes such as Sudan III, Sudan IV, Trypan blue, and Congo red are known to be toxic and carcinogenic. It would therefore be prudent to adopt similar safety precautions with sirius red.

3. *Toluidine blue O* is a hazardous quinone-imine dye. It is a combustible powder and should not be handled close to heat or a naked flame. It is an animal mutagen and an eye irritant. The toxicity of toluidine blue in humans has not been quantified, but it has been proved to be highly toxic in laboratory animals.
4. *Fast green FCF* is an animal carcinogen, and similar safety precautions to those used for toluidine blue should also be observed.
5. *Picric acid* is a strong oxidizing agent and reacts violently with combustible material and reducing agents. It is toxic and can be absorbed into the body by inhalation of the vapor or ingestion of the liquid. It is an irritant to the eyes, skin, and respiratory tract. It is a neurotoxin and can cause convulsions. The powder is explosive when dry and should always be stored under water in an air-tight storage container.
6. *Phosphotungstic acid* is an eye irritant and mildly corrosive.
7. *Ponceau de Xylidene and acid fuchsin* are suspected carcinogens.
8. *Xylene* is a moderately flammable liquid and a mild eye and mucous membrane irritant. It is a primary skin irritant and a central nervous system depressent, it will defat skin, and it may cause dermatitis. In acute cases exposure can result in narcosis, headache, nausea, fatigue, and dizziness. Chronic exposure results in neurological impairment; overexposure can lead to death caused by respiratory failure.
9. *Ethanol* is a flammable liquid and should never be handled close to heat or a naked flame. The vapor is heavier than air and can travel for a considerable distance along the ground to a source of ignition and flashback. Ethanol, however, is regarded as one of the safest industrial solvents. Although it possesses narcotic properties, a vapor concentration sufficient to produce narcosis is rarely if ever reached in a medical laboratory. Ethanol is rapidly oxidized in the body to carbon dioxide and water and does not produce permanent damage to the central nervous system.
10. *Methanol* is a flammable liquid and should never be handled close to heat or a naked flame. The vapor is heavier than air and can travel for a considerable distance along the ground to a source of ignition and flashback. It has a mutagenic effect on animals and should never be handled by staff who are pregnant. It is an eye, skin, and mucous membrane irritant and a central nervous system depressant; it is a narcotic and can cause death. It defats skin, and can cause dermatitis. It can be absorbed through the skin in doses large enough to cause narcosis. The vapor is also toxic and an irritant. Ingestion of 800–1000 ppm is sufficient to cause blindness. Prolonged exposure at 50,000 ppm for 1–2 h will cause death.
11. *Isopropyl alcohol* is a flammable liquid and should never be handled close to heat or a naked flame. The vapor is heavier than air and can travel for a considerable distance along the ground to a source of ignition and flashback. It is a severe eye, skin, and mucous membrane irritant and a central nervous system depressant; death may occur from respiratory paralysis. In cases of acute exposure to isopropyl alcohol, lachrimation, narcosis, eye damage, respiratory paralysis, and coma have been reported. Chronic exposure to isopropyl alcohol results in permanent corneal damage and death.

12. *Formaldehyde* is a moderately flammable liquid when exposed to heat or a naked flame. It is a proven animal carcinogen, and a strong eye, skin, and mucous membrane irritant and skin sensitizer. Death has been reported in workers exposed to high levels of formalin vapor.
13. *Chloroform* is an animal carcinogen and is suspected of having the same effect upon humans. It is an embryotoxin and should never be handled by staff who are pregnant. It is highly toxic by all routes of exposure and can be absorbed through the skin in doses large enough to cause toxicity. It is an anesthetic and a skin, eye, and respiratory tract irritant. It affects the central nervous system, liver and kidney damage may occur, and death can result from cardiac arrest. Ingestion of alcoholic drinks enhances the toxicity of chloroform. Persons with pre-existing liver, kidney, or heart disease may be at increased risk from exposure. In acute cases it causes headaches, nausea, jaundice, narcosis, liver, and kidney damage and loss of appetite. Chronic exposure results in liver and kidney damage and disturbances in the gastrointestinal tract.
14. *Acetic acid* is a corrosive substance and will cause severe damage to exposed skin; it is an eye and mucous membrane irritant.
15. *Formic acid* is a strong corrosive, a flammable chemical, and a suspected carcinogen. It is also an irritant to skin, eyes, and mucous membranes. The vapor is also an irritant and corrosive. Severe burns can result from exposure, and also chronic bronchitis, painful breathing, nausea, vomiting, and dental erosion can occur.
16. *Methyl benzoate* is a colorless combustible liquid with a characteristic unpleasant odor; it is harmful if swallowed, inhaled, or absorbed through the skin. It is irritating to the eye, mucous membranes, and upper respiratory tract and may cause allergic, respiratory, and skin reactions.
17. *Tricresyl phosphate* is a colorless, odorless, noncombustible liquid but may cause eye, skin, digestive, and respiratory tract irritation. Acute exposure leads to nausea, vomiting, and diarrhea.
18. *Immunohistology substrates*. Some substrates such as diaminobenzidene (DAB) are well-established carcinogens, and clearly appropriate safety precautions should be observed. It would be prudent to treat all immunohistology substrates with the same caution as recommended above for the use of histology dyes.

3.1.3. General Comments on Tissue Processing

Histochemical processing of connective tissues consists of five main stages, fixation, decalcification, processing, sectioning, and staining.

3.1.3.1. Fixation

The first stage in histochemical processing is the fixation step, which aims to preserve tissues permanently in as life-like a state as possible. Clearly this is also dependent on the procurement of the tissue specimens as soon as possible after death. Hydration of the specimens should be maintained when they are in transit before they are placed in fixative. Drying of the specimen will result in an artifact, which will become apparent after processing. Fixation is best carried out at a neutral pH between 6.8 and 7.4. Hypoxia of tissues lowers the pH, so there must be sufficient buffering capacity in the fixative to counter this; formalin can also break down to formic acid on prolonged storage. At least a 20:1 ratio of fixative to tissue should be used for fixation (*see* **Note 6**).

3.1.3.2. Decalcification

Cartilage specimens containing adjacent bony tissues require decalcification before the specimen can be processed further. Traditional decalcification agents such as hydrochloric, nitric, and sulphuric acids have been used for the demineralization of bone specimens but are not suitable for the decalcification of cartilage/bone specimens because of the hydrolysis of cartilage matrix components that occurs. Decalcification with mineral acids also leads to an impairment in the staining properties of the cartilage, nucleic acids generally stain poorly with hematoxylin and other cationic dyes, and the cytoplasm may be overstained by the briefest of exposures to anionic dyes such as eosin. Chelating agents such as ethylenediaminetetraacetic acid (EDTA) have also been employed for decalcification, but the process is considerably slower and may take months to achieve complete decalcification of large specimens compared with a few days for the mineral acids. Chelating agents, however, have some advantages when time is not as critical as the optimal preservation of cellular morphology and detail. Organic acids such as formic acid represent a compromise between the strong acids and chelators in terms of their speed of decalcification (~1 wk for specimens of similar size to those examined in this study) and the avoidance of undesirable effects on tissue morphology and staining.

Osteochondral specimens destined for immunohistochemical examination may be particularly sensitive to the decalcification procedure undertaken. This step may therefore require modification in an effort to preserve cartilage antigenic epitopes. It is important to remove specimens from decalcifying fluid as soon as they are decalcified to avoid damage from overexposure (*see* **Note 7**). A simple chemical method can be used to determine the end point of decalcification. A sample of decalcifying fluid is neutralized with sodium hydroxide and mixed with an equal volume of saturated ammonium oxalate solution. Any fine white precipitate that forms after a 30-min stand represents calcium oxalate and indicates the presence of free calcium in the decalcifying fluid.

3.1.3.3. Processing

After fixation and decalcification, the next step in histochemical processing is embedding. Embedding mechanically supports the tissue, converting it into a form that can be physically cut into microscopic sections with preservation of native tissue structure. The most common embedding medium is paraffin wax. Aqueous tissues, however, cannot be directly infiltrated with paraffin.

First the water must be removed from the tissues (*see* **Note 8**). This is accomplished by taking the tissues through a series of alcohols from 70 to 100%. Then a "clearing" agent is used to remove the dehydrating medium using a solvent that is also miscible with the embedding medium (*see* **Note 9**). Xylene is commonly employed for this purpose in paraffin-embedded specimens. Paraffins of different melting points with various hardnesses are available depending on the histotechnologist's requirements and the prevailing climatic conditions (warm vs cold). Paraplast wax also contains added plasticizers, which make the paraffin blocks easier to cut (*see* **Note 10**). A vacuum can be applied for the tissue infiltration stage. Some specimens can also be double embedded for added mechanical support: in this chapter celloidin (nitrocellulose) was also infiltrated into the tissue specimen.

3.1.3.4. Sectioning

The next stage in tissue processing is sectioning with a microtome. A thorough knowledge of the practice of histology and the cutting equipment's capabilities, plus manual dexterity, are all essential attributes for the cutting of a good, thin paraffin section. The result obtained depends not only on the skill of the histotechnologist but also on the quality of the equipment and chemicals used. It is important to have a properly fixed and embedded tissue block and a sharp microtome blade or many artifacts can be introduced during sectioning. Common artifacts at this stage include tearing, ripping, holes, folding, or wrinkling of the tissues. The orthopedic specimen will always be harder than the wax it is embedded in, thus it must be appropriately positioned in the paraffin block to minimize this factor and also to facilitate its ease of cutting with the microtome. The blocks must also be slowly and carefully trimmed to avoid damaging the specimen by pulling all or part of it out of the wax block. After the initial trimming, the paraffin blocks are soaked in a softening solution for 30 min, retrimmed, and then soaked again before sectioning (*see* **Note 10**). Once cut, the sections are floated on a warm water bath just below the melting point of the wax, which helps to remove wrinkles. Then the sections are picked up onto microscope slides and heated in an oven to dry, melt the wax, and cause the sections to adhere to the slide. Adherence of cartilage sections to slides can be problematic but clearly is very important in ensuring the success of any subsequent histological procedure (*see* **Notes 11** and **12**).

3.1.3.5. Staining

Before staining of the tissue section can be accomplished, the whole embedding procedure must be reversed to remove the embedding medium and return the tissue section to aqueous conditions conducive to staining with histochemical dyes or with primary and secondary antibody systems in immunohistological procedures. This is accomplished by deparaffinizing the sections in xylene, followed by graded alcohol washes back to water. Specific details of the stains and immunohistological procedures used in this study are provided below in **Subheadings 3.2.5.** and **3.2.6.**

3.1.3.6. Mounting

Mounting represents the final step in histochemical processing and is essential to prevent the tissue section from being scratched and also to provide better optical qualities for microscopic examination. The stained slide, however, must first be taken through a series of alcohol solutions again to remove the water, and then through clearing agents to a point at which a permanent resinous mounting substance can be applied beneath a glass cover slip (*see* **Notes 13** and **14**). The prepared microscope slide can then be added to existing archival material.

3.2. Processing of Ovine Cartilage

3.2.1. Tissue Sampling and Fixation

1. Ideally fix the cartilage within 30 min of sacrifice of the animal or keep it on ice until this is possible (up to 24 h).
2. Trim off all soft tissues external to the stifle (knee) joint, leaving the joint capsule intact.
3. Cut the exposed femur and tibia above and below the joint capsule with a bone saw.
4. Open the joint capsule, excise the cruciate ligaments, and expose and saw the tibial plateau and femoral condyles using a bandsaw into approx 3-mm-thick osteochondral slabs so that they fit into the processing cassettes (**Fig. 2**). Then place the specimens in at least 50 mL of 10% neutral buffered formalin and fix for 48 h. Transfer the specimens into 70% ethanol until a sufficient number have accumulated to decalcify and process them as a single batch (*see* **Note 6**).

3.2.2. Decalcification and Preparation of Tissue Blocks for Histological Processing

1. Prepare coronal osteochondral slabs of the mid-weight-bearing regions of the fixed stifle joints as shown in **Fig. 2** and then decalcify in 10% formic acid, 5% formalin for 8 d with constant agitation at room temperature using a Lipshaw bone decalcifier apparatus; the heat function is not used. Change the decalcification solution daily (*see* **Note 7**).
2. Equilibrate the cartilage/bone tissue slabs in 70% ethanol, in which they may be stored until a batch of specimens is available for the tissue processor dehydration step.

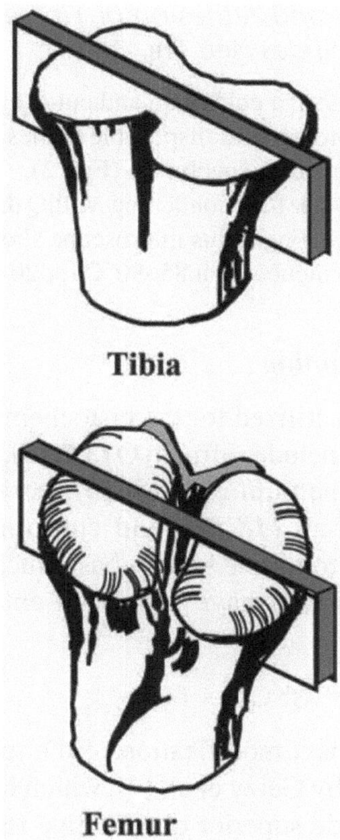

Fig. 2. Schematic representation depicting how midcoronal osteochondral tissue slabs were sampled from the mid-weight-bearing regions of the unilaterally meniscectomized and the sham operated ovine stifle joints for histochemical processing.

3.2.3. Dehydration and Processing of Tissues for Double Embedding

1. On d 1, immerse the tissue sections in 70% ethanol (2 × 1 h) to ensure equilibration, and then in 80% ethanol (3 h), 95% ethanol (3 h), and 100% ethanol (4 × 3 h) in an automatic tissue processor.
2. On d 2, transfer the sections to tightly sealed glass containers and equilibrate in methyl benzoate for 24 h (*see* **Note 1**).
3. On d 3, equilibrate the sections in a mixture of 1% celloidin and 1.5% tricresyl phosphate in methyl benzoate for 24 h.
4. On d 4–6, equilibrate the sections in 5% celloidin and 1.5% tricresyl phosphate in methyl benzoate for 3 d.
5. On d 7–8, wash the sections in chloroform (3 × 20 min) to remove excess celloidin, and then vacuum-infiltrate with Paraplast wax using four changes of 2 h, 3 h, overnight, and 3 h; on d 8, embed the specimens in Paraplast wax.

3.2.4. Cutting, Flotation, and Adhesion of Tissue Sections to Microscope Slides (see **Fig. 3**)

1. Cool the paraffin blocks on a cold plate and cut 4-μm sections using a Reichert-Jung 2035 rotary microtome with disposable blades (*see* **Note 10**). Coronal sections are made of the cartilage specimens (**Fig. 2**).
2. Float out sections on a water bath containing MilliQ distilled water at approx 52°C.
3. Pick up sections on SuperFrost Plus microscope slides (*see* **Note 12**) and immediately place them in an incubator at 85–90°C for 20–30 min and then 55°C overnight.

3.2.5. Histochemical Staining

Several dyes have been utilized for the histochemical visualization of cartilage proteoglycans; these include safranin O *(3,9,10)*, alcian blue *(11,12)*, toluidine blue-O *(3,9,10)*, ruthenium red *(13–15)*, acridine orange *(16,17)*, the carbocyanine dye Stains-all *(18,19)*, and cuprolinic (cupromeronic) blue *(20,21)*. Combinations of toluidine blue O/basic fuchsin *(22)*, alcian blue/safranin O/thionine/resorcin *(23)* have also been employed to stain cartilage proteoglycans.

3.2.5.1. Toluidine Blue O/Fast Green FCF

The method described is a modification of the toluidine blue O/fast green FCF procedure described by Getzy et al. *(9)*, which has been shown to be more reproducible and to provide superior quantitative results than the safranin O/ fast green FCF procedure *(3,10)*. This may partly be owing to impurities in some dye preparations *(24)* (*see* also comments in **Note 5**).

Procedure.

1. Thoroughly deparaffinize the sections in several washes in xylene (3 × 5 min) and then take them through graded alcohols to 70% v/v ethanol.
2. Stain the sections in 0.04% w/v toluidine blue O in buffer B for 10 min at room temperature.
3. Rinse the sections briefly in running tap water.
4. Counterstain slides in 0.1% w/v aqueous fast green FCF for 2 min.
5. Rinse slides briefly in running tap water.
6. Dehydrate slides rapidly in two changes of 99% isopropyl alcohol.
7. Clear slides in two changes of xylene.
8. Mount slides with Eukitt or another resinous mounting medium.

Results.

Tissue proteoglycans stain metachromatically with toluidine blue O, giving a vivid blue-purple color (*see* **Note 15**). Fast green FCF is a useful counterstain for the delineation of adjacent areas in the tissue section that are either devoid of or contain depleted proteoglycan levels compared with control tissues; these

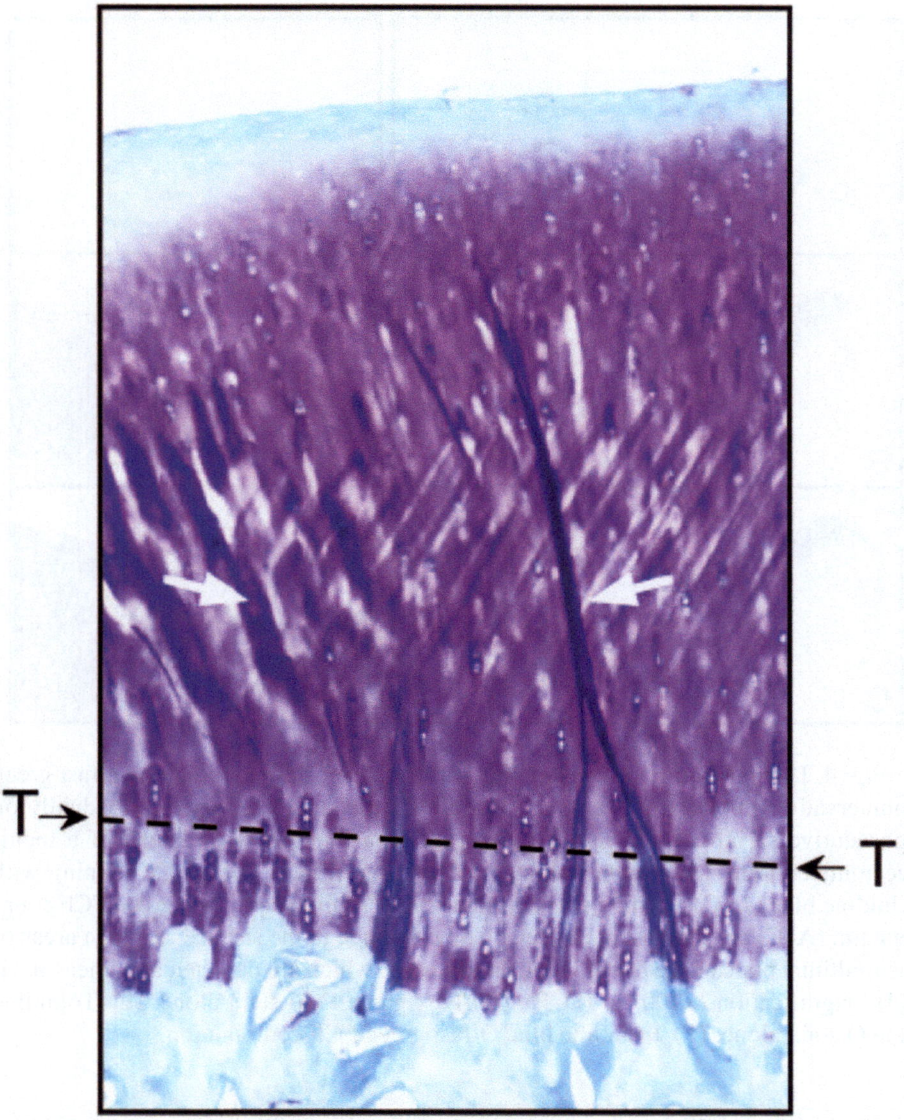

Fig. 3. Demonstration of several processing artifacts (arrows) on a toluidine blue/fast green-stained cartilage section from a femoral condyle, zone 2 of a laterally meniscectomized joint. The section has lifted from the microscope slide because of abnormal tissue swelling during flotation, resulting in folding or wrinkling of the specimen and entrapment of stain, which does not diffuse from the specimen as fast as adjacent areas; hence these areas appear darker on the section (white arrows). A cutting artifact is also evident in this section: the specimen has a series of parallel rips that have not stained in the procedure (T, tidemark). The calcified cartilage and subchondral bone, however, appear to be normal in this specimen.

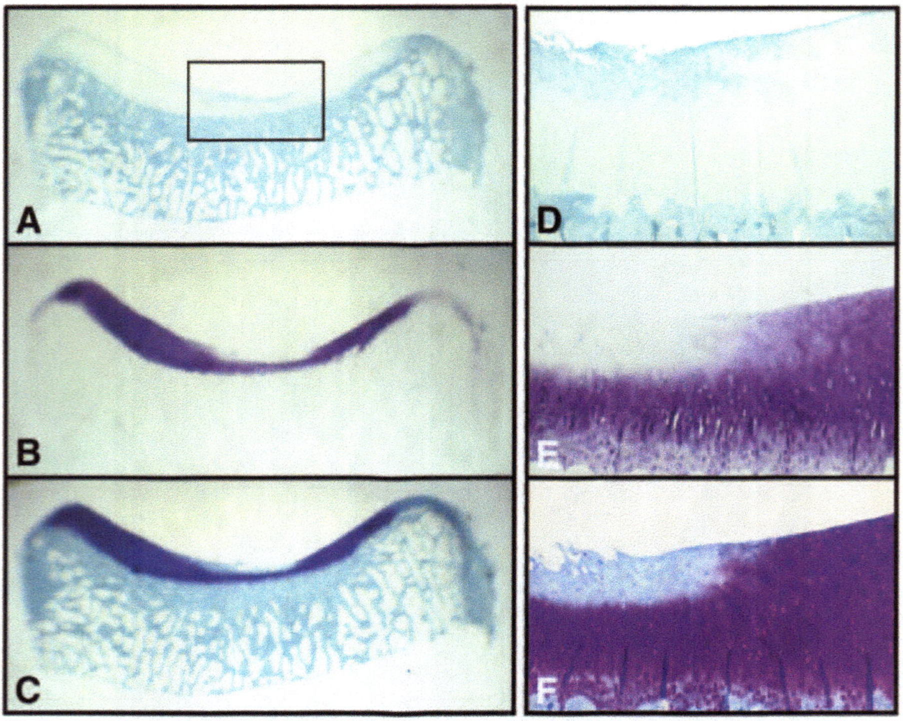

Fig. 4. Demonstration of the superior performance of the toluidine blue/fast green counterstain combination over each of these stain components used individually on consecutive serial coronal tissue sections from a lateral tibial plateau of a meniscectomized joint. **(A)** Single staining with fast green FCF. **(B)** Single staining with toluidine blue O. **(C)** Staining with toluidine blue O followed by fast green FCF counterstain. (A–C) are macroscopic views. Some damage to the surface cartilage areas of the midtibial plateau is evident in the boxed areas, which are depicted at higher (original) magnification (×100) in (D–F). **(D)** Fast green FCF stain alone. **(E)** Toluidine blue O stain alone. **(F)** Toluidine blue O/fast green FCF combination.

areas and bone stain green. The green-purple color combination provides good contrast for photographic reproduction (*see* **Figs. 3–5**).

3.2.5.2. Masson's-Trichrome

Procedure.

The method described is a modification of the original method of Masson ***(25)*** and a later modification ***(26)***.

1. Thoroughly deparaffinize the sections using several washes in xylene (2 × 5 min), and then take them through graded alcohols to water (*see* **Note 9**).

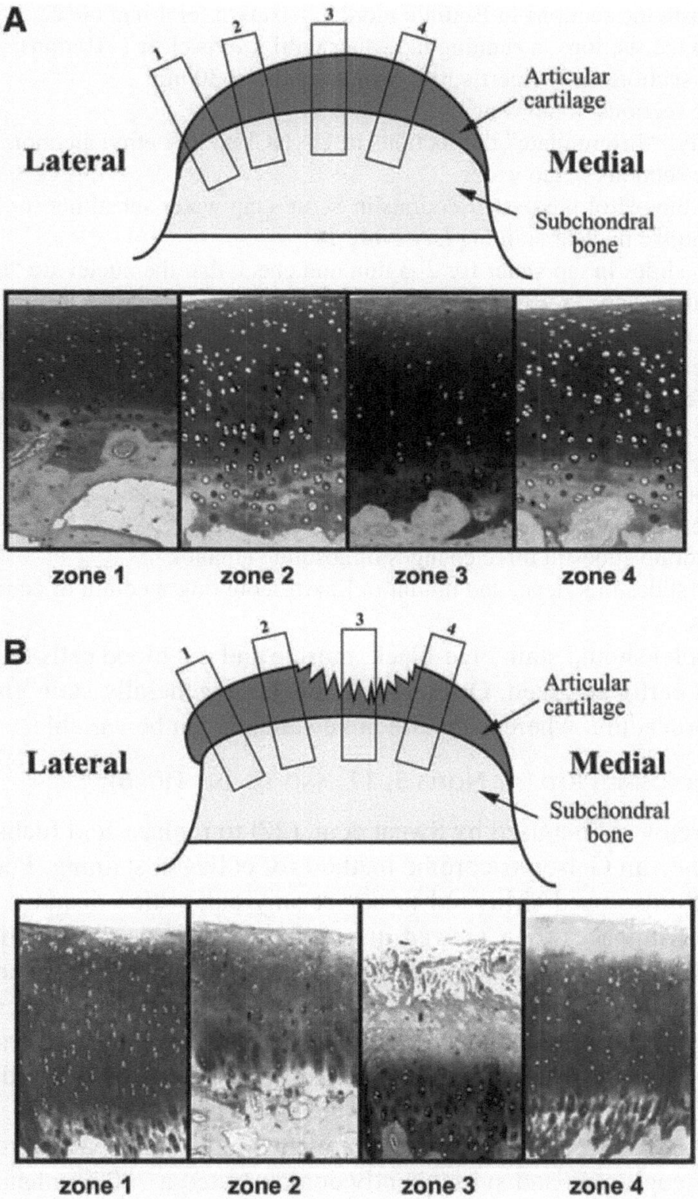

Fig. 5. Toluidine blue O/fast green FCF staining of specific regions (zones 1–4) of the midcoronal osteochondral tissue slabs prepared as depicted in **Fig. 2** viewed in the coronal plane. Sham operated (**A**) and unilaterally laterally meniscectomized (**B**) stifle joints from a 2-yr-old sheep. Low-power views are depicted (original magnification ×16) encompassing the full depth of the articular cartilage, calcified cartilage, and underlying subchondral bone.

2. Incubate the sections in Bouin's mordant/fixative for 1 h at 60°C.
3. Wash the sections in running tap water until it runs clear (~10 min).
4. Stain sections in Weigert's iron hematoxylin for 30 min.
5. Rinse sections in tap water.
6. Briefly, "differentiate" the sections in 1% HCl in 70% ethyl alcohol.
7. Rinse sections in tap water.
8. Alter the pH of the tissue sections in Scott's tap water substitute for 2–3 min to accentuate nuclear staining (*see* **Note 16**).
9. Wash slides in tap water for 2–3 min and check that the nuclei are "blue" using the microscope (*see* **Note 16**). Repeat if necessary.
10. Stain sections in Ponceau de Xylidene: acid fuchsin working mixture for 10 min.
11. Rinse sections briefly in distilled water.
12. "Differentiate" the slides in 5% w/v phosphotungstic acid solution until collagen is decolorized (~5 min) (*see* **Note 16**).
13. Rinse slides briefly in distilled water.
14. Counterstain with 2% w/v fast green FCF in 1% acetic acid (2 min).
15. Rinse slides in absolute ethanol.
16. Dehydrate slides in three changes of absolute ethanol.
17. Clear slides in xylene, and mount in Eukitt mounting medium or equivalent.

Results.

The nuclei should stain blue-black, muscle and red blood cells red, and collagen and cartilage green. Osteoid and new bone generally stain green in the Masson procedure, whereas mature bone staining can be variable.

3.2.5.3 Picrosirius Red (*see* **Notes 5, 17,** and **18** and **Fig. 6**)

Sirius red was first used by Sweat et al. *(27)* to replace acid fuchsin, which fades in the van Geison trichrome method for collagen staining. Puchtler and Sweat *(28)* also used sirius red to detect amyloid, which displays an apple-green birefringence when viewed under polarized light. Sirius red was also noted to enhance the normal birefringency of collagen fibers in tissue sections. Junquiera et al. *(29)* refined this method further with the use of picric acid in conjunction with polarization microscopy to detect collagen fibers in tissue sections. They also demonstrated that proteoglycans associated with the collagen fibrils compromised their staining properties with sirius red. Junquiera et al. *(29)* introduced an enzymatic treatment step using papain to remove the tissue proteoglycans and subsequently demonstrated a 700% enhancement in the birefringency of collagen when stained with sirius red. The role of picric acid in this staining procedure is not known; however, if it is omitted from the staining solution then all tissue components stain red. Picric acid therefore seems to prevent the indiscriminate staining of noncollagenous structures by sirius red in this procedure. Kiraly et al. *(30)* used a lengthy (18-h) predigestion step with testicular hyaluronidase to remove the tissue proteoglycans prior to

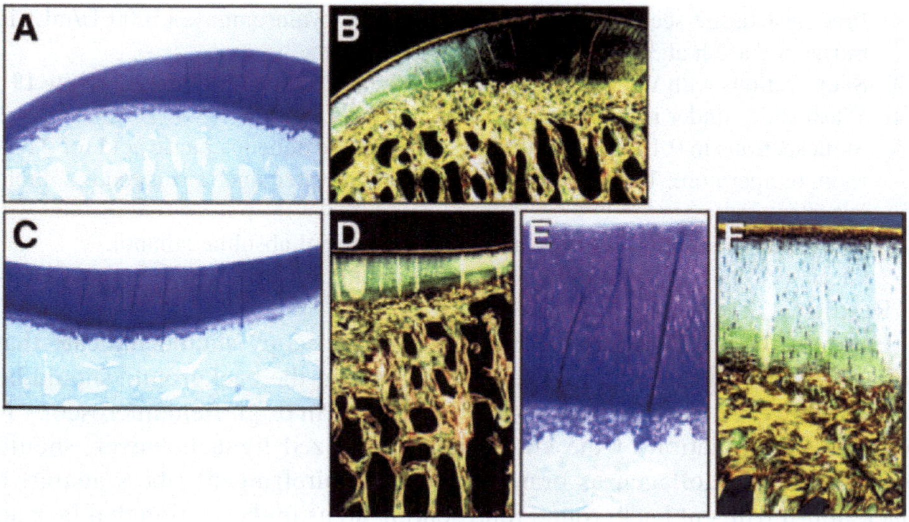

Fig. 6. Histological examination of coronal sections of the weight-bearing regions of the lateral femoral condyle (**A,B**) and tibial plateau (**C–F**) of a control sham operated ovine stifle joint from a 7-yr-old sheep. Toluidine blue O/fast green FCF-stained sections (A, C, E) and picrosirius red-stained sections (B, D, F) viewed under polarized light. Toluidine blue staining demonstrates a uniform proteoglycan distribution throughout the articular cartilage and delineation of the tidemark and calcified cartilage in the femoral condyle and tibial plateau (A, C, E). Picrosirius red staining of equivalent joint regions demonstrates differences in the collagen organization at different cartilage depths and within the trabeculae of the subchondral bone (B, D, E). Particularly prominent is a highly refractile surface lamina at the articulating joint surface and a dark, poorly refractile region underlying this. The surface lamina contains tangentially arranged collagen fibers; in the mid to deep and calcified cartilage zones the collagen fibers are thicker and are arranged parallel to the plane of the polarized light used for microscopic examination. Chondrocytes appear as blackish dots with picrosirius red staining. Original magnifications ×16 in (A–D) and ×50 in (E, F).

sirius red staining. Using these prolonged digestion conditions, we had difficulty in maintaining adherence of the cartilage sections to the microscope slides. We therefore employed a shorter hyaluronidase digestion step (2 h), which results in removal of approx 85% of the cartilage proteoglycans based on safranin O staining ***(30)*** and used an extended sirius red staining step (2 h) to ensure optimal collagen staining.

Procedure.

1. Thoroughly deparaffinize the sections in xylene (3 × 5 min) then take them through graded alcohols to water (*see* **Note 9**).

2. Predigest tissue sections with bovine testicular hyaluronidase (1000 U/mL) in buffer A for 2 h at 37°C.
3. Stain sections with Wiegert's iron hematoxylin for 30 min (optional; *see* **Note 19**).
4. Wash slides under running tap water.
5. Stain sections in 0.1% sirius red F3BA in saturated aqueous picric acid for 2 h at room temperature. The sections are not rinsed in water since sirius red is soluble in water.
6. Dehydrate the sections rapidly in several changes of absolute ethanol.
7. Clear sections in xylene and mount in Eukitt or equivalent.

Results.

Examination of the slides by brightfield microscopy should indicate that collagen has stained red and nuclei gray to brown; the background should be yellow. However, not all that is visibly stained red in brightfield microscopy is collagen. Examination of the slides under polarized light, however, should demonstrate the collagen as orange/red highly birefringent fibers against a black non-refringent background representing areas in the section that lack an organized tertiary collagenous structure (**Fig. 7**).

3.2.6. Immunohistochemical Procedures

Tissues were processed as outlined above in **Subheadings 3.2.1.** to **3.2.4.** (*see* **Note 20**). The immunolocalizations were undertaken using a Sequenza vertical cover plate immunostaining system (Shandon).

Procedure.

1. Initially deparaffinize the sections in xylene (2 × 5 min) and then take them through graded alcohols to water.
2. With specimens destined for the horseradish peroxidase (HRP) detection system, block the endogenous peroxidase activity by incubating the tissue sections with 3% aqueous H_2O_2 for 5 min and wash the tissue in distilled water.
3. Predigest the type II collagen immunolocalizations with proteinase K for 6 min at room temperature using a proprietary proteinase K reagent (DAKO cat. no. S03020) following the manufacturer's instructions. This is followed by a testicu-

---

Fig. 7. Histological examination of coronal sections of the weight-bearing regions of the lateral femoral condyle (**A**, **B**, **E**, **G**) and tibial plateau (**C**, **D**, **F**, **H**) of a laterally meniscectomized stifle joint from a 7-yr-old sheep sampled 6 mo post meniscectomy. Toluidine blue O/fast green FCF-stained sections (A, C, E, H) and picrosirius red-stained sections (B, D, F, G) viewed under polarized light. Toluidine blue staining demonstrates a focal loss of proteoglycan and surface fibrillation of the articular cartilage in the weight-bearing region of the joint; the tidemark and calcified cartilage of the femoral condyle and tibial plateau are also prominently delineated (A, C, E, H). Cell death within regions of fibrillated cartilage and cell cloning in adjacent deeper joint regions are also clearly evident (E, H). Picrosirius red staining of equivalent joint

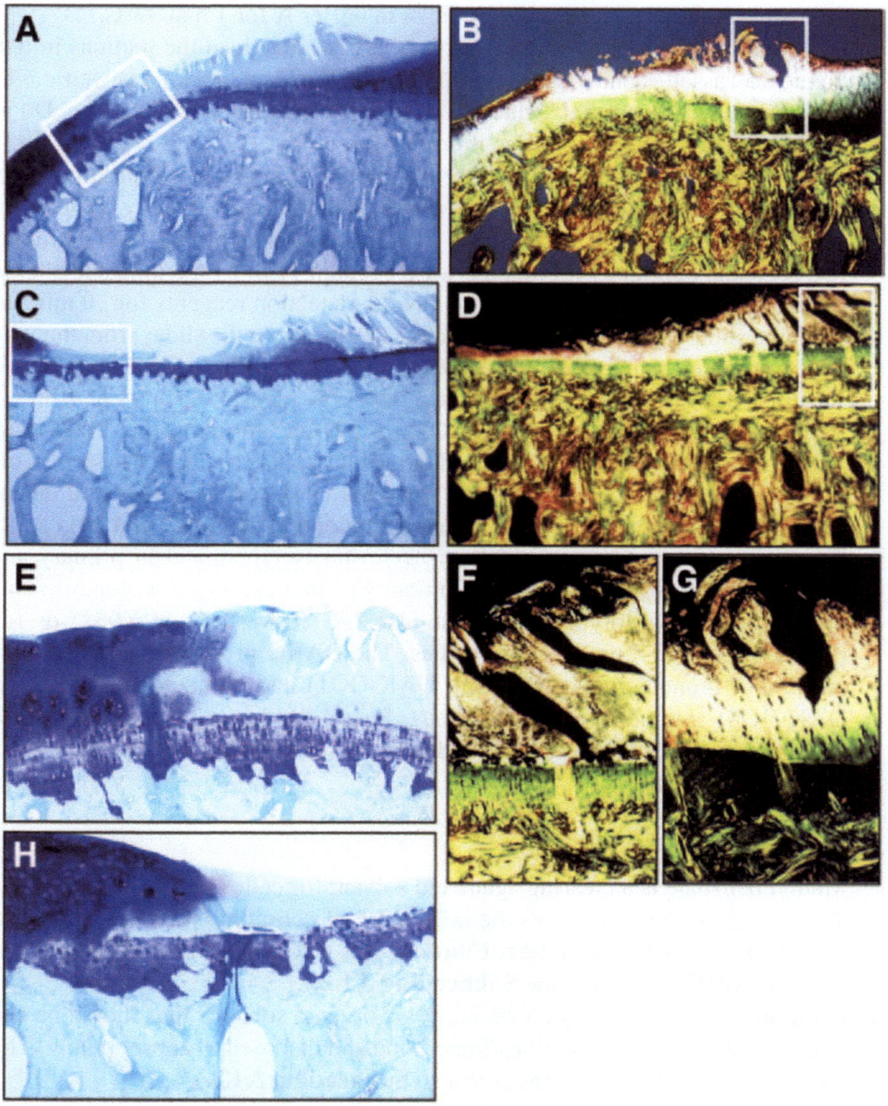

Fig. 7. (*continued*) regions demonstrates distinct differences in the collagen organization at different cartilage depths and within the trabeculae of the subchondral bone (B, D, F, G) as well as significant differences from equivalent regions of the sham operated control joint tissues presented in **Fig. 6**. Particularly prominent is the surface fibrillation in the weight-bearing joint regions in response to meniscectomy, as well as loss of the highly refractile surface lamina at the articulating joint surface and the dark poorly refractile region underlying this. The boxed regions in (A–D) are also presented at higher magnification in (E–H), respectively. Original magnification ×16 in (A–D) and ×100 in (E–H).

lar hyaluronidase digestion (1000 U/mL) in buffer A for 1 h at 37°C.

4. Following the enzymatic epitope retrieval procedures, load the sections into the Sequenza cassettes and wash for 5 min in TBS-T. Then block nonspecific binding sites with 10% normal swine serum for 10 min at room temperature. Do not wash the slides prior to addition of primary antibody.
5. Incubate with the antitype II collagen primary antibody (1/100 dilution) overnight at 4°C in the Sequenza vertical cover plate immunohistology chamber.
6. Then wash the slides in TBS-T for 5 min, incubate with biotinylated antimouse IgG secondary antibody for 30 min, wash again in TBS-T for 5 min, add alkaline phosphatase or HRP-conjugated streptavidin detection reagents for 30 min, and wash the slides again in TBS-T for 5 min. Then remove the slides from the vertical cover plate chamber and place in horizontal racks. Use NovaRED or DAB as substrates for the HRP detection system. Use new fuchsin, fast red, or 4-bromo-3-chloro-1 indolyl phosphate (BCIP)/nitroblue tetrazolium (NBT)/iodo nitrotetrazolium violet (INT) for the alkaline phosphatase detection system. Color development with each substrate was allowed to proceed for the optimal incubation periods recommended by each manufacturer (*see* **Notes 13** and **14**).
7. Prepare control sections in which an irrelevant isotype-matched primary antibody is substituted for the primary antibody of interest. For this step, use commercial (DAKO) isotype-matched mouse IgG (DAKO Code X931) or IgM (DAKO Code X942) control antibodies. The DAKO products X931 and X942 are mouse monoclonal IgG_1 (clone DAK-GO1) and monoclonal IgM (clone DAK-GO8) antibodies directed against *Aspergillus niger* glucose oxidase, an enzyme that is neither present nor inducible in mammalian tissues.

Results (*see* **Fig. 8**).

4. Notes

1. Methyl benzoate is a clearing agent and solvent for celloidin.
2. Tricresyl phosphate improves the infiltration of celloidin into tissue specimens for effective double embedding. **Caution:** it is noxious and should be used with adequate ventilation (also *see* **Subheading 3.1.2.**).
3. **Caution:** xylene and chloroform are toxic organic solvents that should be used with proper ventilation facilities/fume-hood and disposed of appropriately. They are potential liver carcinogens (*see* also **Subheading 3.1.2.**).
4. **Caution:** formic acid is a corrosive chemical and should be used with care employing eye protection, rubber gloves, and long-sleeved lab coat or equivalent protective clothing.
5. It may be useful to use only a single batch of dye to standardize procedures. Impurities in some dye preparations can lead to difficulties with reproducible staining *(9)*. More than one colored product may be present in some batches of dye products; furthermore, other compounds are also often added to commercial dye products to aid in their precipitation properties and also to adjust their color intensity.

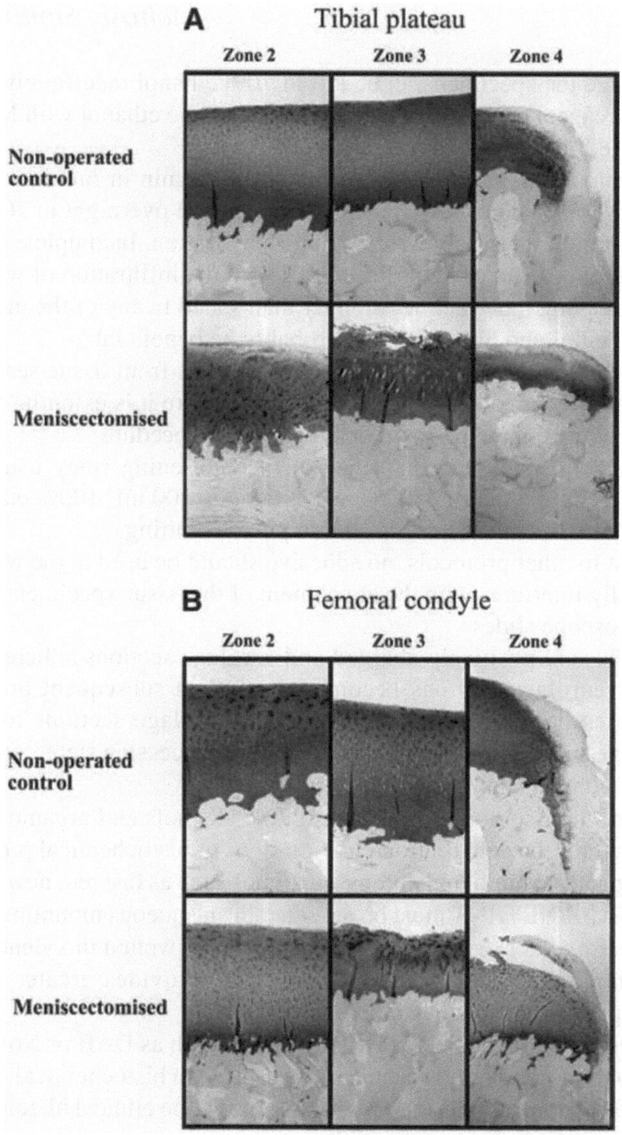

Fig. 8. Immunolocalization of type II collagen in coronal sections of nonoperated control and unilateral laterally meniscectomized stifle joints from a 2-yr-old sheep. Medium-power views (×50) are provided of particular zones within sections prepared from the lateral tibial plateau and femoral condyles. These tissue zones correspond to a midlesion area (zone 3) and adjacent areas adjacent located laterally (zone 2) and medially (zone 4) to the lesion site. These are similar to the zones depicted in diagramatically in **Fig. 5B**. Equivalent zones of nonoperated control joints are also depicted for comparison. Type II collagen levels are generally depleted in the meniscectomized joints, particularly so in focally disrupted surface areas in zone 3.

6. At this stage the specimen can be left in 70% ethanol indefinitely without damage. This reagent should be made up from absolute ethanol with MilliQ distilled water of 18.2 mΩ resistivity.
7. After decalcification, wash the specimen for 30 min in running tap water, and then in several changes of 70% ethanol, and leave overnight in 70% ethanol.
8. It is very important to achieve complete dehydration. Incomplete dehydration of tissue specimens can present difficulties with the infiltration of wax during processing. Leaving the specimens longer than stated in any of the methyl benzoate solutions will do no harm and will probably be beneficial.
9. Xylene is commonly used for removal of paraffin from tissue sections. Paraffin is strongly birefringent in polarized light; therefore it is essential that it be thoroughly removed in the picrosirius red staining procedure.
10. If the paraffin blocks need further surface softening (they usually do), then immerse them in a mixture of 50 mL ammonia, 300 mL 100% ethanol, 300 mL glycerin, and 300 mL water for 30 min prior to cutting.
11. In contrast to other protocols, no adhesive should be used in the water bath since this actually interferes with the attachment of the tissue specimens to SuperFrost Plus microscope slides.
12. These slides are positively charged and cartilage sections adhere well to them. Very few cartilage sections become detached in subsequent processing steps using these slides. Adequate adherence of cartilage sections to conventional microscope slides through extended histology processing steps can present a significant technical challenge.
13. Because of their solubility properties in the alcohols and organic solvents commonly used for the dehydration/clearing steps of histochemical processing, alkaline phosphatase immunohistology substrates such as fast red, new fuchsin BCIP/NBT, or BCIP/NBT/INT must be mounted in an aqueous mounting medium such as Aquaperm. After drying, the slide may then be wetted in xylene and mounted in a resinous mountant such as Eukitt. This provides greater resolution for microscopy than an aqueous mountant.
14. Substrates commonly used for HRP histology such as DAB or NovaRED are not soluble in the alcohols and organic solvents used in histochemical processing and are therefore more straightforward for use in routine clinical histological applications. However, they do not provide as attractive colors as the new fuchsin and fast red alkaline phosphatase substrates.
15. Carboxylated and sulfated polymers react metachromatically with toluidine blue. Metachromasia is a phenomenon exhibited when negatively charged entities (polyanions) such as the glycosaminoglycan side chains of proteoglycans react with certain cationic dyes (toluidine blue) to form a dye polymer complex that has a different absorption maxima from the normal dye monomer (blue) and thus displays a different color emission (purple-red). Entitities that stain with toluidine blue (nuclei) without inducing metachromasia (i.e., stain blue) are said to be orthochromatic.

16. The nuclei should be "overstained" at this stage since the earlier decalcification steps and subsequent phosphotungstic acid treatment steps in the Masson procedure diminish nuclear staining.
17. Sirius red F3BA is a relatively large dye molecule containing six sulfonic acid groups; it assumes an elongated conformation approx 46 Å long. This dye causes an increase in birefringence when it binds parallel to collagen. Staining and birefringence is, however, significantly improved by prior removal of proteoglycans from tissue sections.
18. There is little standardization between manufacturers in the naming of dyes; consequently the same chemically identical dye may be obtained from different suppliers under a wide range of names. Sirius red is not yet one of the dyes certified by the biological stain commission. Care should therefore be taken that the correct sirius red dye is purchased. Sirius red F3BA is also known as sirius red F3B Direct red 80, or color index 35780, although CI 35782 is also given in some references. Sirius red F3BA should not be confused with other direct sirius red cotton dyes such as sirius red 4B (CI 28160, direct red 81). Sirius red 4B was originally used with the van Gieson procedure and also stains collagen, basement membrane, and reticulin fibres. Sirius red F3BA (which is essentially a dimerized form of sirius red 4B) is made by 25 different manufacturers and has many alternative trade names. These include Chlorantine fast red 7BLN, Durazol brilliant red B (ICI), Pontamine fast red 7BNL, red or fast red B or 5B to 8B. Full technical information on dye products are frequently not forthcoming from the manufacturers. Furthermore, the direct cotton dye manufacturing process necessarily generates more than one colored product. To further complicate this issue, other compounds are also often added to commercial dye products as fillers to aid in the precipitation properties of the major dye components or to adjust their color intensities. The sirius red dye F3BA used in this study was a Gurr dye obtained from BDH but still has no certification or an assigned CI number. See Conn et al. ***(31)*** for technical information on specific dyes.
19. Nuclei should be "overstained"; otherwise the subsequent picric acid staining step will decolorize them unduly.
20. The decalcification and fixation conditions may have to be varied to improve epitope detectability and obviously depend on the sensitivity of the respective antibody epitopes to these procedures. Various epitope retrieval procedures (enzymatic, heat, pH) may also be adopted to improve epitope detection.

References

1. Lillie, R. D. (1965) *Histopathologic Technic and Practical Histochemistry.* McGraw-Hill, New York.
2. Bancroft, J. D. and Stevens, A. eds. (1996) *Theory and Practice of Histological Technique.* Churchill-Livingstone, New York.
3. Hyllested, J. L., Veje, K., and Ostergaard, K. (2002) Histochemical studies of the extracellular matrix of human articular cartilage—a review. *Osteoarthritis Cartilage* **10,** 333–343.

4. An, Y. H. and Martin, K. L. eds. (2003) *Handbook of Histology Methods for Bone and Cartilage*. Humana Press, Totowa, NJ.
5. Little, C., Smith, S., Ghosh, P., and Bellenger, C. (1997) Histomorphological and immunohistochemical evaluation of joint changes in a model of osteoarthritis induced by lateral meniscetomy in sheep. *J. Rheumatol.* **24,** 2199–2209.
6. Ghosh, P., Numata, Y., Smith, S., Read, R., Armstrong, S., and Johnson, K. (1993) The metabolic response of articular cartilage to abnormal mechanical loading induced by medial or lateral meniscectomy in *Joint destruction in Arthritis and Osteoarthritis* (Van den Berg, W., et al., eds.), Birkhauser, Verlag, Basel.
7. Burgeson, R. E. and Hollister, D. W. (1979) Collagen heterogeneity in human cartilage: identification of several new collagen chains. *Biochem. Biophys. Res. Commun.* **87,** 1124–1131
8. Woods, A. E. and Ellis, R. C. (1994) *Laboratory Histopathology: A Complete Reference*. Churchill Livingstone, New York.
9. Getzy, L. L., Malemud, C. J., Goldberg, V. M., and Moskowitz, R. W. (1982) Factors influencing metachromatic staining in paraffin embedded sections of rabbit and human articular cartilage: a comparison of the safronin O and toluidine blue O techniques. *J. Histotechnol.* **5,** 111–116.
10. Naumann, A., Dennis, J. E., Awadallah, A., et al. (2002) Immunochemical and mechanical characterisation of cartilage sub-types in rabbit. *J. Histochem. Cytochem.* **50,** 1049–1058.
11. Mason, R. M. (1971) Observations on the glycosaminoglycans of aging bronchial cartilage studied with Alcian Blue. *Histochem. J.* **3,** 421–434.
12. Goldstein, D. J. and Horobin, R. W.(1974) Surface staining of cartilage by Alcian blue, with reference to the role of microscopic dye aggregates in histological staining. *Histochem. J.* **6,** 175–184
13. Shepard, N. and Mitchell, N. (1977) The use of ruthenium and p-phenylenediamine to stain cartilage simultaneously for light and electron microscopy. *J. Histochem. Cytochem.* **25,** 1163–1168.
14. Davis, W. L., Jones, R. G., Knight, J. P., and Hagler, H. K. (1982) Cartilage calcification: an ultrastructural, histochemical, and analytical x-ray microprobe study of the zone of calcification in the normal avian epiphyseal growth plate. *J. Histochem. Cytochem.* **30,** 221–234
15. Hunziker, E. B., Ludi, A., and Herrmann, W. (1992) Preservation of cartilage matrix proteoglycans using cationic dyes chemically related to ruthenium hexaammine trichloride. *J. Histochem. Cytochem.* **40,** 909–917.
16. Shepard, N. and Mitchell, N. (1981) Acridine orange stabilization of glycosaminoglycans in beginning endochondral ossification. A comparative light and electron microscopic study. *Histochemistry* **70,** 107–114
17. Brandes, G. and Reale, E. (1990) The reaction of acridine orange with proteoglycans in the articular cartilage of the rat. *Histochem. J.* **22,** 106–112.
18. Green, M. R. (1975) Simultaneous differential staining of nucleic acids, proteins, conjugated proteins and polar lipids by a cationic carbocyanine dye. *J. Histochem. Cytochem.* **23,** 411–423

19. Hasty, K. A., Smith, G.N., Jr., and Kang, A. H. (1983) Histochemical identification of sulfation position in chondroitin sulfate in various cartilages. *J. Histochem. Cytochem.* **31,** 1367–1374
20. Guerra, D., Frizziero, L., Losi, M., Bacchelli, B., Mezzadri, G., and Pasquali-Ronchetti, I. (1996) Ultrastructural identification of a membrane-like structure on the surface of normal articular cartilage. *J. Submicrosc. Cytol. Pathol.* **28,** 385–393.
21. Orford, C. R., Gardner, D. L., O'Connor, P., Bates, G., Swallow, J. J., and Brito-Babapulle, L. A. (1986) Ultrastructural alterations in glycosaminoglycans of dog femoral condylar cartilage after surgical division of an anterior cruciate ligament: a study with cupromeronic blue in a critical electrolyte concentration technique. *J. Anat.* **148,** 233–244.
22. Inoue, N., Ikeda, K., Aro, H. T., Frassica, F. J., Sim, F. H., and Chao, E. Y. S. (2002) Biologic tendon fixation to metallic implant augmentaed with autogenous cancellous bone graft and bone marrow in a canine model. *J. Orthop. Res.* **20,** 957–966.
23. Balogh, G., Kovacs, P., and Csaba, G. (1982) ASTRIN—a new trichrome staining technique. *Z. Mikrosk. Anat. Forsch.* **96,** 138–144.
24. Horobin, R. W. (1969) The impurities of biological dyes: their detection, removal, occurrence and histological significance—a review. *Histochem. J.* **1,** 231–265.
25. Masson, P. (1929) Some histological methods. Trichrome stainings and their preliminary technique. Bulletin of the International Association of Medicine. *J. Tech. Methods* **12,** 75.
26. Bancroft, J. D. and Cook, H. C., eds. (1994) *Manual of Histological Techniques and their Diagnostic Application*. Churchill Livingstone, New York, p. 42.
27. Sweat, F., Puchtler, H., and Rosenthal, S. I. (1964) Sirius red F3BA as a stain for connective tissue. *Arch. Pathol.* **78,** 69–72.
28. Puchtler, H. and Sweat, F. (1964) Histochemical specificity of staining methods for connective tissue fibres: resocin-fuchsin and Van Giesens picro-fuchsin. *Histiochimie* **4,** 24–34.
29. Junquiera, L. C., Bignolas, G., and Brentani, R. R. (1979) Picrosirius staining plus polarisation microscopy, a specific method for collagen detection in tissue sections. *Histochem. J.* **11,** 447–455.
30. Kiraly, K., Hyttinen, M. M., Lapvetelainen, T., et al. (1997) Specimen preparation and quantification of collagen birefringence in unstained sections of articular cartilage using image analysis and polarising light microscopy. *Histochem. J.* **29,** 317–327.
31. Conn, J. H. (1961) *Biological Stains*, 7th ed. Williams & Wilkins, Baltimore.

4

Histochemical Visualization of the Cartilage Hyaladherins Using a Biotinylated Hyaluronan Oligosaccharide Bioaffinity Probe

James Melrose and Susan Smith

Summary

Hyaluronan (HA) binding proteins (HABPs) were localized in cartilaginous ovine tissues (articular cartilage, intervertebral disc) using a biotinylated HA (bHA) oligosaccharide bioaffinity probe. The bHA oligosaccharide probe was prepared by partial digestion of HA with ovine testicular hyaluronidase, and the oligosaccharides were labeled with biotin hydrazide and purified by a combination of aggrecan G1 domain and avidin affinity chromatography. Hyaladherins were prominently visualized in tissue sections using the bHA oligosaccharide probe as pericellular components in hypertrophic epiphyseal and vertebral growth plate chondrocytes and in the enlarged cells of the cartilaginous end plate of the intervertebral disc. Weaker extracellular staining was also evident in the matrix of the ovine newborn hip and knee joint cartilages. The bHA oligosaccharide probe also visualized intracellular HABPs (IHABPs) in the hypertrophic growth plate chondrocytes of the primary ossification centers. Monolayer cultures of ovine chondrocytes rapidly internalized the bHA oligosaccharide affinity probe to discrete cytoplasmic, nuclear, and perinuclear regions, which were visualized by indirect fluorescent microscopy. This bHA oligosaccharide affinity probe may be useful in future investigations designed to characterize these novel cartilage IHABPs and the role that HA endocytosis plays in cellular regulatory processes in cartilage homeostasis.

Key Words: Hyaluronan; hyaluronan binding proteins; hyaladherins; intracellular hyaluronan binding proteins; cartilage; intervertebral disc.

1. Introduction

In relatively acellular connective tissues such as cartilage, hyaluronan (HA) performs specific interactions extracellularly via the matrix hyaladherins ***(1–7)***. These have also been termed the hyalectans ***(8,9)*** or lecticans ***(10)***, emphasizing the functional role these proteins play in matrix assembly and stabilization. The interaction of aggrecan with HA facilitates the assembly of massive extra-

From: *Methods in Molecular Medicine, Vol. 101: Cartilage and Osteoarthritis, Volume 2: Structure and In Vivo Analysis*
Edited by: F. De Ceuninck, M. Sabatini, and P. Pastoureau © Humana Press Inc., Totowa, NJ

cellular macromolecular arrays, which are entrapped within the type II collagen network in hyaline cartilage. The interplay of these matrix components provides viscoelastic and hydrodynamic properties to hyaline cartilage that are essential for correct joint function. The interaction of aggrecan with HA is mediated via an amino-terminal globular domain that extends from the aggrecan core protein known as the G1 domain or hyaluronan binding region (HABR), which shares sequence homology with a small matrix glycoprotein termed link protein *(2,3)*. Link protein displays affinity for HA and the G1 domain of aggrecan, which facilitates the formation of HA-link-aggrecan ternary complexes in the cartilage extracellular matrix *(2–4,11)*. The formation of such complexes is defective in osteoarthritic articular cartilage, which compromises normal joint function (*see* **Note 1**).

In the present study we have prepared a biotinylated HA (bHA) oligosaccharide bioaffinity probe and utilized it for histochemical visualization of extracellular matrix, cell surface, and intracellular hyaladherins in a number of ovine cartilages (**Figs. 1** and **2**). This probe may be useful in investigations of these cartilage intracellular HABPs (IHABPs), which still await characterization, and also for studies examining HA endocytosis/IHABPs and chondrocyte regulatory processes in cartilage homeostasis.

2. Materials

2.1. Equipment and Chemicals

1. Standard histology processing equipment: tissue processor, microtome, and Sequenza vertical cover plate system for antibody incubations.
2. Standard tissue culture equipment for isolation and culture of chondrocytes: laminar flow hood, and CO_2-humidified incubator.
3. Fast protein liquid chromatography (FPLC; Pharmacia HR 10/30) and standard chromatography columns for affinity chromatography.
4. Fluorescent microscope, e.g., Leica DMLB MPS60 photomicroscope system, equipped with filters for assessment of fluorescein labeling.
5. 170-kDa Hyaluronan (Fidia SpA, Abano Terme, Italy).
6. 1000 U/mg Ovine testicular hyaluronidase (Boehringer-Mannheim, N. Ryde, NSW, Australia).
7. Fractogel TSK HW 50(S) FPLC gel (Selby Biolab, Gladesville, NSW, Australia).
8. Immobilized avidin affinity chromatography kit, biotin hydrazide (Pierce, Rockford, IL).
9. Epoxy-activated sepharose (Pharmacia AMRAD Biotech, N. Ryde, NSW, Australia).
10. Fetal calf serum (Trace Bioscience, NSW, Australia).
11. Tissue culture plasticware (Falcon, Becton-Dickinson).
12. Secondary detection reagent kits: streptavidin-alkaline phosphatase, streptavidin horseradish peroxidase conjugates LSAB+, $LSAB_2$; new fuchsin, nitroblue tetrazolium (NBT)/5-bromo-4-chloro-3-indolyl phosphate (BCIP)/iodo nitrotetra-

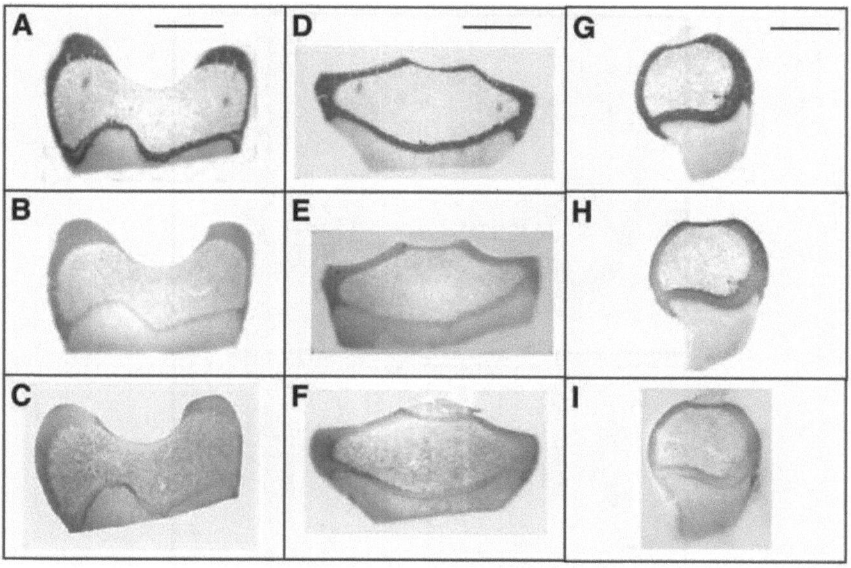

Fig. 1. Histochemical comparison of the distribution of proteoglycan (toluidine blue O/fast green FCF staining; (**A**, **D**, **G**), type II collagen (**B**, **E**, **H**), and hyaluronan binding proteins (bHA oligosaccharide staining; **C**, **F**, **I**) in vertical midcoronal sections of a femoral condyle (A–C) and tibial plateau (D–F) of an ovine knee (stifle) joint and in midsagittal section of a head of femur (G–I) of a hip joint from a 5-d-old sheep. The images are macroscopic views. Streptavidin horseradish peroxidase detection and NovaRED substrate were used for visualization. Scale bar, 1 cm in (A), (D), and (G); applies to all panels.

zolium (INT) diaminobenzidene histology substrates; Protein block-serum free, X0909 (DAKO AUSTRALIA, Botany, NSW, Australia).

13. NovaRED™ histology substrate (Vector, Burlingame, CA).
14. Avidin (14.8 U/mg protein), 2-(4'-hydroxyazobenzene)-benzoic acid (HABA), 1-ethyl-3-[3-dimethylamino)-propyl]-carbodi-imide (EDC), DNAase I, clostridial collagenase, Dulbecco's modified Eagle's medium (DMEM)-F-12, 1:1 mix, L-glutamine and D-biotin (Sigma).
15. Formic acid (analytical grade) for decalcification of osteochondral and vertebral-intervertebral disc specimens.
16. Organic solvents for fixation, dehydration, and deparaffinization of histology specimens (ethanol, xylene).
17. 10% Neutral buffered formalin for fixation of histology specimens.
18. SuperFrost® Plus microscope slides (Menzel-Glaser).
19. Permafluor aqueous mounting medium (Immunon, Pittsburgh, PA).
20. Kodak Ektachrome P1600 Daylight (EPH 135-36) 35-mm slide film for fluorescent microscopy.

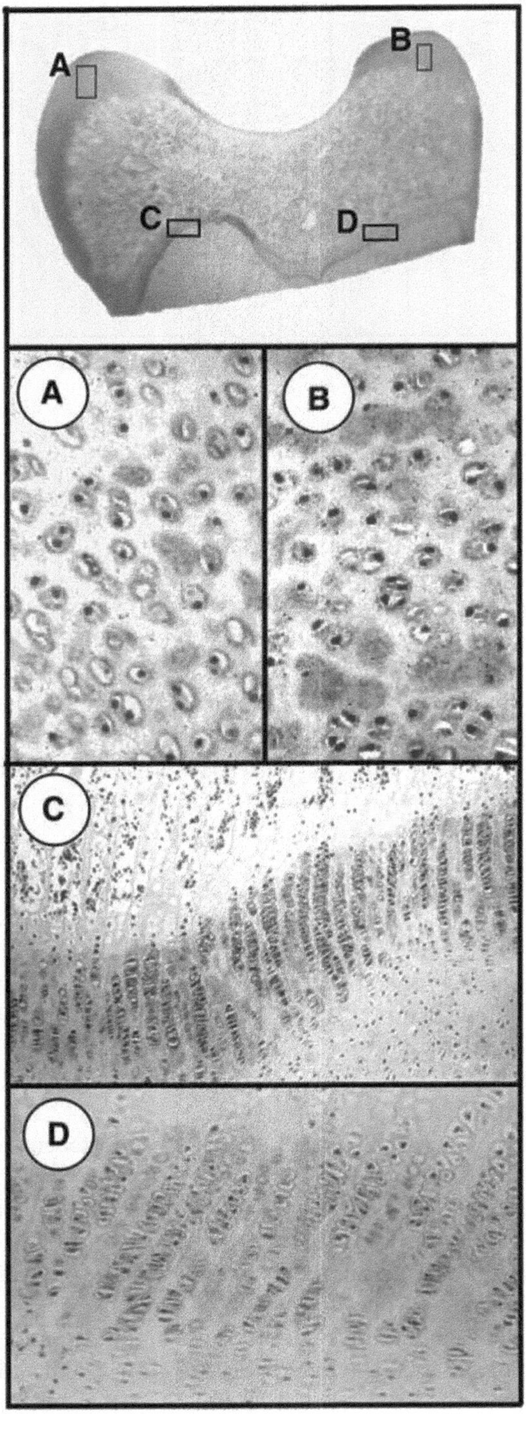
A
B
C
D
A
B
C
D

2.2. Buffers, Tissue Fixative, and Culture Media

1. Buffer A, testicular hyaluronidase digestion buffer: 0.1 *M* sodium phosphate buffer, pH 5.0, containing 0.15 *M* NaCl.
2. Buffer B, FPLC elution buffer: 0.2 *M* ammonium acetate buffer, pH 6.8.
3. Buffer C, HA oligosaccharide biotinylation labeling buffer: 0.1 *M* 2-*N*-morpholino ethanesulphonic acid (MES) buffer, pH 5.5.
4. Buffer D, aggrecan G1 domain affinity chromatography equilibration and starting buffer: 20 m*M* Tris-HCl, pH 7.2.
5. Buffer E, aggrecan G1 domain affinity chromatography elution buffer: 4 *M* GuHCl buffered with 20 m*M* Tris-HCl, pH 7.2.
6. Buffer F, Tris-buffered saline (TBS): 50 m*M* Tris-HCl, pH 7.6, containing 0.15 *M* NaCl and 0.05% Tween-20.
7. Tissue fixative: 10% neutral buffered formalin in phosphate buffer, pH 7.0.
8. Culture media: 1:1 mixture of DMEM-F12 media supplemented with 2 m*M* L-glutamine and 10% fetal calf serum buffered to pH 6.8 with 15 m*M* N-2-hydroxyethyl piperazine-*N'*-2-ethanesulphonic acid (HEPES) and 0.12% w/v sodium bicarbonate.
9. Decalcification solution: 10% formic acid, 5% formalin.

3. Methods (*see* Note 2)

3.1. Preparation of the bHA Oligosaccharide Bioaffinity Probe

1. Dissolve Fidia 170-kDa HA (1 g) in buffer A (50 mL) and digest for 6 h at 37°C with ovine testicular hyaluronidase (100 U/mL).
2. Subject the HA oligosaccharides to Fractogel TSK HW 50(S) FPLC. Elute the column with buffer B at 30 mL/h and monitor fractions for hexuronic acid content. Pool fractions of K_{av} 0.2–0.7 and lyophilize *(12)*.
3. Redissolve 70 mg of the FPLC HA oligosaccharide pool in 4 mL of buffer C and add 0.35 mL of a 17-mg/mL suspension of biotin hydrazide in buffer C with thorough mixing.
4. Add 255 μL of a 120 mg/mL EDC solution in buffer C to this mixture and stir at room temperature for a further 16 h.
5. Apply the bHA oligosaccharide preparation to a 10-mL aggrecan-G1 domain affinity column eluted with 10 bed vol of buffer D. Elute the bound oligosaccharide

---

Fig. 2. (*opposite page*) Composite figure depicting a macroscopic view (top) of a newborn ovine femoral condyle in midcoronal section (with the boxed areas A–D presented at higher power views below) stained with the bHA oligosaccharide probe to visualize the HABPs. The HABPs have a pericellular distribution and are also present more diffusely in extracellular locations throughout the articular cartilage (**A**, **B**), whereas in the epiphyseal growth plates (**C**,**D**) the HABPs are strongly pericellularly localized in the columnar hypertrophic chondrocytes. Original magnification ×200 in (A) and (B); ×50 in (C); ×100 in (D).

fractions from the column with 2 bed vol of buffer E and precipitate overnight with 9 vol of absolute methanol at 4°C.

6. Collect the precipitated bHA oligosaccharides by centrifugation (10 min at 10,000*g*), redissolve it in 2 mL of buffer D, and perform avidin affinity chromatography following the manufacturer's instructions to remove any nonbiotinylated HA oligosaccharide.
7. Rechromatograph the bound oligosaccharide pool from the avidin affinity chromatography on the Fractogel TSK HW 50(S) FPLC column as indicated above in **step 2** and monitor fractions for hexuronic acid and biotin colorimetrically by displacement of avidin from a preformed avidin-HABA complex using D-biotin as a standard *(13*; *see* **Note 3**).
8. Pool fractions of K_{av} 0.2–0.7 and lyophilize twice to remove all traces of buffer B (*see* **Note 4**).

3.2. Preparation of an Aggrecan G1 Domain Affinity Column

1. Prepare hyaluronan binding aggrecan fragments by limited tryptic digestion of powdered bovine nasal cartilage *(14)*.
2. Extract the G1 aggrecan fragments from the washed tissue residue using buffer E and isolate by HA affinity chromatography *(14)*.
3. Immobilize the G1 aggrecan fragments on epoxy-activated sepharose following the manufacturer's instructions *(15)*.

3.3. Isolation and Culture of Ovine Articular Chondrocytes

3.3.1. Tissue Collection and Dissection

1. Isolate articular chondrocytes from six 2-yr-old pedigree merino wethers (desexed males), obtained from our university sheep breeding colony *(16)*.
2. Trim off excess muscle and other soft tissues extraneous to the stifle (knee) joint capsule, spray the specimens with 70% ethanol in a laminar flow hood, and allow to air-dry.
3. Open the joint capsule with sterile instruments and wash the articulating surfaces of the joint with sterile isotonic saline; wipe dry with sterile gauze.
4. Collect aseptically full-thickness cartilage from the femoral condyle and tibial plateau joint surfaces omitting the joint margins using fresh instruments.

3.3.2. Tissue Digestion

1. Digest diced articular cartilage in sterile 0.1% w/v pronase, 0.01% w/v DNAase I in DMEM-F12-FCS at 37°C for 90 min (15 mL/joint).
2. Spin down the tissue residue and add 15 mL of sterile 0.05% w/v collagenase, 0.01% w/v DNAase I in DMEM-F12-FCS and continue incubation for a further 16 h at 37°C.
3. Filter the solubilized tissue samples through 70-μm cell sieves and spin down the cells (800*g* for 10 min); this typically yields approx 24–30 million cells per joint.

3.3.3. Monolayer Culture of Articular Chondrocytes

For further details, *see* **ref. *16***.

1. Disperse cell pellets from the tissue dissociation protocols in DMEM-F12-FCS media supplemented with 2 m*M* L-glutamine, and establish them in monolayer cultures in 75-cm^2 canted neck culture flasks at a density of 3 million cells/flask in 20 mL of DMEM-F12-FCS, 2 m*M* L-glutamine media at 37°C under an atmophere of 5% CO_2 in air with 98% humidity.
2. Once the cells have reached confluence, detach them by trypsinization, spin down the cells, and conduct viability assays on them using trypan blue exclusion and a hemocytometer.
3. Re-establish the cells in culture in square Petri dishes (10 × 10 cm) at a density of 50,000 cells/mL in DMEM-F12-FCS, 2 m*M* L-glutamine (10 mL). Allow the cells to attach to SuperFrost® Plus microscope slides for 8 h (*see* **Note 5**) and then change the media. Grow the attached cells for a further 48 h, after which the media is replaced with fresh media supplemented with the bHA oligosaccharide affinity probe (10 µg/mL).

3.4. Preparation of Tissues for Histological Procedures

For further details, *see* **refs. 12** and **17** and **Fig. 3**.

1. Fix en bloc 2-d-old lumbar ovine intervertebral discs (IVDs) with adjacent vertebral bodies still attached in 10% neutral buffered formalin for 2 d and then decalcify in daily changes of 10% formic acid in 5% neutral buffered formalin with constant agitation for 5 d (*see* **Note 6**).
2. Cut vertical sagittal slabs (4–5 mm thick) of the decalcified vertebral body-IVD specimens and dehydrate in graded alcohols by standard histology procedures, embed in Paraplast wax, and cut 4-µm vertical sagittal sections.
3. Mount the tissue sections on SuperFrost Plus glass slides, deparaffinize in xylene (2 changes × 5 min), and rehydrate through graded ethanol washes (100–70% v/v) to water.
4. Fix whole ovine knee (stifle) and hip (head of femur) joints in 10% neutral buffered formalin for 48 h, decalcify for 5 d, and then prepare midcoronal osteochondral slabs (3–4 mm). Embed these tissue slabs in paraffin and process as indicated above; then prepare 4-µm tissue sections and mount on SuperFrost Plus slides.

3.4.1. Histochemical Localization of HABPs

For further details, *see* refs. **12** and **14** and **Fig. 4**.

1. Predigest tissue sections with bovine testicular hyaluronidase (1 mg/mL) in buffer A for 1.75 h at 37°C.
2. If specimens are destined for the horseradish peroxidase detection system, then block endogenous peroxidase activity at this stage by incubating the tissue sec-

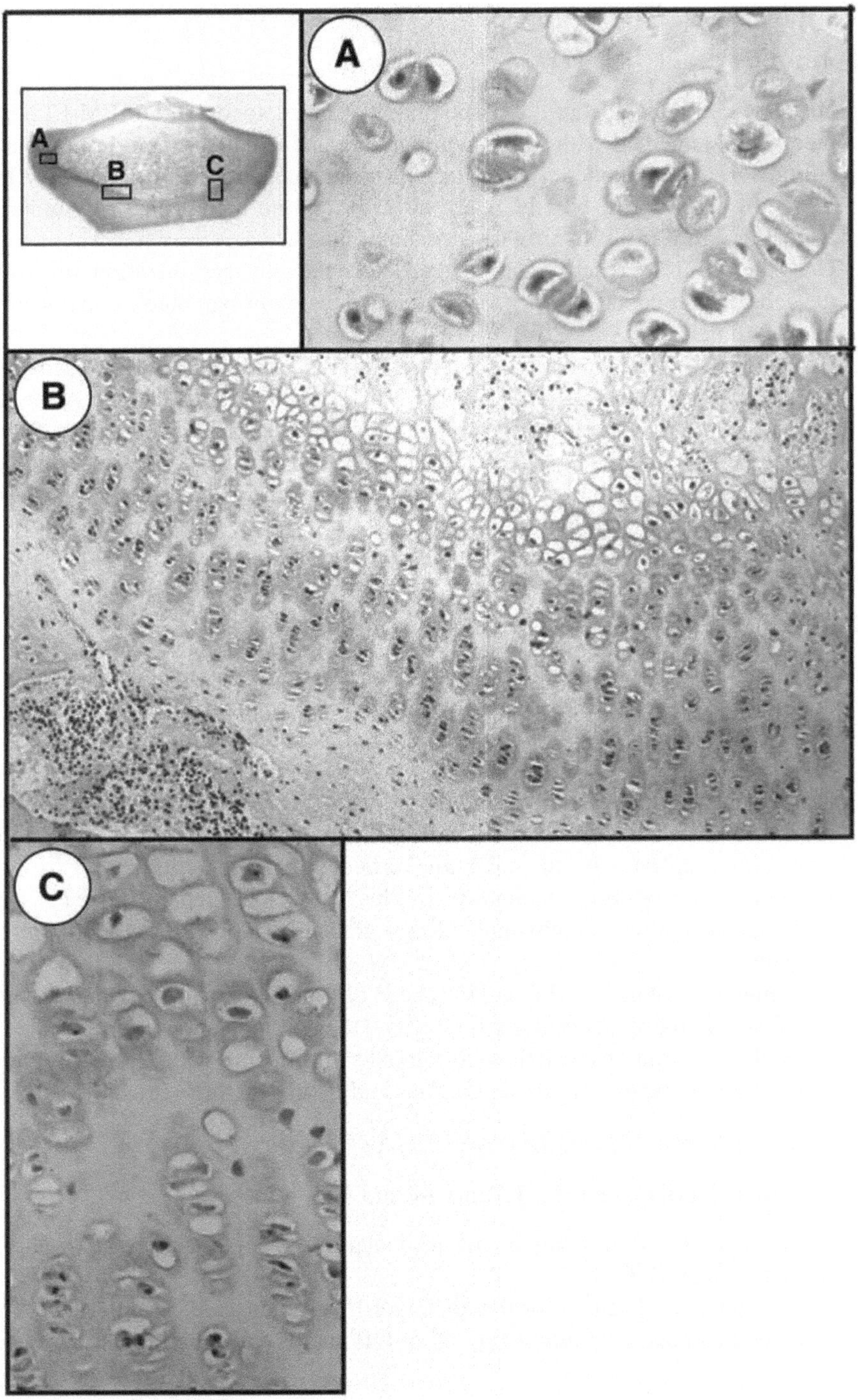
A
B
C
A
B
C

tions with 3% H_2O_2 for 5 min and rinse in water and then in buffer F prior to loading the slides in the Sequenza immunoblotting chamber.

3. Block nonspecific binding for 10–15 min at room temperature using a proprietary, serum-free blocking agent (DAKO Protein block-serum free, X0909; *see* **Note 7**).
4. After the slide is drained, add the bHA oligosaccharide (10 μg/mL) probe in buffer F and keep overnight at 4°C.
5. Use streptavidin alkaline phosphatase conjugate (DAKO $LSAB_2$, K1018) or streptavidin horseradish peroxidase conjugate (DAKO LSAB+, K1015) for the detection step (30 min at room temperature) using the chromogenic substrates new fuchsin or NBT/BCIP/INT for alkaline phosphatase; or NovaRED or diaminobenzidene for the horseradish peroxidase detection system.
6. Negative control samples do not receive the hyaluronidase predigestion step; also preincubate additional control samples with an excess of competing nonlabeled HA oligosaccharide (200 μg/mL) prior to addition of the affinity probe.

3.4.2. Indirect Fluorescent Visualization of the bHA Oligosaccharide Internalized by the Cultured Ovine Chondrocytes

See **Fig. 5**.

1. After 48 h in monolayer culture, supplement the DMEM-F12-FCS, 2 m*M* L-glutamine media with 10 μg/mL of the bHA oligosaccharide probe.
2. After an additional 2, 10, and 30 min in culture, remove selected slides, wash three times in cold PBS, fix in ice-cold acetone (2 min), and air-dry.
3. Also, process control slides in a similar manner but with the omission of the bHA oligosaccharide probe or with the addition of the bHA probe and an excess of competing nonlabeled HA oligosaccharide (200 μg/mL).
4. Add (5 μg/mL) avidin fluorescein isothiocyanate (FITC) in buffer F and incubate the slides at room temperature for 30 min.
5. Wash the slides twice in buffer F and mount in Permafluor mounting medium prior to examination by fluorescent microscopy (*see* **Note 8**).
6. Take 35-mm slides of the fluorescein localization in the chondrocyte monolayers using Kodak Ektachrome P1600 Daylight (or equivalent) high-speed film. Scan the 35-mm slides with a slide scanner (Microtek 35t plus) using Adobe version

---

Fig. 3. (*opposite page*) Higher power views depicting the distribution of HABPs visualized using the bHA oligosaccharide probe in discrete regions of a newborn ovine tibial plateau sectioned midcoronally. A macroscopic view is presented at the top left of this composite figure to act as a key for the boxed zones **(A–C)**, which are depicted at higher magnification. Although some diffuse extracellular staining for HABPs was evident, they have a predominantly pericellular distribution in hypertrophic chondrocytes adjacent to (A) or in the chondrocyte columns in the growth plates (B, C). Original magnification ×400 in (A) and (C); ×200 in (B).

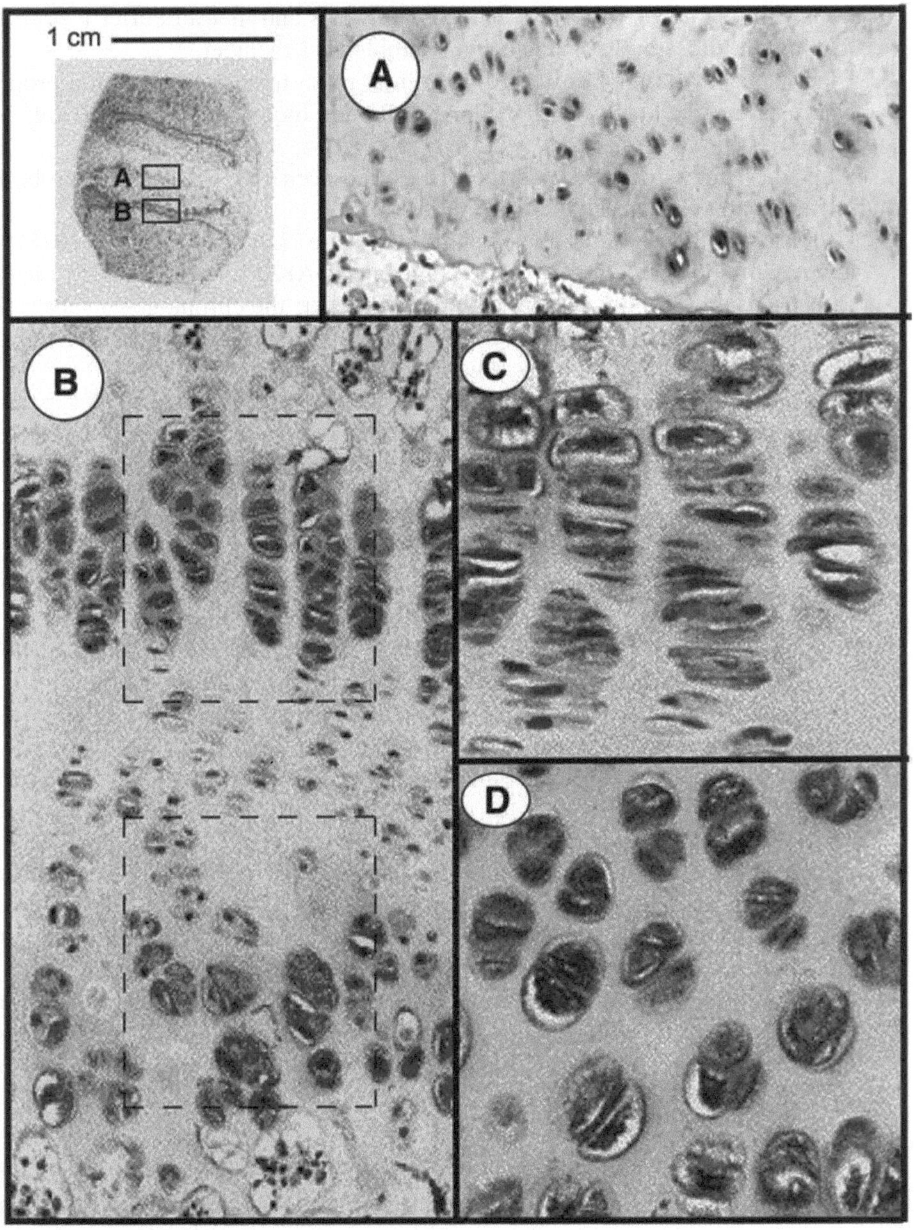

Fig. 4. Higher power views depicting the distribution of HABPs in the cartilaginous end plate of the intervertebral disc **(A)** and vertebral growth plates **(B)** in vertical midsagittal sections of a 2-d-old newborn sheep. A macroscopic view is presented as a key at the top left of the figure. Strong expression of HABPs in the hypertrophic cells at each poles of the vertebral growth plates is clearly evident. The boxed areas in the

5.0 software and import the digitized images into a drawing package for assembly of the composite histology figures.

4. Notes

1. The interested reader is referred to the web site "Science of Hyaluronan Today" (http://www.glycoforum.gr.jp/science/hyaluronan/hyaluronanE.html) for further information. This web site is a useful source of current information on hyaluronan and hyaluronan binding proteins, and additional reviews are added regularly (also *see* Chap. 3).
2. Further details on the histology procedures and associated consumables are covered in Chapter 3.
3. This procedure should confirm that the HA oligosaccharide preparation is biotinylated, provide a measure of its level of polydispersity and the relative distribution of the biotin in the labeled product, and also demonstrate that free biotin has been separated from the labeled probe.
4. Ammonium acetate is a volatile buffer and may be removed by freeze drying; however, the pellet from the first freeze-drying step should be redissolved in MilliQ distilled water and this procedure repeated to ensure that all traces of buffer are removed.
5. The cells attach rapidly (within 2–3 h) to Superfrost Plus microscope slides.
6. It is important that disc specimens be fixed and decalcified en bloc to avoid any distortion in native tissue architecture, which can happen when the softer connective tissues undergo the dehydration-rehydration steps of the histochemical processing. Also, see related comments in Chapter 3.
7. At this point in an immunohistology procedure, it is normal for the nonspecific binding in the tissue sections to be blocked using a mammalian serum differing from that in which the secondary antibody was raised. Serum, however, may contain a range of hyaluronan binding proteins that can potentially interfere with the procedures conducted with the bHA oligosaccharide probe. A proprietary non-serum-blocking agent (DAKO Protein block-serum free, X0909) is therefore used for this step.
8. Permafluor mountant has antifading properties that help to preserve the fluorescence of the slides; however, they should also be wrapped in silver paper and stored in the dark.

Fig. 4. (*continued*) macroscopic view are also depicted elsewhere at higher magnification in (A) and (B). The hypertrophic cells of the caudal and cranial poles of the vertebral growth plate (B) are also presented at higher magnification (**C**, **D**). Strong pericellular expression of HABPs is clearly evident in the hypertrophic cells depicted, as well as some intracellular HABP staining. Original magnification ×200 in (A); ×400 in (B); ×800 in (C) and (D).

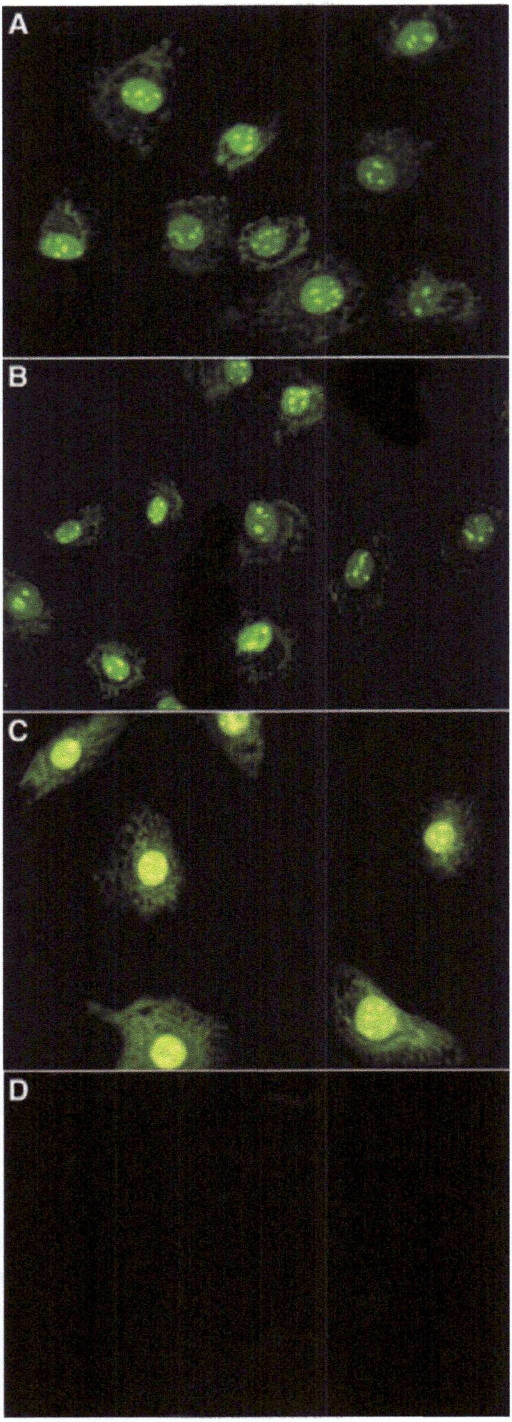
A
B
C
D

References

1. Asari, A., Miyauchi, S., Miyazaki, K., et al. (1992) Intra- and extracellular localisation of hyaluronic acid and proteoglycan constituents (chondroitin sulfate, keratan sulfate and protein core) in articular cartilage of rabbit tibia. *J. Histochem. Cytochem.* **40,** 1693–1703.
2. Hardingham, T. E. (1998) Cartilage: aggrecan-link protein-hyaluronan aggregates http://www.glycoforum.gr.jp/science/hyaluronan/HA05/HA05E.html.
3. Hascall, V. C. and Heinegård, D. (1974) Aggregation of cartilage proteoglycans. The role of hyaluronic acid. *J. Biol. Chem.* **249,** 4232–4241.
4. Knudson, C. B. (1993) Hyaluronan receptor-directed assembly of chondrocyte pericellular matrix. *J. Cell. Biol.* **120,** 825–834.
5. Lammi, P., Lammi, M. J., Tammi, R. H., Helminen, H. J., and Espanha, R. H. (2001) Strong hyaluronan expression in the full thickness rat articular cartilage repair tissue. *Histochem. Cell Biol.* **115,** 301–308
6. Parkkinen, J. J., Häkkinen, T. P., Savolainen, S., et al. (1996) Distribution of hyaluronan in articular cartilage as probed by a biotinylated binding region of aggrecan. *Histochem. Cell Biol.* **105,** 187–194.
7. Watanabe, H., Cheung, S. C., Itano, N., Kimata, K., and Yamada, Y. (1997) Identification of hyaluronan-binding domains of aggrecan. *J. Biol. Chem.* **272,** 28,057–28,065.
8. Iozzo, R. V. (1998) Matrix proteoglycans. From molecular design to cellular function. *Annu. Rev. Biochem.* ***67,*** 609–652.
9. Iozzo, R. V. and Murdoch, A. D. (1996) Proteoglycans of the extracellular envi-

Fig. 5. (*opposite page*) Demonstration of intracellular HABPs by visualization of the bHA oligosaccharide bioaffinity probe internalized by subconfluent articular chondrocytes grown in monolayer culture after 2 (**A**), 10 (**B**), and 30 min (**C**) of exposure to the affinity probe. The chondrocytes were initially allowed to attach to SuperFrost Plus microscope slides in monolayer culture for 48 h, the media was then supplemented with bHA oligosaccharide probe (10 μg/mL) for up to 30 min, and then the cells were washed, fixed in acetone, and air-dried. Avidin-FITC conjugate was subsequently used for detection of the bHA oligosaccharide probe by indirect fluorescent microscopy. In the negative control panel (**D**), the cells were preincubated with a 20-fold excess of nonlabeled HA oligosaccharide for 30 min prior to addition of the bHA oligosaccharide probe, and the slide was fixed after a further 30 min of incubation. Strong staining for the bHA oligosaccharide probe is evident in the nucleus and in nuclear condensations, which appear to be the nucleoli, as well as in discrete cytoplasmic vacuoles and the ruffled borders of the chondrocytes, in microspikes at the cell margins, and in filopodia and lamellopodia. This is consistent with intracellular HA's documented role in cellular locomotory processes via intracellular HABPs. Original magnification ×400 in all panels.

ronment: clues from the gene and protein side offer novel perspectives in molecular diversity and function. *FASEB J.* **10,** 598–614.
10. Yamaguchi, Y. (2000) Lecticans: organizers of the brain extracellular matrix. *Cell. Mol. Life. Sci.* **57,** 276–289.
11. Caterson, B. and Baker, J. (1978) The interaction of link proteins with proteoglycan monomers in the absence of hyaluronic acid. *Biochem. Biophys. Res. Commun.* **80,** 496–503.
12. Melrose, J., Tammi, M. and Smith, S. (2002) Visualisation of hyaluronan and hyaluronan binding proteins within ovine vertebral cartilages using biotinylated aggrecan G1-link complex and biotinylated hyaluronan oligosaccharides. *Histochem. Cell Biol.* **117,** 327–333.
13. Green N. M. (1970) Spectrophotometric determination of avidin and biotin. *Methods Enzymol.* **128,** 418–424
14. Melrose, J. (2001) Cartilage and smooth muscle cell proteoglycans detected by affinity blotting using biotinylated hyaluronan, in *Methods in Molecular Biology*, vol. 171, *Proteoglycan Protocols* (Iozzo, R. V., ed.), Humana, Totowa, NJ, pp. 53–66.
15. Le Glëdic, S., Përin, J.-P., Bonnet, F., and Jollës, P. (1982) Interaction between the hyaluronic acid binding region and the common tryptic fragment of the link proteins from bovine nasal cartilage complex. An affinity chromatography study. *Biochem. Biophys. Res. Commun.* **104,** 1298–1305
16. Melrose, J., Smith, S., Ghosh, P., and Taylor, T. K. F. (2002) Comparison of the morphology and growth characteristics of intervertebral disc cells, synovial fibroblasts and articular chondrocytes in monolayer and alginate bead cultures. *Eur. Spine J.* **12,** 57–65.
17. Melrose, J., Knox, S., Smith, S., and Whitelock, J. (2002) Perlecan, the multidomain proteoglycan of basement membrane is also a prominent pericellular component of hypertrophic chondrocytes of ovine vertebral growth plate and cartilaginous end plate cartilage. *Histochem. Cell Biol.* **118,** 269–280.

5

Methods for Cartilage and Subchondral Bone Histomorphometry

Philippe Pastoureau and Agnès Chomel

Summary

This chapter presents the histological assessment of cartilage and bone of tibial plateaus, by procedures that have been applied and validated in two animal models of osteoarthritis: meniscectomized rats and guinea pigs. It starts from bone sampling, followed by all the steps of sample preparation from embedding to sectioning (without prior decalcification), staining, and mounting. Depending on the cartilage or bone components to be visualized, two dyes are described: safranin O and Goldner's trichrome. On these stained sections, various histomorphometric parameters are then quantified using the dedicated programs of an image analyzer. The following parameters are evaluated at the medial side of the tibia and are described at the levels of both cartilage (cartilage thickness, fibrillation index, proteoglycan content ratio based on safranin-O staining intensities and chondrocyte density) and bone (subchondral bone plate thickness).

Key Words: Cartilage; histology; bone; histomorphometry; safranin O; Goldner's trichrome; image analysis; thickness; fibrillation; proteoglycan; chondrocyte density; subchondral bone plate.

1. Introduction

Osteoarthritis (OA) is a major joint disease of humans and various animals in which articular cartilage degenerates over a period of time, causing denudation of the joint surface *(1)*. It is also characterized by concomitant changes in subchondral bone *(2)*. In animal models of OA, the histological assessment of articulations is the best way to analyze properly all the lesions characteristic of the disease at the cartilage and bone levels. The OA-affected tibias are sampled, fixed, and embedded in methyl methacrylate without prior decalcification. Then, after precise positioning of the embedded bone in order to reach the lesion area at the medial tibial plateau, coronal sections are cut by a microtome

From: *Methods in Molecular Medicine, Vol. 101: Cartilage and Osteoarthritis, Volume 2: Structure and In Vivo Analysis*
Edited by: F. De Ceuninck, M. Sabatini, and P. Pastoureau © Humana Press Inc., Totowa, NJ

using a tungsten carbide blade. Nonconsecutive sections are stained with safranin O or Goldner's trichrome (for further analysis). Histomorphometric parameters can be quantified using special programs of an image analyzer. The following parameters are evaluated on the medial side of the operated tibia: cartilage thickness (CT), fibrillation index (FI), proteoglycan content ratio based on safranin O staining intensities (PC),chondrocyte density (CD), and subchondral bone plate thickness (SBPT). The degree of user interaction varied from manually tracing objects to almost complete computer automation.

2. Materials

2.1. Equipment

1. Microtome polycut E (Reichert-Jung, Cambridge Instruments, Germany).
2. Tungsten carbide blade, 16 cm long with a 60°-facet angle (*see* **Note 1**).
3. Microscope with various objectives (2.5×, 4×, 10×, and 25×).
4. Tri-CCD color camera (Sony).
5. Personal computer, linked to the microscope by the tri-CCD camera and equipped with special software (*see* **Note 2**).
6. Rotating wet-sander (**Fig. 1**) with abrasive discs (grain = 80).
7. Refrigerator for methyl methacrylate storage.
8. Small glass flasks with hermetic caps (vol = 11.5 mL).
9. Disposable scalpels.
10. Microscope slides.
11. Microscope cover glasses.
12. Staining trays.
13. Curved forceps.
14. Grinder (Autosharp 5, Shandon; *see* **Fig. 2** and **Note 3**).
15. Cigaret paper.

2.2. Chemicals

2.2.1. Embedding

1. 37% Formaldehyde solution.
2. Absolute ethanol.
3. Toluene.
4. Methyl methacrylate (MMA).
5. Aluminum oxide.
6. Dibutyl phthalate.
7. Benzoylperoxide.

2.2.2. Staining

1. Safranin O (Merck cat. no. 15948) .
2. Light green (Fluka cat. no. 62110).
3. Acetic acid (glacial).

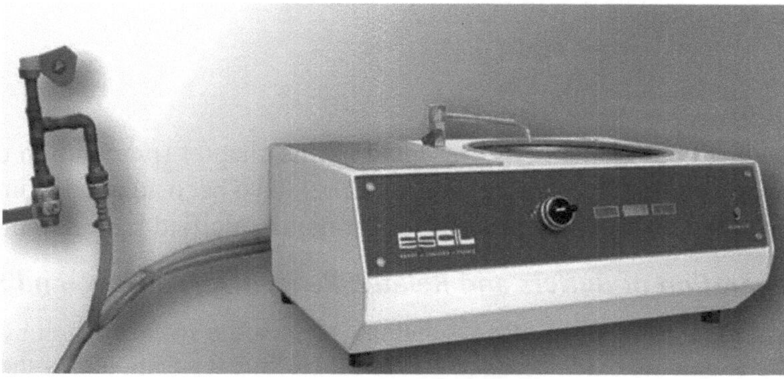

Fig. 1. Rotating wet-sander with an abrasive disc (working under running tap water), used to expose the embedded tibia along the right plane for cutting.

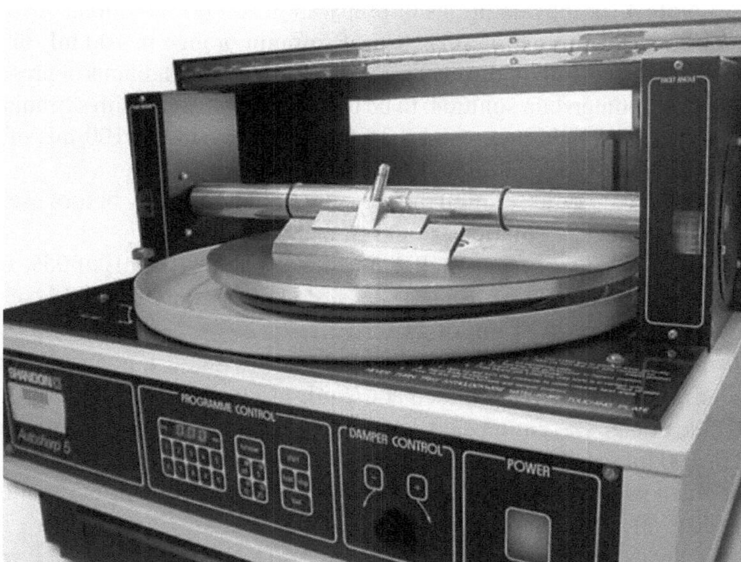

Fig. 2. Grinder used to sharpen the tungsten carbide blades.

4. Methylcyclohexan.
5. Entellan mounting medium (Merck cat. no. 7961).
6. Hematoxylin (Merck cat. no. 1.04303).
7. Iron(III) chloride hexahydrate.
8. Hydrochloric acid (37%).
9. Acid fuchsin (Merck cat. no. 5231).
10. Ponceau S (Merck cat. no. 1.15927).

11. Orange G (Merck cat. no. 1.15925).
12. Molybdatophosphoric acid.

3. Methods

All the histological methods presented in this chapter (preparation of buffers, bone embedding, sectioning, and staining) have been adapted from previously described histological procedures for nondecalcified bone samples *(3)*.

3.1. Preparation of Buffers and Related Reagents, Fixatives, and Stains

1. Preparation of the three MMA solutions: prepare the stock solution by adding 200 g aluminum oxide beads to 1 L of MMA. Stir for 15 min, and then filter. Repeat twice.
   a. MMA1 solution: add 1 vol of dibutyl phthalate to 3 vol of stock solution.
   b. MMA2: add 1% benzoylperoxide (w/v) to MMA1 solution.
   c. MMA3: add 2.5% benzoylperoxide (w/v) to MMA1 solution.
   See **Note 4** for the conditions of preparation and preservation.
2. Safranin O dye solution: dissolve 1 g of safranin orange in 100 mL of absolute ethanol; then add 50 mL of distilled water (*see* **Note 5** for conditions of preservation).
3. Light green counterstain solution, to be used in combination with safranin O staining: add 0.2 g of light green and 0.35 mL of acetic acid to 100 mL of distilled water (*see* **Note 5** for conditions of preservation).
4. Weigert's hematoxylin solution: prepare this solution freshly before use, by mixing equal volumes of solutions A and B, and then filter.
   a. Solution A: add 1 g of crystallized hematoxylin to 100 mL of 95% ethanol.
   b. Solution B: add 4 g of iron(III) chloride hexahydrate to 95 mL of distilled water, and then add 1 mL of 24% HCl.
5. Fuchsin ponceau solution: add 0.5 g acid fuchsin and 2 g ponceau S to 1 L of distilled water. Dissolve, and then add 2 mL of glacial acetic acid.
6. Molybdic orange G solution: add 2 g of orange G and 4 g of molybdatophosphoric acid to 100 mL of distilled water. Dissolve, and then filter.
7. Light green solution: solubilize 0.1 g of light green in 100 mL of distilled water; then add 2 mL of glacial acetic acid.
8. Acetified water: add 1 mL of glacial acetic acid to 100 mL of distilled water (*see* **Note 5** for preservation of all of these solutions).

3.2. Bone Sampling and Embedding

1. Sacrifice the animals and sample tibias (from healthy or diseased joints; *see* **Note 6**).
2. Section the diaphysis at the insertion site of the fibula (**Fig. 3**).
3. Place each bone in a flask containing the 10% formaldehyde solution for 24 h (*see* **Note 7**).
4. Discard the formaldehyde solution, and then add 80% ethanol (three successive baths of 1 wk each).

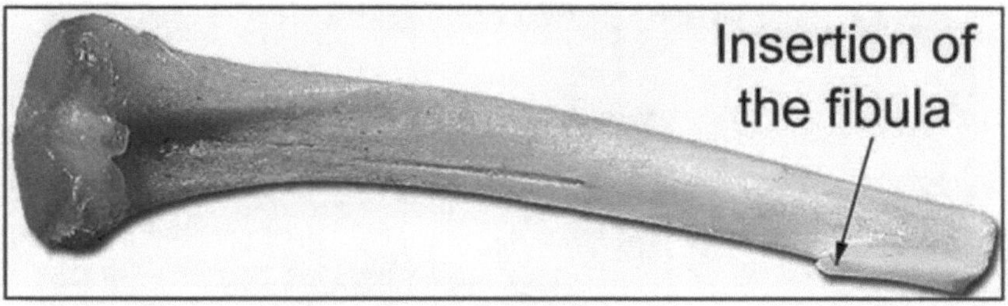

Fig. 3. Proximal part of the tibia sectioned after sacrifice at the insertion site of the fibula.

5. Dehydrate in absolute ethanol (two baths of 3 d each).
6. Substitute ethanol with toluene for 48 h.
7. Soak with prepared MMA solutions at 4°C, for 1 wk in each solution (MMA1, MMA2, and MMA3).
8. Just before embedding (in MMA3), put the tibia in the flask, with the proximal extremity at the bottom. Then place the flask with a hermetic cap in the incubator at 37°C to obtain a solid block containing the bone (for a better but slower embedding, *see* **Note 8**).
9. Remove the block from the flask by breaking the glass with a hammer (*see* **Note 9**).
10. In order to take into account the focal nature of the OA process, and to be sure that all the sections are cut along the same plane, first sand each embedded tibia on a rotary abrasive disk (**Fig. 1**) until the right angle and location for cutting are obtained (arrow in **Fig. 4**).

For instance, in the case of meniscectomized guinea pigs, the tibia is sectioned along the coronal plane for optimal exposition of the central part of the medial tibial plateau where OA lesions first appear *(4)*. Correct sectioning can be confirmed, at an early stage, by checking for equal proportions of lateral and medial cartilage areas separated by a central ligament and the presence of the fibula insertion on the lateral part of the tibia (**Fig. 5**).

3.3. Sectioning

1. Place and tighten the block on the microtome. The sanded surface of the block must be horizontal (*see* **Fig. 6** and **Note 10**).
2. Start cutting at medium speed in order to reach the desired level of sectioning (*see* **Subheading 3.2., step 10**).
3. Adjust the thickness of the sectioning to 8 μm and reduce the speed.
4. Slowly collect the sections using a humidified cigaret paper (*see* **Fig. 7** and **Note 11**).
5. Remove the section (**Fig. 8**) and place it in a glass container with distilled water (*see* **Note 12**).

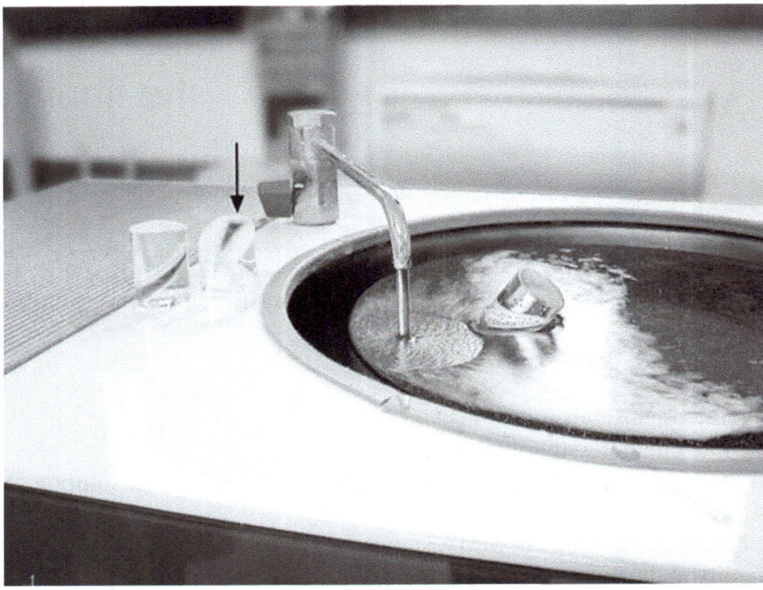

Fig. 4. Wet-sanding of an embedded tibia on the rotating sander. See a block eroded (arrow) along the right plane for cutting.

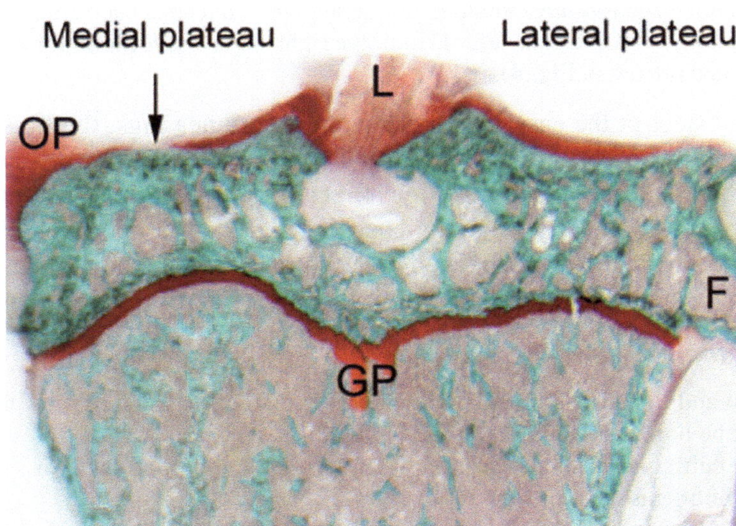

Fig. 5. Histological section of a left tibia from a meniscectomized guinea pig. Site of measurement of histomorphometric parameters: medial tibial plateau (arrow). Safranin O staining; original magnification ×8. OP, osteophyte; L, ligament; GP, growth plate; F, fibula insertion.

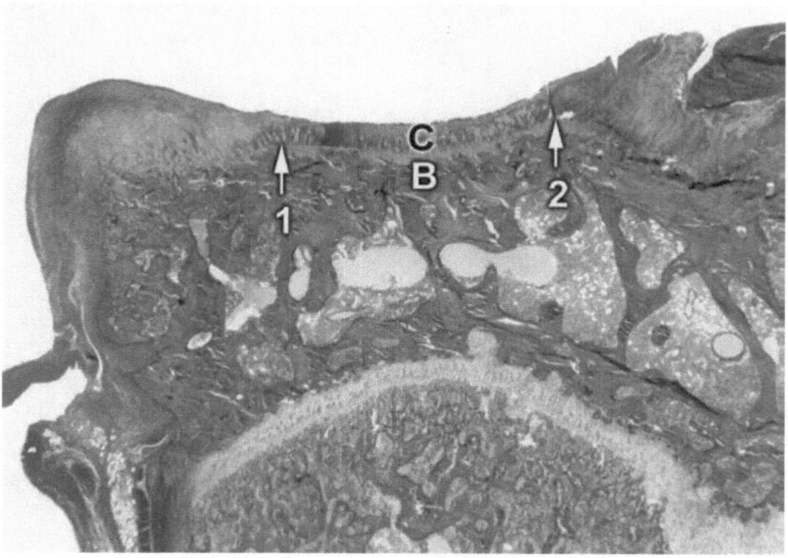

Fig. 6. Embedded tibia placed in a microtome showing the surface sanded along the cutting plane, positioned horizontally before sectioning.

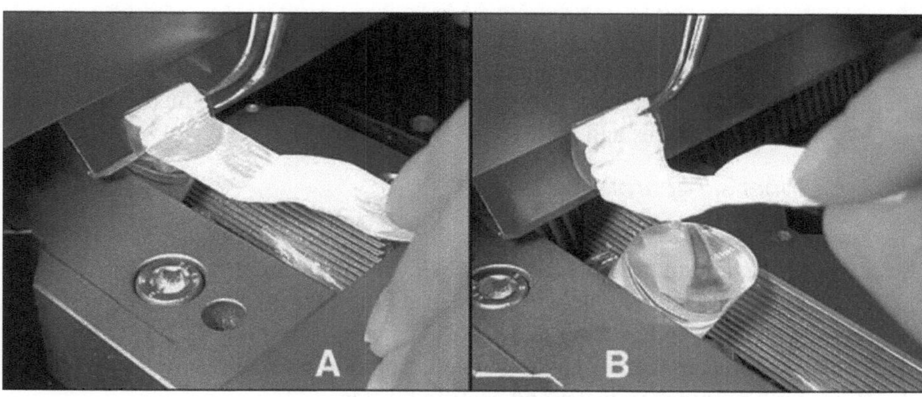

Fig. 7. Two steps of the section collection with a humidified cigaret paper laid on the embedded block (**A**), facilitating the collection of the section on the blade (**B**).

3.4. Staining

3.4.1. Safranin O Staining Counterstained With Light Green

1. Put the sections in the safranin O staining solution for 10 min.
2. Rinse with running tap water.
3. Counterstain in the light green solution for 5 min.
4. Rapidly rinse with running tap water.

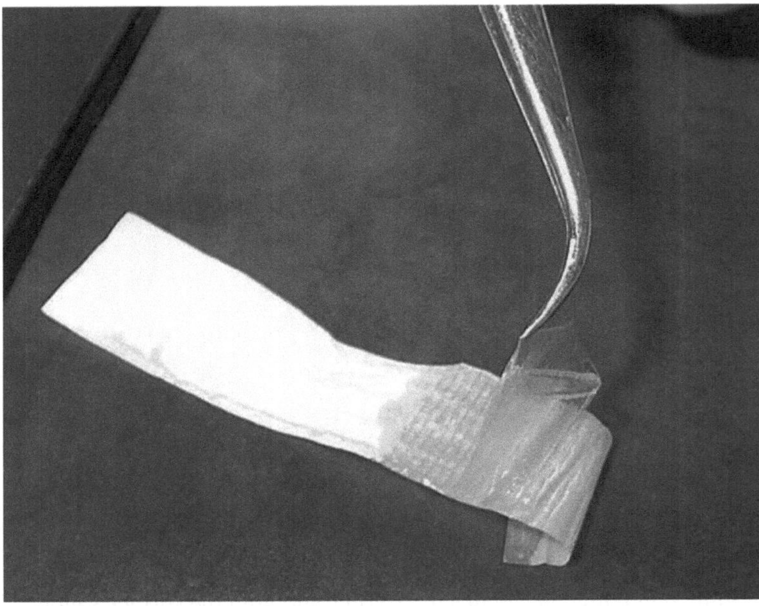

Fig. 8. The section can easily be removed from the cigaret paper.

5. Dehydrate in two baths of absolute alcohol and one bath of methylcyclohexan.
6. Mount the stained sections with a drop of entellan mounting medium between two microscope slides and let dry (*see* **Note 13**).

3.4.2. Goldner's Trichrome Staining

1. Put the sections in Weigert's hematoxylin solution for 10 min.
2. Rinse with running tap water and then with acetified water.
3. Place the sections in the fuchsin ponceau solution for 20 min.
4. Rinse with running tap water and acetified water.
5. Put the sections in the molybdic orange G solution for 6 min.
6. Rinse with running tap water and acetified water.
7. Place the sections in the light green solution for 15 min.
8. Rinse with running tap water and acetified water.
9. Dehydrate the sections in three consecutive baths of absolute alcohol and two baths of methylcyclohexan.
10. Mount the stained sections with a drop of mountant (Entellan) between two microscope slides and let dry (*see* **Note 14**)

3.5. Measurement of Histomorphometric Parameters

An image analysis system, using dedicated software, has been validated for the measurement of histological parameters reflecting osteoarthritic features at the cartilage and bone levels, in the meniscectomized guinea pig model of OA *(4)*. Special software can easily be designed "in house" according to precise criteria of measurements that have been defined for the following histological parameters.

3.5.1. Cartilage Thickness

1. Use sections stained with Goldner's trichrome at a 80× magnification.
2. Measure the thickness between the two morphological indicators positioned as shown in **Fig. 9**.
3. Manually outline the cartilage area between reference marks 1 and 2 (area C in **Fig. 9**) and the subchondral bone.
4. The designed software should be able to segment this region of interest automatically, using, for example, a threshold for black and white extraction with a green image.
5. Calculate the thickness of cartilage as the mean length of all the segments generated from each pixel situated on the border of the corresponding cartilage area

3.5.2. Fibrillation Index

1. Use sections stained with Goldner's trichrome at a 80× magnification.
2. Position the area of measurement centrally between reference marks 1 and 2 (**Fig. 9**).
3. The designed software must perform a segmentation of both cartilage and bone using a threshold for black and white extraction with a green image.
4. On the upper limit of the segmented area, integrate automatically the length of the superficial border (*L* in **Fig. 10**).
5. Calculate the fibrillation index by dividing *L* by the width (*W*) of the measured area (**Fig. 10**).

3.5.3. Proteoglycan Content Ratio

The proteoglycan content ratio (PCR) is calculated by measuring the safranin O staining intensity (SOI) in the superficial and deep zones of the histological sections stained with safranin O.

1. Use sections stained with safranin O at a 80× magnification
2. Use the same area of measurement as for the fibrillation index (*see* **Subheading 3.5.2.**)
3. Segment the cartilage automatically as for the measurement of the cartilage thickness.
4. Outline the superficial (S) and the deep (D) zones of the cartilage by manually drawing the upper margin of the D zone (**Fig. 11**)
5. The corresponding designed software must evaluate the optical density calculated on a gray scale obtained in the red component of the light crossing the section.

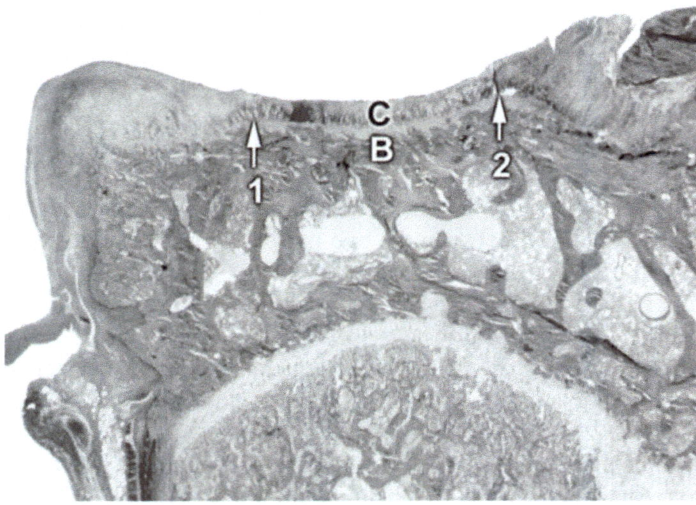

Fig. 9. Histological section of a medial tibial plateau stained with Goldner's trichrome in the guinea pig. Area of measurement of the cartilage thickness is defined by two manually set points (1 and 2) at the margin of the cartilage (C) and bone (B). Original magnification ×32.

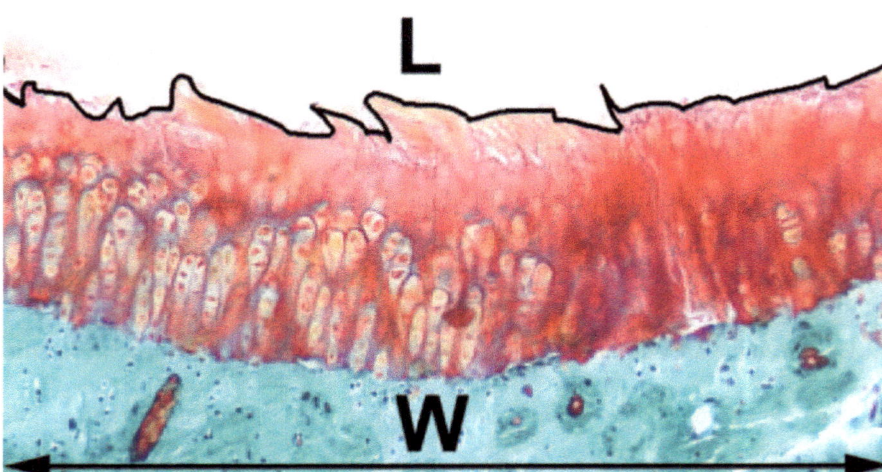

Fig. 10. Histological section of a medial tibial plateau stained with the Goldner trichrome in the guinea pig. Measurement of the fibrillation index (FI). FI is calculated by dividing the length of the fibrillated area (L) by the width (W) of the measured area. Original magnification ×80.

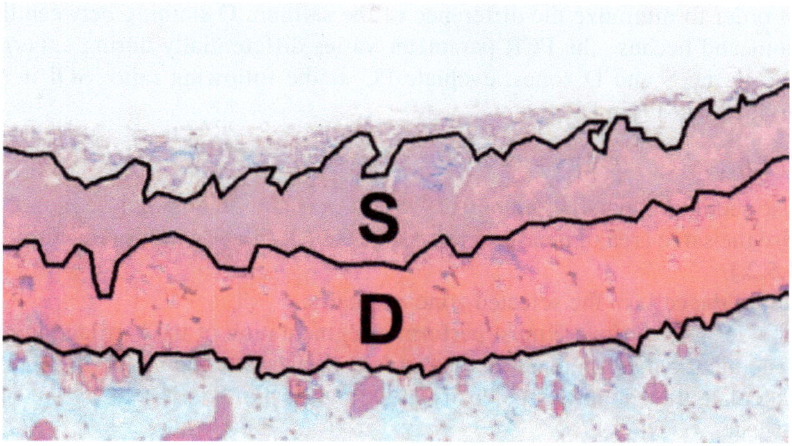

Fig. 11. Histological section of a medial tibial plateau stained with safranin O in the guinea pig. Evaluation of the proteoglycan content ratio (PCR) by measuring the safranin O staining intensity (SOI) in the deep (D) and superficial (S) zone of the articular cartilage after manual delimitation of the D and S zones. PCR of the cartilage is expressed as SOI in S divided by SOI in D. Original magnification ×80.

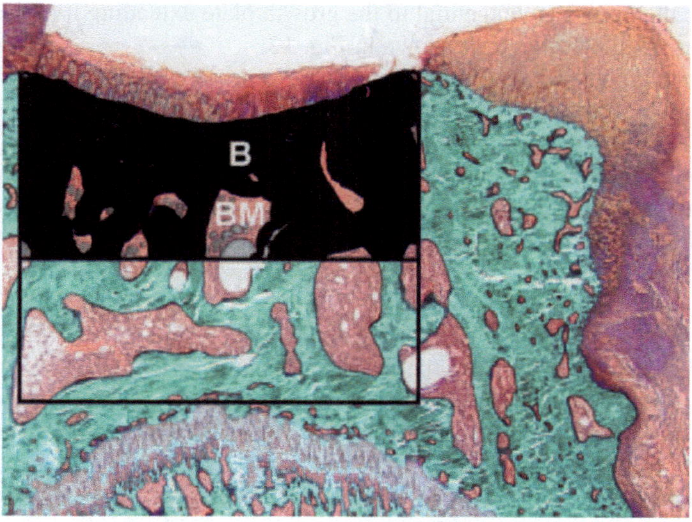

Fig. 12. Histological section of a medial tibial plateau stained with Goldner's trichrome in the guinea pig. The subchondral plate area is generated in the superior half (dark area) above the median of the delimited rectangle. Subchondral bone plate thickness results from the mean distance between each pixel of the upper limit of the bone (B) and its corresponding point at the margin of the bone marrow (BM). Original magnification ×32.

6. In order to minimize the difference of the safranin O staining between the sections and because the PCR parameter varies differentially during experimental OA in the S and D zones, evaluate PC as the following ratio: SOI in S zone divided by SOI in D zone.

3.5.4. Chondrocyte Density

1. Use sections stained with Goldner's trichrome at a 200× magnification.
2. Use the same area of measurement as for the fribrillation index (*see* **Subheading 3.5.2.**).
3. Count the cells in the selected zone manually.
4. The designed software must perform a segmentation of the cartilage in order to generate the measurement of the cartilage surface automatically.
5. Calculate the chondrocyte density, dividing the number of cells by the cartilage surface.

3.5.5. Subchondral Bone Plate Thickness (SBPT)

The designed software must perform an automatic segmentation of the bone in the superior half of the epiphysis (**Fig. 12**).

1. Use sections stained with Goldner's trichrome at a 20× magnification.
2. Perform the segmentation of the bone using a threshold for black and white extraction on red images.
3. Isolate the bone area tangential to the growth plate extending it perpendicularly to the articular cartilage, as shown in **Fig. 12**.
4. The subchondral area can automatically be generated in the superior half above the median of the delimited rectangle (*see* **step 3**).
5. Calculate the SBPT as the mean distance between each pixel of the upper limit of the bone and its corresponding point at the margin of the bone marrow. Depending on the precision of the measurements, at least four nonconsecutive sections must be measured per parameter and per animal. Furthermore, all the sections must be read blindly.

4. Notes

1. Handle with care because of the risk of cutting oneself.
2. Each software should be designed according to the principle of measurements developed in **Subheading 3.5.** and the type of equipment available (microscope, camera, computer, and so on).
3. For a homogeneous quality in a whole series of sections, blades should be sharpened regularly using a specific grinder, as shown in **Fig. 2**.
4. MMA1 solution can be stored at 4°C. MMA2 and MMA3 solutions should be freshly prepared before use.
5. These solutions can be kept for months at ambient temperature in the dark.
6. Ethical guidelines for experimental investigations in animals must be followed. In particular, the experimental procedure for euthanasia must be discussed and accepted by the local ethics committee for animal experimentation.

7. A piece of paper carrying the identification number of the corresponding animal can be included. It will remain intact even after embedding. This will avoid any confusion between samples.
8. To avoid the entrapment of air bubbles within the block during embedding, this phase can be done more slowly, letting the solution catalyze in the flask at ambient temperature rather than 37°C.
9. For safety reasons, avoid the projection of glass splinters by wrapping the flasks in a thick rag before hammering.
10. Always position the block on the microtome in order to start the sectioning from the cortical diaphyseal part of the embedded tibia, to obtain intact sections.
11. At least one section per staining should be taken for each level of sectioning.
12. To collect the histological section without deterioration, detach it from the paper by immersing in distilled water.
13. The success of this staining should result in red or pink cartilage and green underlying bone.
14. This staining results in red chondrocyte cytoplasm, black nucleus, orange matrix collagen, and green calcified cartilage and bone.

References

1. Pelletier, J. P., Martel-Pelletier, J., and Howell, D. S. (1997) Ethiopathogenegis of osteoarthritis, in *Arthritis and Allied Conditions. A Textbook of Rheumatology*, 13th ed. (Koopman, W. J., ed.), Baltimore. Williams & Wilkins, pp.1969–1984.
2. Radin, E. L. and Rose, R. M. (1986) Role of subchondral bone in the initiation and progression of cartilage damage. *Clin. Orthop.* **213,** 34–40.
3. Meunier, P. J. (1983) Histomorphometry of the skeleton, in *Bone and Mineral Research Annual 1*, (Peck, W. A., ed.), Excerpta Medica, Amsterdam, pp. 191–222.
4. Pastoureau, P., Leduc, S., Chomel, A., and De Ceuninck, F. (2003) Quantitative assessment of articular cartilage and subchondral bone histology in the meniscectomized guinea pig model of osteoarthritis. *Osteoarthritis Cartilage* **11,** 412–423.

6

Laser-Mediated Microdissection As a Tool for Molecular Analysis in Arthritis

Martin Judex, Elena Neumann, Steffan Gay, and Ulf Müller-Ladner

Summary

Most current approaches to the analysis of gene expression in arthritic tissue samples are based on RNA isolated either from cultured synovial cells or from synovial biopsies. However, this strategy does not distinguish between specific gene expression profiles of cells originating from separate tissue areas. Therefore, we established the combination of laser-mediated microdissection and RNA arbitrarily primed polymerase chain reaction (RAP-PCR) for differential display to analyze profiles of gene expression in histologically defined areas of arthritic tissue. Cryosections derived from synovial tissue were used to obtain cell samples from different tissue areas using a microbeam laser microscope. RNA was isolated and analyzed using nested RAP-PCR to generate a fingerprint of the expressed gene sequences. Differentially expressed bands were isolated, cloned, and sequenced. Differential expression of identified sequences was confirmed by *in situ* hybridization and immunohistochemistry.

Key Words: Laser-mediated microdissection; fingerprint; gene expression analysis; synovium; synovial tissue; rheumatoid arthritis; osteoarthritis.

1. Introduction

The sequencing of the human genome and the development of powerful and sensitive analytical tools were the basis for studying intracellular mechanisms of cell activation on a molecular level. To achieve a better understanding of the pathogenesis and the course of arthritic joint diseases such as osteoarthritis (OA) and rheumatoid arthritis (RA), and to facilitate long-term monitoring of the effects of antiinflammatory and disease-modifying drugs, it is desirable that this molecular analysis be performed on specific cell populations that are crucial for the disease and that can be obtained from their native or diseased environment.

Current methods to identify genes that are differentially expressed from RA and related arthritic diseases—such as OA—are usually based on RNA iso-

From: *Methods in Molecular Medicine, Vol. 101: Cartilage and Osteoarthritis, Volume 2: Structure and In Vivo Analysis*
Edited by: F. De Ceuninck, M. Sabatini, and P. Pastoureau © Humana Press Inc., Totowa, NJ

lated either from cultured cells or from synovial biopsies. In both cases, the examined cells consist of a mixed population of all cell types from the different areas and compartments of the synovium. In general, this problem can result in gene expression profiles that are most likely superimposed on each other.

To address this issue and to obtain detailed insights into the molecular processes occuring in exactly defined histological areas of the synovium, we adapted laser-mediated microdissection (LMM) *(1)* for the analysis of RA synovium *(2)*. This method has recently been developed for molecular oncology *(3)* and is also being used in our laboratory for examination of gene expression profiles of colonic crypts and (pre)malignant stages of colon carcinoma *(4)*. Based on these experiences, it can be stated that LMM can easily be adapted to other types of articular tissue samples including synovia derived from OA joints and other arthritides and, as is currently being established in our laboratory, even to low-cell-number cartilage specimens.

Following the protocol mentioned below, LMM allows isolation of histologically clearly defined regions of a cryosection *(1)*. After RNA isolation, subsequent nested RNA arbitrarily primed polymerase chain reaction (RAP-PCR) *(5,6)* amplifies a subpopulation of the expressed RNA sequences isolated from the dissected tissue. The "fingerprints" generated by this strategy can then be compared to identify genes that are differentially expressed between two distinct and histologically defined areas of the same synovial tissue or between the same areas of different tissue samples. This initial identification should be followed by histological confirmation on both the RNA and the protein level using *in situ* hybridization and immunohistochemistry.

2. Materials

2.1. Preparation of Tissue Sections

1. Synovial tissue samples.
2. Embedding medium (TissueTek® O.C.T. medium, VWR Scientific Products, Corporation, San Diego, CA).
3. Custom-made aluminum mold (aluminum foil modeled into a mold by wrapping it around the end of a text marker; about 3 cm deep: autoclaved)
4. Cryostat (Reichert-Jung 2800 Frigocut, IMEBINC, San Marcos, CA or equivalent).
5. Polyethylene naphthalate (PEN) membrane (P.A.L.M., Wolfratshausen, Germany).
6. RNase Zap (Ambion, TX).
7. Poly-L-lysine (0.01% poly-L-lysine in sterile, diethyl pyrocarbonate [DEPC]-treated H_2O).
8. UV crosslinker (UV Stratalinker 2400, Stratagene, San Diego, CA or equivalent).

9. Hematoxylin solution: dissolve 1 g hematoxylin, 0.1 g sodium iodate, 50 g potassium aluminum sulfate in 1 L DEPC-treated H_2O. Add 50 g chloral hydrate and 1 g crystalized citric acid, sterile filter, and store in the dark.

2.2. Laser Microdissection

1. Robot Microbeam laser microscope (P.A.L.M., Germany or equivalent).
2. Autoclaved laser pressure catapulting (LPC) microcentrifuge tubes (clear, 500 μL volume; P.A.L.M).

2.3. RNA Extraction and RAP-PCR

1. RNeasy spin column purification kit (Qiagen, Hilden, Germany) or other RNA isolation kit.
2. DNase I (Qiagen).
3. Arbitrary 10–12-mer oligonucleotide primers (for examples, *see* **Subheading 3.6.1.** below and ref. *5*).
4. 10X Reverse transcription (RT) buffer: 500 m*M* Tris-HCl, pH 8.3, 750 m*M* KCl, 30 m*M* $MgCl_2$, 200 m*M* dithiothreitol (DTT).
5. 100 m*M* dNTP mix.
6. Murine moloney leukemia virus (MMLV) reverse transcriptase.
7. 10X RAP-PCR buffer: 100 m*M* Tris-HCl, pH 8.3, 100 m*M* KCl, 40 m*M* $MgCl_2$.
8. AmpliTaq® DNA polymerase Stoffel fragment (Perkin Elmer, Norwalk, CT).
9. [α-^{32}P]dCTP (3000 Ci/mmol).
10. Thermocycler (model 9700, Applied Biosystems, Foster City, CA or equivalent).

2.4. Gel Electrophoresis and Cloning

1. Agarose and sequencing gel equipment.
2. Gel dryer (model 583, Bio-Rad, Hercules, CA or equivalent).
3. Gel loading buffer: (0.25% bromophenol blue, 0.25% xylene cyanol FF, 30% glycerol).
4. Tris-borate ethylenediaminetetraacetic acid (EDTA) buffer (TBE): 90 m*M* Tris-borate, 2 m*M* EDTA.
5. 8 *M* Urea, 5% polyacrylamide sequencing gel, prepared with TBE buffer.
6. Running buffer: 1X TBE.
7. Single-strand conformation polymorphism (SSCP) gel: 25 mL 2X mutation detection electrophoresis (MDE) gel solution (FMC, Rockland, MD), 6 mL 10X TBE, 10 mL 98% glycerol, H_2O to 100 mL, polymerized with 400 μL APS, and 40 μL *N*,*N*,*N*′,*N*′-tetramethylethylenediamine (TEMED).
8. SSCP running buffer: 0.6X TBE.
9. SSCP loading buffer: 0.25% bromophenol blue, 0.25% xylene cyanol FF, 30% glycerol, 50% formamide.
10. BioMax X-ray film (Kodak, Stuttgart, Germany) or equivalent.

11. TOPO TA Cloning® Kit DUALPromoter (Invitrogen, De Schelp, Netherlands) or other TA cloning system.

3. Methods

3.1. Tissue Preparation and Embedding

1. Rinse fresh rheumatoid synovial tissue samples in cold buffered saline to remove excess fibrin and clotted blood.
2. Remove adipose tissue as much as possible.
3. Dissect the tissue specimens into individual segments no larger than 5 mm^3 using a sterile scalpel.
4. Fill a custom-made aluminum mold with TissueTek embedding medium, and place tissue segments in the mold so they are completely submerged in embedding medium; the target surface of the tissue section should lie flat and face down to facilitate easier identification of the target tissue compartment for cryocutting.
5. Lower this mold slowly into liquid nitrogen to prevent inhomogenous freezing, which would generate ice crystals in the sample; this ultimately leads to cracks within the frozen embedding medium and reduced quality of the tissue sections.
6. Label all cryoblocks with a cryomarker, wrap them tightly in aluminum foil, and store at –80°C until sectioning. Ideally, tissue harvesting and processing should be performed as rapidly as possible to prevent excessive RNA degradation (*see* **Note 1**).

3.2. Preparation of the Slides

1. Clean glass slides with ethanol and RNase Zap® to remove any residual RNases.
2. Carefully mount a piece of PEN membrane of about the same dimensions as the slide on the slide with tweezers (*see* **Note 2**).
3. Flatten the membrane using sterile cotton swabs to prevent the occurrence of creases.
4. Fix the membrane by using a small piece of autoclave tape on the barcode label side of the slide.
5. Dip the slide in 100% ethanol and let it air-dry in a vertical position.
6. Smooth out creases and tape the membrane on the slide area opposite from the barcode. Slides prepared in this way can be stored in a clean, closed container for several weeks at room temperature.

3.3. Preparing the Tissue Sections

1. Immediately before use, treat the slides with an ultraviolet (UV) crosslinker (1200 $\mu J/cm^2$) and coat them with poly-L-lysine under RNase-free conditions by dipping them into 0.01% poly-L-lysine dissolved in DEPC-treated H_2O. This treatment facilitates adherence of tissue sections to the membrane. After air-drying, the coated slides can be stored in an RNase-free container at 4°C for up to 2 wk.
2. Place the tissue in the cryostat for about 10 min prior to cutting to allow adjustment to the cutting temperature.

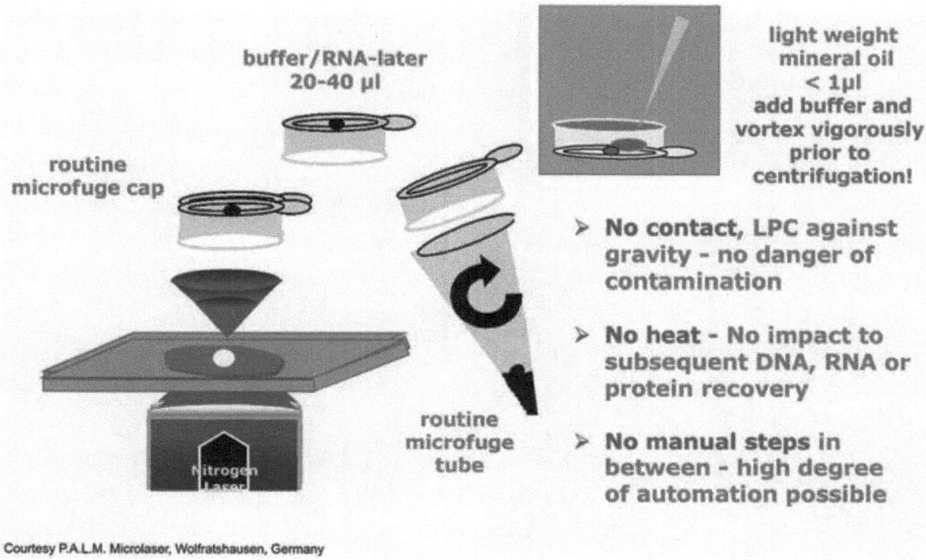

Fig. 1. Schematic diagram of the LMM procedure LPC, laser pressure catapulting. (Generously provided by P.A.L.M. Microlaser, Wolfratshausen, Germany.)

3. Prepare cryosections (7–8 µm) under RNase-free conditions (*see* **Note 3**).
4. After a short drying phase, fix the slides in 95% ethanol/5% acetic acid at –20°C for 5–10 min.
5. Air-dry slides thoroughly and incubate in hematoxylin solution for up to 5 min to facilitate later identification of tissue areas by light blue cellular staining (*see* **Note 4**).
6. Discolor slides in DEPC-treated tap water (not in deionized water) and dehydrate in an ascending ethanol sequence (75, 95, and 100% ethanol). Dipping the slides in ethanol for a few seconds is sufficient.
7. Finally, the slides have to be dried again, because residual ethanol interferes with laser dissection. To minimize RNA degradation, the time span between staining and microdissection needs to be kept as short as possible.

3.4. Laser Microdissection

3.4.1. Principle

The Robot MicroBeam laser microscope uses a pulsed nitrogen laser with a wavelength of 337 nm (**Fig. 1**). The small beam focus of the UV laser allows very accurate photoablation: in this process the focused laser beam cracks molecules at the cutting line to the atomic or low molecular level. Because of its short wavelength, this type of nonthermic ablation avoids energy dispersion into adjacent cells and therefore preserves RNA integrity in the target cells and

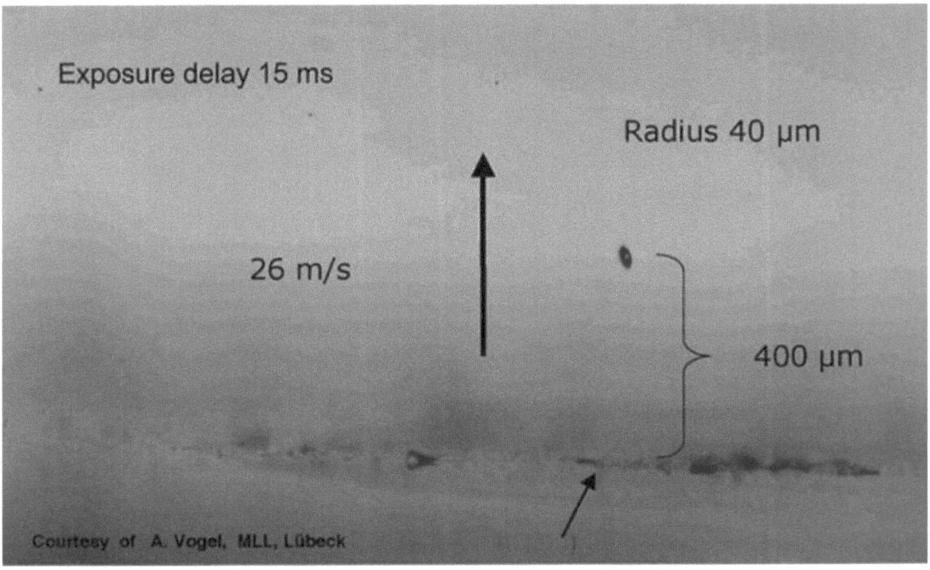

Fig. 2. Catapulting of a tissue fragment toward the cap of a microcentrifuge tube. (Laser pressure catapulting [LPC] was a generous gift of Dr. A. Vogel, MLL, Lübeck, Germany.) Longer arrow, movement vector of catapulted fragment; shorter arrow, origin of catapulted fragment.

tissues. LMM is a rapid, reliable, and precise technique. In addition, physical contact of the investigator with the tissue is negligible, which results in minimized contamination problems. Also, multiple areas of similar tissue can be harvested from the same section because surrounding tissue is left intact by the procedure. Dissected areas are collected in the cap of a microcentrifuge tube via LPC. LPC catapults the object of interest vertically off the membrane-coated slide using a high-energy, defocused, short-duration laser pulse (**Fig. 2**). Alternatively, larger pieces of tissue (e.g., sublining) can be picked up with a 27-gage needle under a stereomicroscope and transferred to the microcentrifuge tube. The cap with the dissected tissue is then placed immediately on the microcentrifuge tube containing lysis buffer, and the tissue is lysed by mixing. This solution should be kept on ice or, for long-term storage, at –80°C.

A critical parameter for the success of the entire procedure is the minimum amount of cells needed to obtain enough RNA to generate a stable fingerprint, i.e., a highly reproducible pattern of amplification products that range from 100 to approx 600 bp in length. This amount varies considerably for tissues of different origins and needs to be determined individually. As a starting point,

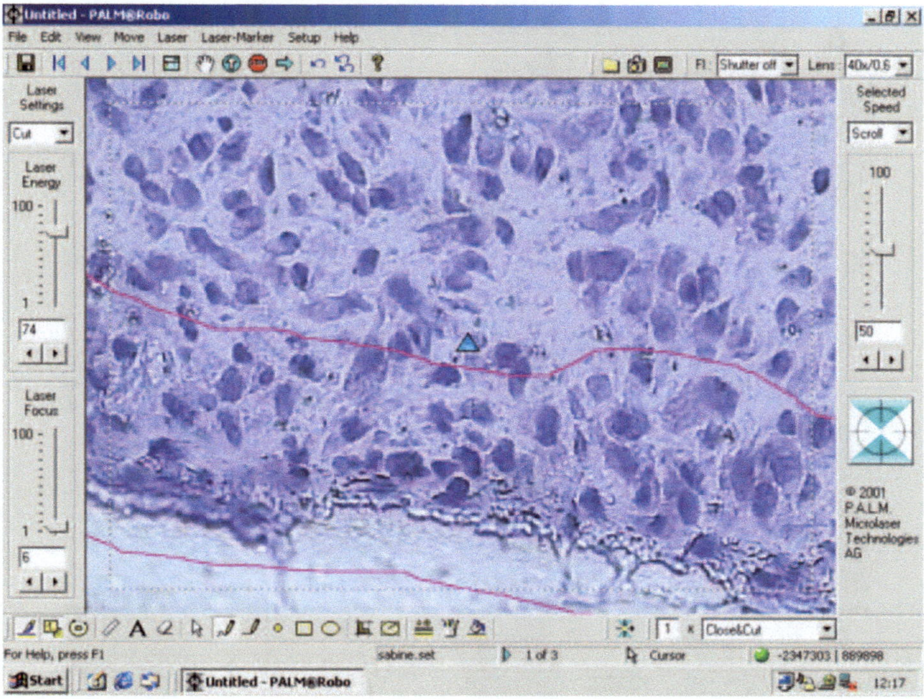

Fig. 3. Selection of the areas of interest (here: lining layer of rheumatoid synovium) using the tissue-marking feature of the PA.L.M. software (red line). Marked areas can thereafter be automatically dissected and sampled by the PA.L.M. program. Note that the high magnification allows inclusion or exclusion of single cells. Blue triangle, starting point of laser beam.

areas containing 150, 300, 450, 600, and 900 cells should be microdissected from different tissue regions and used for RNA isolation (*see* **Note 5**).

3.4.2. Microdissection

1. Count 150 cells of the region of interest.
2. Circle the respective area using the tissue-marking function of the P.A.L.M. software (**Fig. 3**).
3. Sample one, two, three, or six fragments of the same size and cell density sequentially by either LPC or picking them up with a sterile needle.
4. Immediately transfer fragments to an LPC microcentrifuge tube containing 300 μL of lysis buffer (RNeasy spin column purification kit or equivalent).
5. **Figure 4** illustrates the same section before and after removal of an inflamed region around a small terminal synovial vessel.

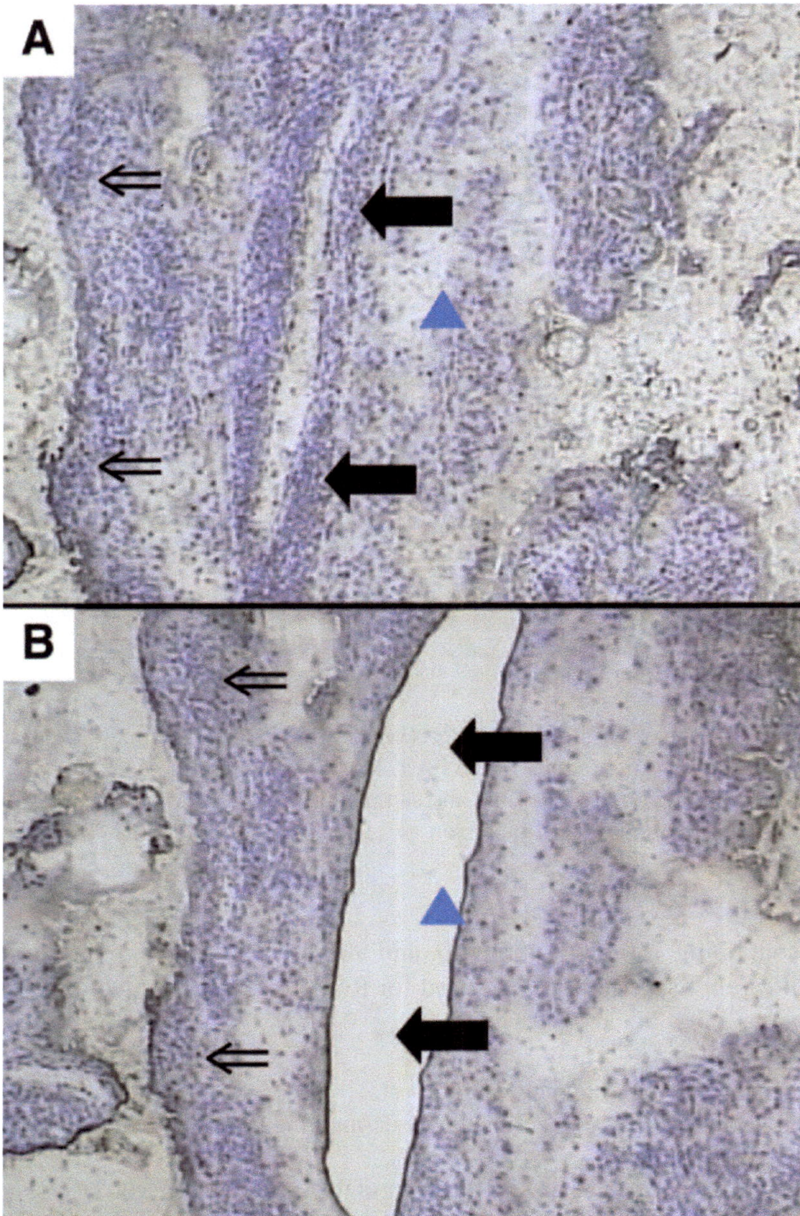

Fig. 4. Same tissue section before **(A)** and after **(B)** LMM of an inflamed region around a terminal vessel in rheumatoid synovium. Open arrow, lining layer; bold arrow, terminal vessel surrounded by inflammatory cells; blue triangle, starting point of laser beam. (Experiment performed in collaboration with Dr. Ulfgren and Prof. Klareskog, Karolinska Institute, Stockholm, Sweden.)

3.5. RNA Extraction

1. Extract RNA by silica gel binding using the RNeasy spin column purification kit or any other method providing DNA-free high-quality RNA.
2. Treat total RNA on the spin column with DNase I (Qiagen) at room temperature for 30 min to remove the remaining genomic DNA (*see* **Note 6**).
3. Perform the extraction according to the instructions of the manufacturer, and elute the RNA with 30 μL of RNase-free water (*see* **Note 7**).
4. Apply the eluate to the column a second time and spin through again to increase yield (*see* **Note 8**).

3.6. RAP-PCR

3.6.1. Principle

RAP-PCR *(4,7)* results in amplification of an arbitrary subset of the total cellular RNA and has several advantages compared with other commonly used amplification methods:

1. Unlike all methods using oligo dT priming, it is not biased toward the 3' end of the RNA. Since the 3' region is often untranslated, it is generally more variable and less informative than the translated part of the mRNA.
2. In a typical RAP-PCR fingerprint, approx 50–100 fragments can be visualized, including relatively rare messages that happen to match with the arbitrary primers. Therefore, rare messages that may not have been detected by other methods can also be detected *(5)*.
3. Finally, RAP-PCR can be finished in a few hours and is a rather robust and easy-to-perfom method.

RAP-PCR consists of two major steps: transcription of total RNA into cDNA using reverse transcriptase (RT reaction) and a first arbitrary primer followed by amplification of a subset of the cDNA (arbitrarily primed PCR, or AP-PCR). This procedure uses short primers (10–12 mers) of an arbitrarily selected sequence and a low annealing temperature of only 35°C. These conditions permit annealing of the primers to regions on the target nucleic acid when they match at least five or six bases at the 3' end, a situation that on average takes place about every few hundred base pairs.

Nested RAP-PCR differs from the original protocol by the introduction of a second AP-PCR step of 35 amplification cycles using a nested primer that is shifted one base to the 3' end, and a reduction of the first PCR step to 15 cycles. As a result, the complexity of the fingerprint is reduced even further, resulting in improved detection of rare messages.

3.6.2. RAP-PCR Fingerprinting

1. Mix RNA (approx 5 μg in 30 μL) with 20 μL RT solution for a final volume of 50 μL containing 1X RT buffer, 0.2 m*M* dNTPs, 2 μ*M* primer, and 100 U MMLV reverse transcriptase (*see* **Note 9**).
2. To exclude DNA contamination, a reverse transcriptase-free reaction should be included in all RAP-PCR experiments.
3. Apply the following reaction conditions:
   a. 5-min Ramp from 25°C to 37°C (primer annealing).
   b. 60 min at 37°C (reverse transcription).
   c. 15 min at 68° (inactivation of enzyme).
4. Purify and concentrate the synthesized cDNA using the Microcon YM-100 kit (Millipore, Billerica, MA) according to the manufacturer's instructions. The final eluate contains the entire amount of cDNA in a volume of only 1–5 μL.
5. Perform AP-PCR for second-strand synthesis using the nested PCR strategy. Preamplify for 15 cycles using the first arbitrary PCR primer (*see* **Note 9**) by mixing the cDNA (approx 5 μg in 1–5 μL, whole volume eluted from the Microcon column) with PCR solution for final concentrations of 1X PCR buffer, 0.2 m*M* dNTPs, 4 μ*M* primer, and 2.5 U AmpliTaq DNA polymerase Stoffel fragment in a volume of 20 μL.
6. Cycling conditions are as follows:
   a. 5 min at 94°C (initial denaturation).
   b. 15 Cycles of 94°C for 30 s, 35°C for 30 s, and 72°C for 60 s.
   c. 7 min at 72° (final extension).
7. Purify the PCR products using the Millipore Microcon YM-100 kit and bring to a total volume of 30 μL with nuclease-free water.
8. Use one-third of the amplified products (10 μL) for the second amplification step with the nested 10-mer arbitrary primer (*see* **Note 9**).
9. The reaction is performed in a volume of 20 μL under the same conditions as before with the addition of 2 μCi [α-^{32}P]dCTP (3000 Ci/mmol).
10. Cycling conditions are the same as indicated above, except that this time 35 cycles are performed.
11. All reactions are carried out in duplicate to test the reproducibility and stability of the RNA fingerprint.

3.6.3. Gel Electrophoresis

1. Mix an aliquot of the PCR reaction 1:1 with loading buffer, denature it (94°C for 3 min and then put on ice immediately), and load onto an 8 *M* urea, 5% polyacrylamide sequencing gel prepared with TBE buffer.
2. Perform electrophoresis at 45°C and 100 W for about 90 min or until the bromophenol blue band reaches the lower third of the gel.
3. Peel the gel away from the glass support using a Whatman filter paper of about the same size as the gel, and cover it with cling film.
4. Dry the gel under vacuum at 80°C for 1–2 h, and expose it to a BioMax X-Ray film (Kodak) overnight.

3.6.4. Band Excision and Elution of Fragments

1. Visually identify differentially expressed bands on the X-ray film.
2. Excise them from the gel by aligning the film with the dried gel, marking the bands of interest with a pin and cutting out the bands using a scalpel (*see* **Note 10**).
3. The corresponding region must also be isolated from the respective control lane, which should contain the product at significantly higher or lower levels.
4. Elute PCR products by soaking the gel fragments, with the Whatman filter paper still attached, in Tris-HCl buffer (10 m*M* Tris-HCl, pH 8.5) at room temperature for 1 min, followed by a centrifugation step.
5. Transfer the supernatant containing the PCR fragments to a fresh tube, and store it at –20°C or use it immediately for reamplification.

3.7. Purification of Differentially Expressed Bands by Gel Electrophoresis

3.7.1. SSCP Gel Electrophoresis: Principle

As these eluates usually contain a mixture of several PCR products of more or less identical molecular weight, further purification by other techniques is required. SSCP gel electrophoresis can be used for this purpose. This method utilizes a characteristic phenomenon of single-stranded DNAs: they fold to form stable and metastable structures that affect their mobility in a non-denaturing acrylamide gel, thereby facilitating differentiation between PCR products of roughly the same molecular weight.

3.7.2. SSCP Gel Electrophoresis

1. Reamplify PCR products for 20 cycles using the same conditions and primers that were used in the second AP-PCR step.
2. Mix 5 µL of this PCR reaction with 15 µL SSCP loading buffer and denature at 95°C, then put on ice immediately.
3. Load samples onto the SSCP gel.
4. Run the gel for 12–15 h at a constant power of 5 W.
5. Peel the gel away from the glass support using Whatman filter paper (*see* **Note 11**), dry it, and expose it to BioMax X-Ray film.
6. Cut out differentially expressed bands and elute PCR products as before. Reamplify the products again, omitting the [α-^{32}P]dCTP.
7. Run the products on an agarose gel.
8. Cut out and elute fragments using the MinElute gel extraction kit (Qiagen).

3.8. Cloning and Sequencing of Differentially Expressed Genes

The eluate can then be used for cloning into the pCRII TOPO® vector using the TOPO TA Cloning Kit DUALPromoter according to the manufacturer's instructions and sequencing by standard methods *(4,7)*. At least five clones should be sequenced per cloning reaction to ascertain that only the desired sequence and not a mixture of different PCR products has been cloned.

3.9. Confirmation of Differential Expression

The differential expression of genes identified by the combination of LMM and RAP-PCR needs to be confirmed by other methods, as there is always a chance that during the miscellaneous reamplification and gel electrophoresis steps an irrelevant gene sequence has been selected.

If an antibody to the respective protein is available, immunohistochemistry is the method of choice. Otherwise, expression of the corresponding mRNA may be confirmed by *in situ* hybridization. As the TOPO TA Cloning DUAL-Promoter vector used for cloning and sequencing already contains SP6 and T7 RNA polymerase promoters, RNA probes for the gene of interest can be easily generated.

4. Notes

1. Frozen tissue should be kept at very low temperatures and well wrapped for as long as possible during the procedure (use dry ice for transportation and other procedures). Because of slow but continuous RNA degradation even at –20°C, tissue specimens should not be used more than three times.
2. The electrostatically charged PEN membrane is very fragile and has to be handled with extra care.
3. Four to 10 cryosections can be cut and placed on the same slide. However, the embedding medium from one section must not touch or overlap tissue from another section.
4. The hematoxylin solution should not be used more than three times. Dyeing takes a shorter time using fresh hematoxylin solution compared with previously used solutions.
5. For RA synovial tissue, an area containing 600 cells (spanning between 200,000 and 2 million μm^2, depending on cell density) was sufficient to obtain the amount of RNA necessary for stable fingerprinting. Therefore, in all our subsequent experiments, tissue areas containing at least 600 cells were used. It is crucial to use only areas that represent a homogenous compartment of the tissue of choice (as opposed to "mixed" areas containing sublining as well as microvasculature, for example). Pilot experiments that are currently performed demonstrated that laser microdissection can also be performed on OA synovial tissue and most likely also on cartilage. However, because of the lower cell density compared with RA and specific properties of cartilage, optimization of the procedure may be required.
6. Although RNA fingerprints are relatively insensitive to DNA contamination, no chances should be taken here. Therefore, a DNAse digest should always be performed.
7. Addition of carrier RNA was tested but showed no improvement in yield and was thus discontinued.

8. To get a feeling for the amount of RNA that can be isolated, the RNA concentration of a few samples can be determined using the RiboGreen RNA Quantitation kit (Molecular Probes, Eugene, OR), which detects RNA in concentrations of down to 1 pg/μL.
9. Of the different arbitrary primers that were tested, for our purposes the combination of OPN23 (5'-CAG GGG CAC C-3') as RT primer and OPN21 (5'-ACCAGGGGCA-3')/OPN21 nested (5'-CCAGGGGCAC-3') for the AP-PCR steps resulted in the most stable and reproducible fingerprints. However, other arbitrarily chosen 10–12-mer primers may work as well or even better for samples of different origin.
10. Cutting the bands from the gel has to be done no later than 2 wk after drying of the gel as the gel will shrink over time, making an exact alignment with the film impossible.
11. Owing to the added glycerol, SSCP gels are very sticky. They are best peeled off from the glass support by bending the Whatman paper 180° and carefully pulling it parallel to the surface of the glass plate.

Acknowledgments

The authors thank Wibke Ballhorn for excellent technical assistance. The experiments were supported by grants from the German Research Society (DFG Mu 1383/1-3 and Mu 1383/3-4).

References

1. Bonner, R. F., Emmert-Buck. M., Cole. K., et al. (1997) Laser capture microdissection: molecular analysis of tissue. *Science* **278,** 1481–1483.
2. Judex, M., Neumann, E., Lechner, S., et al. (2003) Laser-mediated microdissection facilitates analysis of area-specific gene expression in rheumatoid synovium. *Arthritis Rheum.* **48,** 97–102.
3. Wild, P., Knüchel, R., Dietmaier, W., Hofstädter, F., and Hartmann, A. (2000) Laser microdissection and microsatellite analyses of breast cancer reveal a high degree of tumor heterogeneity. *Pathobiology* **68,** 180–190.
4. Lechner, S., Müller-Ladner, U., Neumann, E., et al. (2001) Use of simplified transcriptors for the analysis of gene expression profiles in laser-microdissected cell populations. *Lab. Invest.* **81,** 1233–1242.
5. Trenkle, T., Welsh, J., Jung, B., Mathieu-Daude, F., and McClelland, M. (1998) Non-stoichiometric reduced complexity probes for cDNA arrays. *Nucleic Acids Res.* **26,** 3883–3891.
6. Welsh, J., Chada, K., Dalal, S. S., Cheng, R., Ralph, D., and McClelland, M. (1992) Arbitrarily primed PCR fingerprinting of RNA. *Nucleic Acids Res.* **20,** 4965–4970.
7. Kullmann, F., Judex, M., Ballhorn, W., et al. (1999) Kinesin-like protein CENP-E is upregulated in rheumatoid synovial fibroblasts. *Arthritis Res.* **1,** 71–80.

7

Analysis of Protein Distribution in Cartilage Using Immunofluorescence and Laser Confocal Scanning Microscopy

Stephan Soeder, Alexander Kuhlmann, and Thomas Aigner

Summary

Protein localization in cartilage sections by antibodies that specifically bind to epitopes of a protein is one of the most powerful technologies in modern cartilage research. Studies using two or more primary antibodies that recognize different protein epitopes allow the colocalization of different gene products in one cartilage section. In addition, specific histochemical stains help to visualize nuclear DNA, mitochondria, and other subcellular compartments. By these immunohistological methods, the distribution of proteins can be analyzed throughout different zones of articular cartilage. In particular, with the use of laser scanning confocal microscopy, subcellular localization of proteins can also be determined (i.e, nuclear, cytoplasmic, membrane-associated, and extracellular). Overall, immunohistochemical methods are fairly simple to handle, and the reagents required are inexpensive, with the exception of basic technical equipment (fluorescence microscope or confocal microscope). However, as with many methodologies, technical knowledge and experience is important to avoid and/or interpret either false-positive or false-negative results.

Key Words: Immunohistochemistry; confocal microscopy; cartilage imaging; fluorescence; fluorochrome; DNA.

1. Introduction

Protein localization in cartilage sections by antibodies that specifically bind to epitopes of a protein is one of the most powerful technologies in modern cartilage research. Basically, the primary antibody (monoclonal or polyclonal) binds to the protein epitope of interest, and subsequent binding of a secondary antibody, conjugated to a reporter molecule, allows localization of the protein by, for example, colorimetric or fluorescence detection methods. Studies using two or more primary antibodies that recognize different protein epitopes allow

From: *Methods in Molecular Medicine, Vol. 101: Cartilage and Osteoarthritis, Volume 2: Structure and In Vivo Analysis*
Edited by: F. De Ceuninck, M. Sabatini, and P. Pastoureau © Humana Press Inc., Totowa, NJ

the colocalization of different gene products in one cartilage section. In addition, specific histochemical stains help to visualize nuclear DNA, mitochondria, and other subcellular compartments. By these immunohistological methods, the distribution of proteins can be analyzed throughout different zones of articular cartilage ***(1,2)***. In particular, with the use of laser scanning confocal microscopy, the subcellular localization of proteins can also be determined (i.e, nuclear, cytoplasmic, membrane-associated, and extracellular). Overall, immunohistochemical methods are fairly simple to handle, and the reagents required are inexpensive, with the exception of basic technical equipment (fluorescence microscope or confocal microscope). However, as with many methodologies, technical knowledge and experience is important to avoid and/or interpret either false-positive or false-negative results. It is always of prime importance, therefore, to include positive and negative controls in each experiment. One limitation of all immunostaining techniques is that the results obtained are considered semiquantitative. Therefore, other technologies are needed for determining absolute values of protein concentrations present in the cartilage.

2. Materials

1. Conventional fluorescence microscope (Leica, Nikon, Olympus, Zeiss).
2. Laser scanning confocal microscope (Leica, Nikon, Olympus, Zeiss).
3. Primary antibodies (mono- or polyclonal; different companies depending on the antigen to be detected).
4. Proteolytic enzymes for pretreatment of specimens:
   a. Protease XXIV (bacterial; Sigma-Aldrich, Taufkirchen, FRG).
   b. Pronase (*Streptomyces griseus*; Roche Diagnostics, Mannheim, FRG)
   c. Hyaluronidase (bovine testis; Roche Diagnostics, Mannheim, FRG).
   d. Trypsin (Sigma-Aldrich, Taufkirchen, FRG).
5. Conjugated secondary antibodies (e.g., Molecular Probes, Eugene, OR) and other labels (e.g., fluorochrome-labeled streptavidin; BioGenex, San Ramon, CA).
6. Tyramides and tyramide buffer (e.g., Molecular Probes).
7. Nuclear counterstains (*see* **Table 1**).
8. 10X phosphate buffered saline (PBS): 1.37 *M* NaCl + 27 m*M* KCl + 75 μ*M* Na_2HPO_4 + 14.7 μ*M* KH_2PO_4.
9. 10X Tris-buffered saline (TBS): 50 m*M* Tris-HCl, pH 7.35, 9% NaCl.
10. Dilution solution (DS): 5 m*M* Tris-HCl, pH 7.35, 0.9% NaCl, 1% bovine serum albumin (BSA), 0.02% NaN_3.
11. PFA: 4% paraformaldehyde in PBS, pH 7.4 (*see* **Note 1**).
12. Triethoxysilylpropylamin (Sigma-Aldrich).
13. SuperFrost® Plus slides (Dakopatts, Glostrup, Denmark).
14. Slides and cover slides (any company).
15. Dimethylsulfoxide (DMSO; Sigma-Aldrich, Taufkirchen, Germany).

Table 1
Absorption and Emission Maxima for Commonly Used Nuclear Counterstains in Immunofluorescence Microscopy

Fluorochrome	Absorption (A_{max} in nm)	Emission (E_{max} in nm)	Laser lines	Manufacturer (among others)
DAPI	358	461	UV-Ar (351 nm)[a]	Sigma, St. Louis, MO
Hoechst 34580	392	440	UV-diode (405 nm)[a]	Molecular Probes, Eugene, OR
Sytox blue	445	470	Ar (457 nm), HeCd (442 nm)[a]	Molecular Probes
Sytox green	504	523	Ar (514 nm)	Molecular Probes
Ethidium bromide	518	605	Ar (514 nm)	Sigma
Propidium iodide	535	617	HeNe (543 nm)	Molecular Probes
Syto 61	620	647	HeNe (633 nm) Red diode (633 nm)	Molecular Probes

[a]Normally not available.

16. Pap-pen (Science Services, Munich, FRG).
17. Series 1000 vibratome (Ted Pella).

3. Methods

3.1. Localization of Proteins by Immunofluorescence

3.1.1. Principles of Fluorescence Immunohistochemistry

The basis of all immunohistochemical methods is the specific binding of antibodies to epitopes. For immunofluorescence, fluorochrome-labeled secondary antibodies are utilized to visualize the primary antibody bound to its epitope (in most cases a protein; for a more detailed overview, *see* **ref. *3***).

Fluorescence is a three-stage process in which a suitable molecule, the fluorochrome, absorbs energy derived from a photon. This creates a molecule in an excited electronic singlet state (S_1'). The fluorochrome then dissipates some of this initially absorbed energy to reach a relaxed electronic singlet state (S_1). Then the fluorochrome returns to ground state (S_0) by emitting a photon. A single molecule can be continuously induced to emit thousands of photons before being irreversibly destroyed by the exciting radiation, a process known as *photobleaching*. The energy dissipated in the transition from the S_1' to the S_1 state means that the emitted photon is of lower energy then the absorbed photon. Therefore the emitted light is of longer wavelength than the exciting radiation. The difference between excitation and emission is called a Stokes shift. Generally, a fluorochrome with a large Stokes shift has a good signal-to-background

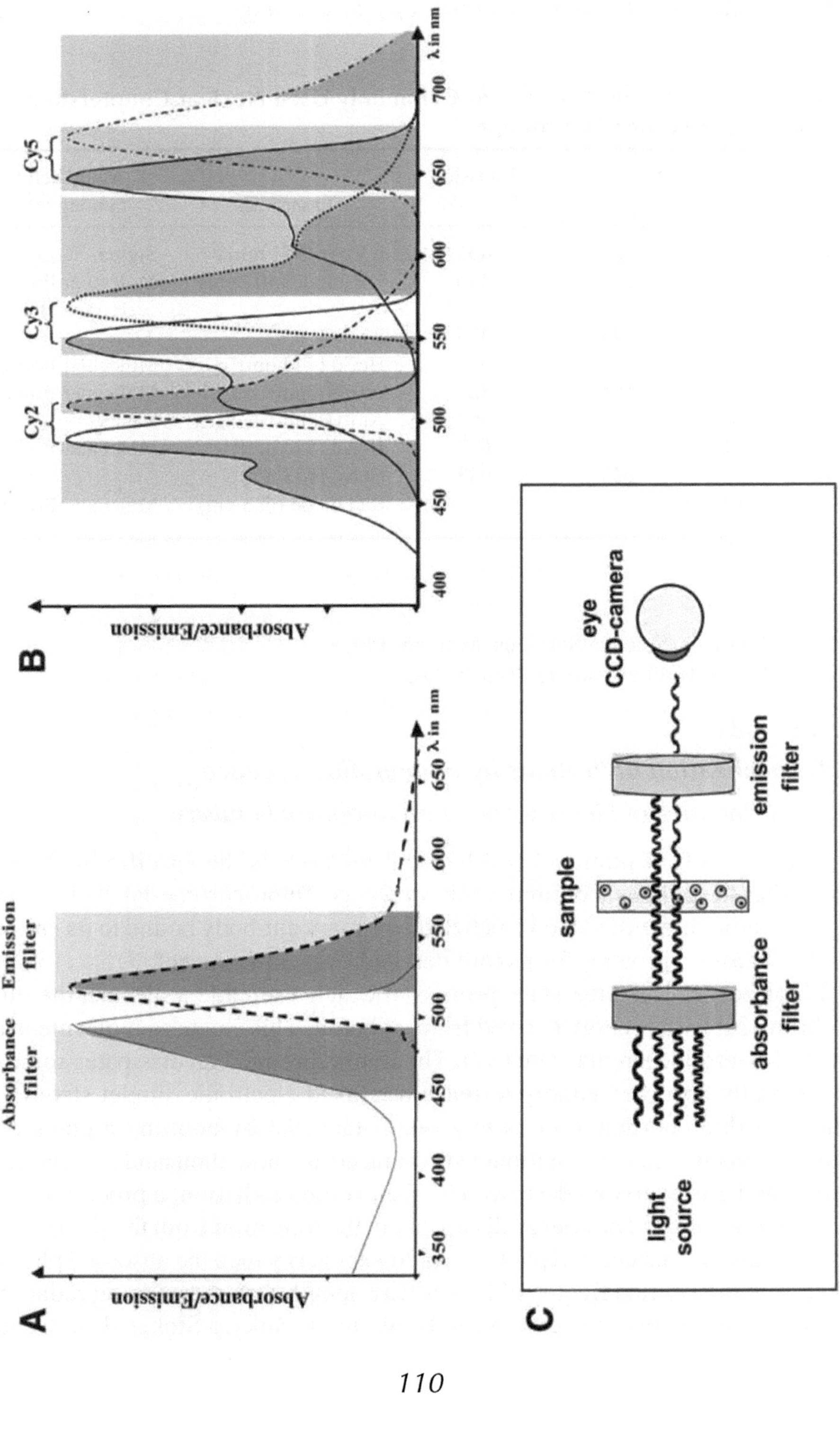
A
Absorbance/Emission
Absorbance filter
Emission filter
350
400
450
500
550
600
650
λ in nm
B
Absorbance/Emission
Cy2
Cy3
Cy5
400
450
500
550
600
650
700
λ in nm
C
light source
absorbance filter
sample
emission filter
eye
CCD-camera

Fig. 1. (**A**) Absorbance and emission spectra for FITC. Both spectra show considerable overlap, but with a suitable filter, the emitted radiation can be detected specifically (e.g., a 450–490-nm absorbance filter and 515–565-nm emission filter). (**B**) For multiple staining only fluorochromes should be used, which have no significant overlap in their emission spectra. The combination of Cy2/Cy3/Cy5, for example, shows a small overlap in the emission spectra, but specific detection is still possible when suitable emission filters are used. (**C**) Only the combination of an absorbance filter and an excitation filter allows detection of fluorochromes. First, the absorbance filter blocks light of any wavelength except for the radiation necessary to excite the fluorochrome. Then, the emission filters blocks the exciting radiation but transmits the emitted photons of the correct wavelength.

ratio. Polyatomic fluorochromes display particularly broad excitation and emission spectra, which, in many cases, show considerable overlap (**Fig. 1A**). For specific detection of emitted radiation, it is necessary to choose excitation and emission filters whose bandpaths do not overlap (**Fig. 1C**). When two or more fluorochromes are used, it is mandatory that one fluorochrome not emit radiation in the emission filter bandpath of the other fluorochromes (**Fig. 1B**). For this reason, fluorochrome labels that differ in their emission spectra should be used for multiple staining of proteins within a section (*see* also **Note 2**).

Immunofluorescence allows specific and sensitive detection of proteins similar to conventional immunohistochemistry. Compared with the latter, the signals obtained by immunofluorescent staining are less stable and can only be analyzed over a certain time (up to months under the correct storage conditions). In particular, exposure to light must be kept to a minimum in order to preserve the signals. The major advantage of immunofluorescence is the ability to use two (or three) different antibodies in the same sample and to be able to detect them simultaneously with the use of secondary antibodies conjugated to different fluorochromes. A further advantage of confocal laser scanning microscopy is the ability to analyze very thick cartilage sections (up to 100 μm) in order to visualize the 3D distribution of proteins.

Either monoclonal or polyclonal primary antibodies can be used in immunohistochemical techniques. Unlike monoclonal antibodies which present a homogeneous immunoglobulin population specific for one epitope, polyclonal antibodies, represent a heterogeneous population that recognize a protein or oligopeptide, but not necessarily a specific epitope. Thus, monoclonal antibodies are generally considered the preferred primary antibody for immunohistochemical methods. However, irrespective of the antibody type, positive and negative controls are always necessary to determine the nonspecific antibody binding that may occur in particular tissue sections (*see* **Note 3**).

3.1.2. Labels

Labels are fluorochromes conjugated to antibodies, proteins, or other molecules (e.g., streptavidin), which are used to detect the primary antibody. **Table 2** lists some of the commonly used fluorochromes. If more than one label is used in the one experiment, then fluorochromes with well-separated emission wavelengths should be used (e.g., Cy3 and Cy5). In tissues with strong autofluorescence such as cartilage, labels with a longer emission wavelength are preferable as they produce less autofluorescent background staining (*see* **Note 4**). Infrared stains such as Cy5, however, are difficult to visualize with the unaided eye and thus are best viewed with a CCD camera. Owing to photobleaching of fluorochromes, light exposure of labeled antibodies, and

Table 2
Commonly Used Fluorochromes for Immunofluorescence

Fluorochrome	Absorption (A_{max} in nm)	Emission (E_{max} in nm)	Laser lines	Manufacturer (among others)
Alexa 350	345	444	UV-Ar (351 nm)[a]	Molecular Probes, Eugene, OR
Alexa 405	399	422	UV-diode (405 nm)[a]	Molecular Probes
Alexa 488	491	515	Ar (488 nm)	Molecular Probes
Cy2	492	510	Ar (488 nm)	Amersham, Buckinghamshire, UK
FITC (Fluorescein)	492	520	Ar (488 nm)	Dianova, Hamburg, FRG; Molecular Probes
Cy3	550	570	HeNe (543 nm)	Amersham
TRITC	550	573	HeNe (543 nm)	Sigma, St. Louis, MO Molecular Probes
Rhodamine red-X	570	590	Kr (568 nm) ArKr (568 nm)	Molecular Probes
Texas red	596	620	HeNe (594 nm)	Dianova Molecular Probes
Alexa 633	622	640	HeNe (633 nm) Red diode (633 nm)	Molecular Probes
Cy5	650	670	HeNe (633 nm) Red diode (633 nm)	Amersham

[a]Normally not available.

stained specimens during processing analysis and storage should be kept to a minimum.

3.1.3. Nuclear Stains

Fluorochromatic nuclear stains (**Table 1**) bind with high affinity to DNA. They are used to visualize the position of the nucleus within the cells relative to the location of the protein of interest (**Fig. 2**). Absorption and emission spectra of the nuclear stains should be different from the other fluorochrome(s) used in the immunostaining experiment in order to avoid nonspecific results. Examples of acceptable nuclear staining and antibody-conjugated fluorochrome pairs are (1) 4,6-diamino-2-phenyindole (DAPI) and Cy3 or Cy5; (2) Sytox Green and Cy5; (3) propidium iodide and Cy5 (with sequential detection protocols only); and (4) Syto 61 and fluorescein isothiocyanate (FITC).

3.1.4. Immunofluorescence: Experimental Protocol

The immunofluororescence staining protocol outlined below is a generalized method that can be altered at various steps to optimize conditions for a particular experiment. For example, pretreatment and dilutions of primary and

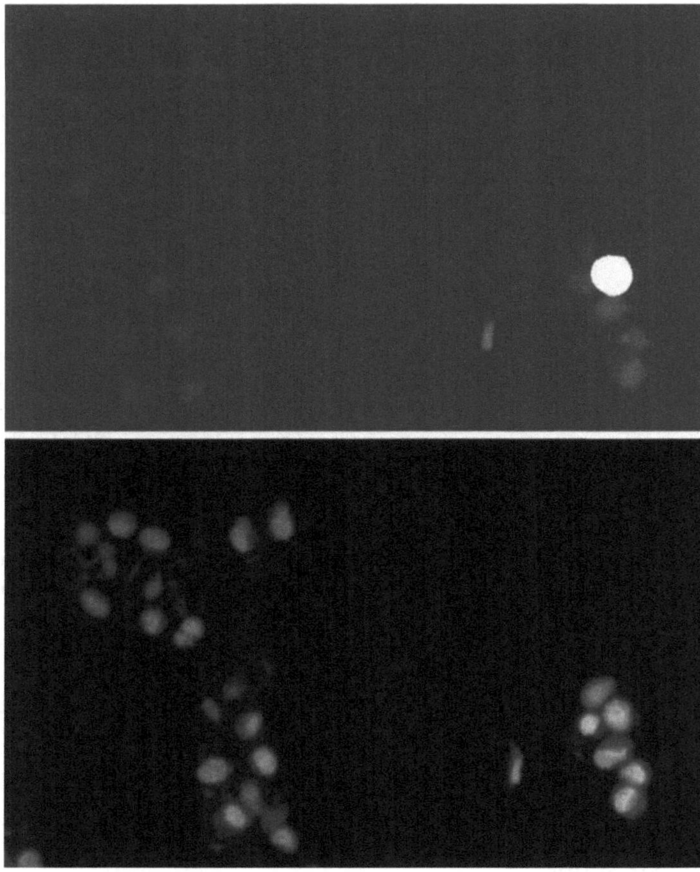

Fig. 2. Localization of the proliferation-associated antigen Ki-67 (**A**, labeled with FITC) in the nucleus (**B**, stained with DAPI) of osteoarthritic chondrocytes within a "brood capsule." As one can easily see, even in these areas of ongoing proliferation most cells are not replicating *(1)*.

secondary antibodies will vary depending on the antibody type as well as the cartilage type. All experimental steps are carried out at room temperature if not otherwise stated.

3.1.4.1. Sectioning

For starting material, *see* **Note 5**, and for use of semithick sections (up to 100 μm) *see* **Note 6**:

1. *Paraffin sections* (for slide pretreatment to increase adhesion of sections, *see* **Note 7**). Cut 2–4-μm-thick sections, remove paraffin, and rehydrate the cartilage sections by processing through 100% xylene (2 × 10 min) followed by decreas-

ing ethanol concentrations (100%, 3 × 5 min; 80%: 1 × 2 min; 50%, 1 × 2 min; H_2O, 5 min).

2. Frozen sections or chondrocyte monolayer cultures. Fix with 4% paraformaldehyde, pH 7.4, for 10 min (or a different fixative depending on the antibody used) and then wash for 10 min in 0.9% NaCl and a further 10 min in H_2O.

3.1.4.2. Enzymatic Pretreatment (If Required)

For alternative pretreatments and a testing approach, *see* **Note 8**.

1. Pretreat sections with the appropriate enzyme for 60 min at 37°C to make the epitope(s) better accessible for binding to the primary antibody. Wash with TBS (3 × 10 min).
2. If a second enzyme pretreatment is required, ensure that the section has been washed thoroughly with TBS (3 × 10 min) before addition of the second enzyme. This will avoid digestion of the second enzyme by the first.

3.1.4.3. Immunodetection

1. Block nonspecific epitopes on the cartilage sections by incubation with 2% BSA or 20% serum (of any unrelated species) in DS for 20 min. Remove the blocking solution by washing in TBS (for significance of the blocking step, *see* **Note 9**).
2. Add the primary antibody diluted in DS to the section and incubate either at 4°C overnight or at 37°C for 1 h in a humidified chamber. Dilutions used depend largely on the starting concentration of the primary antibody as well as the sensitivity level of the detection method to be used. Primary antibody dilutions from 1:10 up to 1:5000 are possible (for antibody testing, *see* **Note 8**; for amounts of diluted antibody to apply to a tissue section, *see* **Note 10**).
3. Wash 3 × 5 min in TBS to ensure complete removal of unbound primary antibody.

After these steps, several methods can be applied to detect the bound primary antibody. The simplest method is addition of a fluorochrome-labeled secondary antibody (dilutions of which will need to be tested) that will bind to the primary antibody on the cartilage section. This protocol describes an additional amplification step using the high-affinity-based streptavidin-biotin detection system. Here, a biotin-labeled secondary antibody ("link") is added to the cartilage section to bind the primary antibody. Detection of the secondary antibody is then carried out by addition of a fluorochrome-labeled streptavidin molecule ("label"; for general remarks on different immunodetection systems *see* **Notes 11** and **12** and for information on signal enhancement by the tyramide system, *see* **Note 13**).

4. Add link antibody to the cartilage section (BioGenex; 1:100 in DS) and incubate in a humidified chamber for 30 min.

Note: To avoid photobleaching of the stainings, all subsequent steps should be performed by avoiding daylight exposure as much as possible. A few minutes of daylight and exposure to lamp light is usually no problem.

5. Wash 2 × 5 min in TBS and add the fluorescent label (e.g., streptavidin-Cy3). Incubate for 30 min.

3.1.4.4. Nuclear Counterstaining

Wash 3 × 10 min in TBS and incubate with the desired nuclear counterstain, e.g., DAPI (0.1 ng/μL in PBS, pH 7.4); propidium iodide (5 ng/mL); Sytox Green (0.5 μ*M* in H_2O) for 10 min. Final wash twice in TBS for 10 min.

3.1.4.5. Final Processing and Storage

1. Apply cover slips over each stained cartilage section using 80% glycerol in H_2O or another embedding medium. (Specialized cover media are usually not needed.) Water or PBS as cover media are unsuitable as the cartilage section will dry out and the fluorochrome will be more unstable.
2. Cover-mounted cartilage sections can be stored in the dark at 4°C for up to several months.

3.1.5. Colocalization of Proteins: Experimental Protocol

It is important that the two primary antibodies used for colocalizing different proteins/epitopes within a cartilage section be raised in two different species (i.e., usually rat, mouse, rabbit, or goat). Double-labeling experiments with antibodies from the same species are possible but are considerably more laborious and requires extensive control experiments to demonstrate conclusively the lack of crossreactivity *(4,5)*. A typical protocol is outlined below, and references will be made to the single-labeling method when applicable. In addition, as with the single-labeling protocol, many variations in methodology are possible.

3.1.5.1. Cartilage Processing and Fixation

See **Subheading 3.1.4.1.**

3.1.5.2. Pretreatment

If both antibodies work with the same pretreatment protocol, one merely follows this method. If both antibodies require different pretreatments (which is rather an exceptional case), they can be carried out sequentially. However, this also requires testing and, in rare cases, it might be impossible to combine two antibodies (e.g., if an enzyme required for one antibody destroys the antigen that the other antibody recognizes).

3.1.5.3. Immunodetection

1. Blocking: *see* **Subheading 3.1.4.3.**
2. Apply both antibodies (e.g., one from rabbit, the other from mouse) to the cartilage section either overnight at 4°C or for 1 h at 37°C in a humidified chamber.

The concentration of antibodies used will be the same as that for the single-labeling experiments.

3. Wash 3 × 10 min with TBS.
4. Apply the first fluorochrome-labeled secondary antibody just like the single-labeling procedure.
5. Wash 2 × 10 min in TBS.
6. Apply second fluorochrome-labeled secondary antibody just like the single-labeling procedure.
7. Wash 2 × 10 min in TBS.

3.1.5.4. Nuclear Counterstaining, Final Processing, and Storage

See **Subheadings 3.1.4.4.** and **3.1.4.5.** Again, make sure that the emission spectrum of the nuclear stain fluorochrome does not overlap with the spectra of the two fluorochromes used for immunodetection.

3.2. Confocal Laser Scanning Microscopy

Confocal laser scanning microscopy (CLSM) is one of the major biological technical advances introduced over the past decade. This technology permits analysis of very thin optical sections through rather thick cartilage samples. Overlapping signals are avoided, thus allowing exact localization of a protein, or other molecule of interest, within the cell or cartilage compartments. In particular, the ability to use multiple labels allows localization of different proteins or cell compartments in one cartilage specimen. In addition, the intensity of staining can be quantified using image analysis software, but only to a limited extent.

3.2.1. Principles, Labels, and Counterstains

CLSM is mainly used for analysis of fluorochrome-labeled sections or cartilage material as described just above. The only limitation is that suitable laser lines need to be available for the fluorochromes of interest. Ultraviolet lasers are not available on many laser microscopes because they are rather expensive. In this case, Hoechst or DAPI as nuclear counterstains would be an unsuitable choice.

The principal advantage of confocal microscopy is that the optical arrangement prevents out-of-focus light from being detected (**Fig. 3**). This gives higher accuracy of focal sectioning, good 3D imaging properties, and improved contrast of the fine image detail. The fluorescent emission created is detected by a photon multiplier tube, and this detection input is reconstructed by computer hardware into an image.

It is useful to overlay images of different fluorochrome-labeled samples so their relative position can be studied through visual inspection.

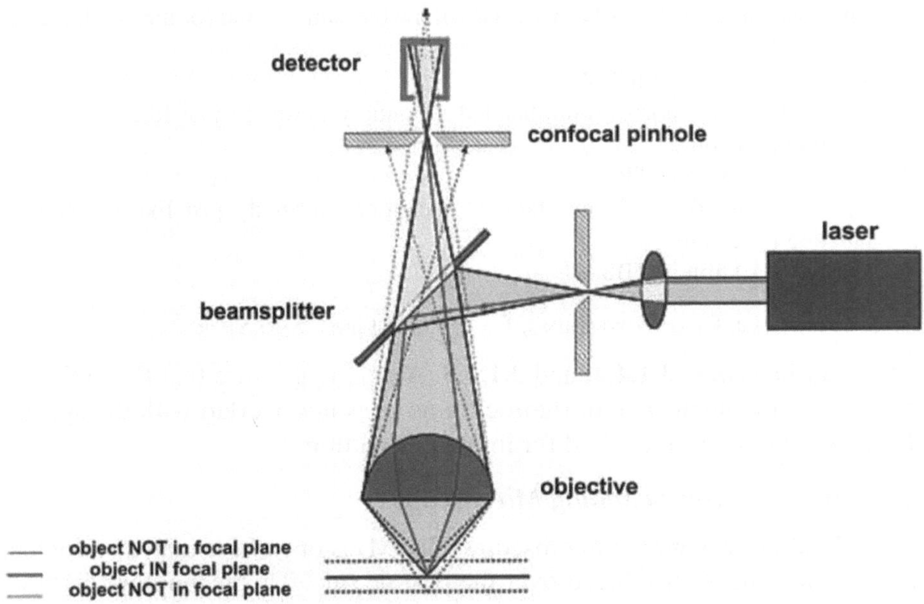

Fig. 3. Basic principles of the confocal microscope. In confocal microscopy, all out-of-focus structures are suppressed during image acquisition. This occurs by an arrangement of diaphragms, which, at optically conjugated points of the path of rays, act as a point of source and as a point detector. Rays from out-of-focus images are suppressed by the detection pinhole. The depth of the focal plane is determined in particular by the numerical aperture of the objective used and the diameter of the diaphragm. The emitted/reflected light passing through the detector pinhole is transformed into electrical signals by a photomultiplier and displayed on a computer monitor screen.

3.2.2. Important Parameters of Confocal Laser Scanning Microscopy

In this chapter we can only emphasize the most important parameters of CLSM, some of which include selection of the correct laser channel as well as the appropriate emission filter settings for the fluorochromes used (for a more detailed overview, *see* **ref. *6***). Proper training of confocal microscopy use through specialists or instruction manuals is necessary to acquire knowledge on the correct methods for analyzing specific samples and to be able to troubleshoot if problems arise. The *laser intensity* can be adjusted according to the needs of the specimen (the higher the power the more sensitive the detection, but the higher also the background and the risk of photobleaching of the specimen).

1. Two scanning modes exist for recording fluorescent signals: the *continuous scan mode* permits permanent recording of images from a single optical level in the

specimen. The continuous scan is best used to optimize the image quality for the first preview scan of a specimen. While the specimen is being scanned continuously, the scan parameters can be modified and the results can be checked directly in the image. However, with bleach-sensitive specimens, it is advisable to restrict the use of the continuous scan function to short time intervals. The *single scan mode* is mostly designed for taking final high-quality photographs and for analyzing bleach-sensitive specimens.

2. The *gain* function allows increased sensitivity of the photodetector. This effect is similar to increasing the laser intensity but without the risk of photobleaching. However, at very high gain levels, the background level is disproportionally increased.
3. The *offset* function permits establishment of a basic threshold level. Only signals higher than the threshold level are displayed on the screen, thus defining a cutoff value and the ability to remove background "noise."
4. The *resolution* of an image is defined by the number of pixels per picture. For preliminary evaluation of a specimen, it is advisable to use a lower resolution image, which takes less time and reduces photobleaching of the specimen. For final documentation a resolution of 1024 × 1024 pixels produces high quality images.
5. *Averaging* allows considerable reduction in background signal, which is important for increasing picture quality. Basically, a specimen can be scanned four to eight times and an average of all the scans documented; the decreased background scatter can be achieved without losing signal.
6. The *pinhole* diameter permits an increase or decrease in the confocal detection procedure: the smaller the diameter of the pinhole, the better the confocal resolution of the image taken (i.e., the thinner the optical section). However, with reduced diameter, there is also a reduction in the amount of photons (i.e., brightness). An optimal setting is usually offered automatically by the confocal software and is usually the best option.

3.2.3. Practical Applications

3.2.3.1. Single Labeling (With and Without Nuclear Visualization)

Detection of a single protein or molecular structure in cells or cartilage sections by a fluorochrome-conjugated seondary antibody can be visualized by CLSM. **Subheading 3.1.4.** describes the immunofluorescence protocol in more detail. A typical example of confocal microscopy analysis is shown in **Fig. 4D** and **E**: the intracellular mediator of bone morphogenetic protein signaling, the receptor-associated Smad 5, is localized in the cytoplasm as well as in the nucleus *(7)*.

3.2.3.2. Colocalization of Two or More Antigens

When performing multilabeling experiments, it is important to choose fluorochromes with excitation and emission spectra that don't overlap, as discussed earlier in **Subheading 3.1.2.** For the experimental procedure of colocalization

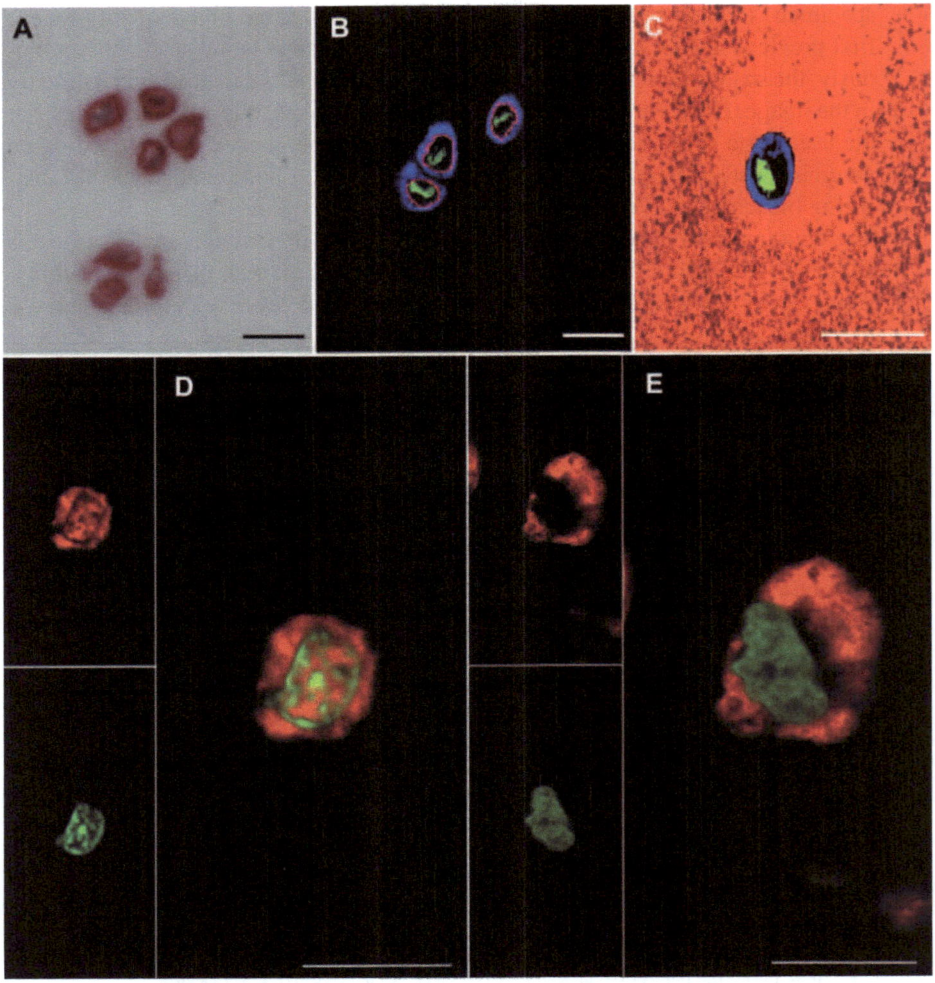

Fig. 4. (**A**) Pericellular staining of type VI collagen in normal articular cartilage by conventional immunohistochemistry. (**B** and **C**) Type VI collagen also detected by LSCM in a double-labeling experiment (blue, collagen type VI; green, nuclear DNA; red, β_1-integrin on the cell membrane). (**C**) also shows type II collagen in the interterritorial cartilage matrix) (**D** and **E**) Laser scanning microscopy of immunolocalized Smad 5 in normal (D) and osteoarthritic (E) cartilage (red, Smad 5; green, nuclear DNA). These results show that most of the Smad 5 is found in the cytoplasm. Notably, the positive nuclear signal is located mostly on the euchromatin and not the heterochromatin. Scale bars, 50 µm in (A–C); 10 µm in (D) and (E). (Courtesy of Leica.)

immunofluorescence, *see* **Subheading 3.1.5. Figure 4B** and **C** show colocalization analysis by confocal microscopy of type VI collagen (pericellular region) with β 1-integrin (membrane-associated) and type II collagen (interterritorial region) ***(4,8)***.

3.2.3.3. z-Scan: 3D Reconstruction

Specimens can be analyzed by acquiring a series of sections along the optical (*z*) axis of the microscope by using the *z*-scan mode ***(9)***. During this process, the microscope is driven by a computer-controlled motor, which analyzes the specimen at different *z* positions to acquire a 3D image. Therefore, after the specimen is processed by 2D imaging techniques, it can then be reconstructed into a 3D volumetric image.

3.3. Concluding Remarks

Immunofluorescence and CLSM provide the unique possibility to colocalize different gene products and cell compartments within cartilage samples and cultured chondrocytes. However, the resolution is insufficient for establishing colocalization at the molecular level (i.e., molecular interactions). In this respect, fluorescence resonance energy transfer (FRET) technology offers an innovative approach to achieve some molecular resolution. In this technology (for review, *see* **refs. *10*** and ***11***), photons emitted from one donor fluorochrome can efficiently excite a second acceptor fluorochrome, given its close proximity (less than about 100 nm). Thus, a positive signal may indicate that both fluorochrome-labeled molecules interact. To date, the labeling of molecules with fluorochromes (mostly green fluorescent protein variants) has been necessary, which made the method laborious end limited to in vitro studies. However, recent protocols have been described employing antibody labeling of molecules ***(12)*** to enable a more widespread use of FRET technology for molecular analysis.

4. Notes

1. To dissolve 4% PFA in PBS, it is usually necessary to heat the solution (not above 60°C) and to add few drops of alkaline solution (e.g., 2 *M* NaOH) to raise the pH. After solubilization, the solution should be readjusted to pH 7.4 with HCl.
2. False-positive detection of fluorochromes owing to overlapping emission spectra represents a significant problem that can often be misinterpreted, especially if both fluorochromes are visualized in a multichannel scanning mode. Thus, scanning should be carried out sequentially using laser channels specific to one type of fluorochrome.
3. Inclusion of appropriate control experiments is essential in all immunostaining procedures, as nonspecific binding of the primary antibodies do frequently occur. (Obviously, it is important to show, by Western blotting, that the antibody can recognize the epitope.) Basically, one can distinguish between three types of control experiments:

a. *Control of the detection system*: here, the primary antibody is replaced by buffer or an isotype-specific pre-immune serum. The process of immunolocalization is carried out as normal. No detection of the epitope of interest should occur. Overall, these controls are negative in any well-established detection system and are thus of little help to ensure the antigen-specific staining pattern of an antibody
b. *Antibody-specific controls*: (1) Pre-immune serum can be used at the same dilution concentration as the primary antibody; (2) also, the primary antibody can be preincubated with a 10-fold molar excess of specific antigen. The latter will block all antibody binding sites such that the epitopes within cells or cartilage sections cannot be recognized. Both control methods should not reveal significant positive staining of the epitope. Low levels of nonspecific binding is tolerable, but expert advice should be taken to ensure that this staining is not real. Overall, the use of pre-immune serum is certainly (if available, which can per definition only be the case for polyclonal antibodies) of great help to detect unspecific pre-existing immunoreactivity against structures within the sections to be investigated. In contrast, the competition assay only confirms that the antibody recognizes its antigen (what it should do anyway, at least if it is affinity-purified).
c. *Immunostaining of cells or tissues known to be positive or negative for the antigen of interest*: the most reliable controls are internal controls. For example, cells know either to react or not to react with the primary antibody are present in the tissue specimen being analyzed. However, if this type of control is not possible (as is often the case when using antibodies against antigens of unknown tissue distribution), then the first two controls mentioned above should be used. Also, one should confirm the obtained data with a different method (e.g., *in situ* hybridization for mRNA expression or Western blotting), which is in all instances a good idea anyway (if feasible).

4. Autofluorescence is a major issue in fluorescence and confocal microscopy. The shorter the wavelength of the light used for excitation, then the higher the autofluorescence; this is not a problem at wavelengths of 600 nm and above. Because cartilage as a collagen-rich tissue shows a very high autofluorescence, dyes with a long excitation wavelength such as Cy5 are very much preferable; classical dyes such as FITC might easily lead to very misleading results.
5. Embedding procedures: the two most common ways of "embedding" cartilage for further analysis are either to fix it and embed it into some sort of paraffin or to freeze it down (within or without freezing media) and to cut frozen sections. The latter can be used straightforwardly after usually a mild fixation (e.g., 5–10 min in 4% PFA or any other suitable fixative). The two advantages of frozen material are that the technology is easier to handle (freezing down in liquid nitrogen and cutting on a cryotome) and that the antibodies potentially work better or only at all in (rather unfixed) frozen material. The clear advantages of paraffin embedding are the better preserved morphology and the ease of obtaining several hundred sections from one block for all kinds of analyses and to store and reuse them for a long period (i.e., several years).

6. Semithick cartilage sections, cut by a Series 1000 vibratome (Ted Pella), preserves cartilage morphology and can also be used in immunostaining procedures. These sections are treated by floating in buffer in small processing tubes (we use Eppendorf caps). Here, the experimental protocol is similar to that for conventional immunostaining of cartilage sections coated on slides. However, predigestion of the thicker sections should be more extensive, and 0.01% saponin (or any other detergent) should be added to antibody and wash solutions to facilitate penetration of the antibodies into the cartilage specimen. In addition, all incubation and washing steps should be performed on a shaking device. These vibratome-cut samples can be easily scanned using CLSM in a 3D manner (*z*-scans).
7. To retain cartilage sections on the glass slides during the immunohistochemical procedure, one should either use specifically processed slides (e.g., SuperFrost Plus slides; Dakopatts) or carry out pretreatment of conventional glass slides using, e.g., triethoxysilylpropylamin (for example, incubate slides for 30 s in acetone, 60 s in 10% triethoxysilylpropylamin in acetone, and then several times in H_2O).
8. Optimized conditions for each antibody should be established in immunostaining procedures.
   a. A suitable antibody dilution to use in an experiment is established by applying a range of antibody concentrations in parallel to the cells or cartilage tissue specimens. An approximate final concentration of 1–2 ng/µL is a good starting point. Final testing of antibody concentration should be done after optimizing the pretreatment conditions.
   b. Basically, two major kinds of pretreatments are in common use for paraffin-embedded material: either incubation of the cartilage section with enzymes or exposure of the specimen to high temperatures. Frozen cartilage sections do often not require pretreatment.
      i. *Hyaluronidase* (e.g., 2 mg/mL in PBS, pH 5) is a common choice of pretreatment enzyme. The specimen should be digested at 37°C for 60 min to eliminate hyaluronic acid and thus improve antigen avail ability in the cartilage. Other common enzymes include *protease XXIV* (0.02–0.2 mg/mL in PBS, pH 7.3, 37°C, 60 min), *pronase* (e.g., 2 mg/mL in PBS pH 7.3), and *trypsin* (0.1–1 mg in PBS, pH 7.3) These enzymes can be stored in 10X buffer for months at –20°C. Any of these enzymes can be tested to find a suitable one that results in strong, specific, positive staining of the epitope.
      ii. *Pretreatment by exposure to heat* can be performed using a micro wave, a pressure cooker, a steamer, or more expensive devices avail able specifically for this purpose. We have found success by apply ing our samples to a steamer at 90°C for 30 min. The major problem with these techniques is that cartilage sections may dislodge from the slides: cartilage tissue is known to swell under such extreme heat conditions.
9. Blocking of nonspecific protein binding sites is usually not required in fixed, paraffin-embedded cartilage specimens if the antibody buffer contains some

albumin as a carrier protein. However, a separate blocking step may be important for frozen sections owing to their shorter fixation incubations. Different blocking solutions (e.g., serum from an unrelated species, albumin, or other commercially available blocking solutions) should be tested to select a suitable, inexpensive blocking agent for the experiment.

10. In general, approx 20–50 μL of diluted antibody is sufficient for covering each section (depending of the size of the section). The smallest volume possible should be used to save on amounts of antibody used per experiment. Encircling the cartilage section with a Pap-pen (Science Services, Munich, FRG) will retain the antibody solution in the area covering the section, so one can use small volumes successfully.
11. Nowadays, for all species detection, antibodies labeled with the correct fluorochromes are available (crossabsorbed to other species): however, if one has, e.g., only fluorochrome-labeled detection antibodies against rabbit antibodies and one intends to use a mouse primary antibody, it is basically no problem to use a rabbit-antimouse secondary antibody, which can than be detected by the fluorochrome-labeled antirabbit antibodies. Most convenient in this respect is the biotin-streptavidin system, which works independently of the species used (the "links" have obviously to be against the right species, but multispecies link cocktails are commercially available ["multilinks"]).
12. "Direct" immunofluorescence utilizes a fluorochrome-labeled primary antibody to detect the localization of an epitope. Direct immunodetection is in practice restricted to very few special applications, such as multidetection fluorescence-activated cell sorting analysis. The direct method is not commonly used in immunofluorescence owing to low detection levels as a result of fewer signal amplification steps and the difficulty of labeling each primary antibody separately.
13. If the fluorescence signal is too weak to be detected, then it can be enhanced with a tyramide amplification. Here, a peroxidase-conjugated label (e.g., BioGenex; 1:200) is added to the sample for 20 min instead of a fluorescence label. The section is then washed with TNT buffer (2 × 5 min). Biotin-tyramide reagent (1:200; Molecular Probes) is added in the appropriate buffer for 20 min at 37°C. After washing with TBS (2 × 10 min) the fluorescent label can then be added (e.g., streptavidin-Cy3 or Cy5).

Acknowledgments

This work was supported by the BMBF (01GG9824). We are grateful to Dr. Audrey McAlinden for professional editing of the manuscript.

References

1. Verschure, P. J., Van Marle, J., Joosten, L. A. B., and van den Berg, W. B. (1994) Localization and quantification of the insulin-like growth factor-1 receptor in mouse articular cartilage by confocal laser scanning microscopy. *J. Histochem. Cytochem.* **42,** 765–773.

2. Verschure, P. J., Van Marle, J., Van Noorden, C. J. F., and van den Berg, W. B. (1997) The contribution of quantitative confocal laser scanning microscopy in cartilage research—chondrocyte insulin-like growth factor-1 receptors in health and pathology. *Microsc. Res. Tech.* **37,** 285–298.
3. Allan, E. (2000) *Protein Localization by Fluorescence Microscopy: A Practical Approach.* Oxford University Press, Oxford.
4. Hambach, L., Neureiter, D., Zeiler, G., Kirchner, T., and Aigner, T. (1998) Severe disturbance of the distribution and expression of type VI collagen chains in osteoarthritic articular cartilage. *Arthritis Rheum.* **41,** 986–997.
5. Negeoscu, A., Labat-Moleur, F., Lorimier, P., et al. (1994) F(ab) secondary antibodies: a general method for double immunolabeling with primary antisera from the same species. Efficiency control by chemiluminescence. *J. Histochem. Cytochem.* **42,** 433–437.
6. Sheppard, D.M., Hotton, D., and Shotton, D. (1997) *Confocal Laser Scanning Microscopy.* Springer Verlag, Berlin.
7. Bau, B., Haag, J., Schmid, E., Kaiser, M., Gebhard, P.M., and Aigner, T. (2002) Bone morphogenetic protein-mediating receptor-associated Smads as well as common Smad are expressed in human articular chondrocytes, but not upregulated or downregulated in osteoarthritic cartilage. *J. Bone Miner. Res.* **17,** 2141–2150.
8. Söder, S., Hambach, L., Lissner, R., Kirchner, T., and Aigner, T. (2002) Ultrastructural localization of type VI collagen in normal adult and osteoarthritic human articular cartilage. *Osteoarthritis Cartilage* **10,** 464–470.
9. Aigner, T., Hemmel, M., Neureiter, D., et al. (2001) Apoptotic cell death is not a widespread phenomenon in normal aging and osteoarthritic human articular knee cartilage: A study of proliferation, programmed cell death (apoptosis), and viability of chondrocytes in normal and osteoarthritic human knee cartilage. *Arthritis Rheum.* **44,** 1304–1312.
10. Gordon, G. W., Berry, G., Liang, X. H., Levine, B., and Herman, B. (1998) Quantitative fluorescence resonance energy transfer measurements using fluorescence microscopy. *Biophys. J.* **74,** 2702–2713.
11. Siegel, R. M., Chan, F. K. M., Zacharias, D. A., et al. (2000) Measurement of molecular interactions in living cells by fluorescence resonance energy transfer between variants of the green fluorescent protein. *Sci. STKE* **38,** 1–6.
12. Sharma, N., Hewett, J., Ozelius, L. J., et al. (2001) A close association of torsina and alpha-synuclein in lewy bodies: A fluorescence resonance energy transfer study. *Am. J. Pathol.* **159,** 339–344.

8

Molecular and Biochemical Assays of Cartilage Components

Caroline D. Hoemann

Summary

The procedure described below is useful for extracting proteins, nucleic acids, and glycosaminoglycans from 5–40 mg of cartilage or tissue-engineered cartilage samples. This extraction method will generate samples compatible with Western blot, RNase protection, dimethyl methylene blue (DMB) assay for glycosaminoglycan, Hoechst DNA assay, and hydroxyproline assay. Most soluble matrix molecules can be extracted from pulverized samples using 4 *M* guanidine HCl, during a 30-min period of vortex agitation at 4°C. Shorter agitation times can give inadequate solubilization. The guanidine HCl-insoluble pellet must be re-extracted with guanidine thiocyanate buffer, to solubilize RNA additionally. The final insoluble pellet can be rinsed with ethanol and digested with papain, to quantify collagen content as well as other insoluble or crosslinked material. Samples between 1 and 5 mg may be directly digested with a small volume of papain buffer for DMB, hydroxyproline, and Hoechst DNA assays.

Key Words: Papain; hydrogel; L-*trans*-hydroxyproline; collagen; glycosaminoglycan; deoxyribonucleic acid; chondroitin sulfate C; standard curve; plate reader; fluorimeter; Hoechst 33258; pulverize; guanidine hydrochloride; guanidine thiocyanate; cartilage. Extraction.

1. Introduction

1.1. Commonly Used Biochemical Assays for Cartilage Components

Adult articular cartilage is a hypocellular tissue, with a stiff, viscoelastic extracellular matrix principally composed of water, collagens (type II, as well as types III, VI, IX, X, XI, XII, and XIV), glycosaminoglycan (GAG)-bearing proteoglycans (aggrecan, biglycan, decorin, and fibromodulin), hyaluronic acid, and noncollagenous proteins (COMP, link). Quantitation of cartilage components will depend on their solubilization, which can be achieved by exhaustive proteolytic digestion. Papain will fully solubilize glycosaminoglycans, by cleaving the core protein *(1)*, and chondrocyte DNA, by degrading nuclear binding proteins *(2)*. Digestion at elevated (60°C) temperatures melts

From: *Methods in Molecular Medicine, Vol. 101: Cartilage and Osteoarthritis, Volume 2: Structure and In Vivo Analysis*
Edited by: F. De Ceuninck, M. Sabatini, and P. Pastoureau © Humana Press Inc., Totowa, NJ

the collagen helix, thereby facilitating collagen proteolysis. Colorimetric assays have been developed to measure GAG content by dimethyl methylene blue (DMB) assay *(1,3,4)* and collagen content by hydroxyproline assay from acid-hydrolyzed samples *(5–7)*. Cartilage cell density can be extrapolated from DNA content measured by the fluorimetric Hoechst 33258 assay *(2)*. Papain-digested cartilage lysates can thus be used for quantitative parallel analysis of DNA, GAG, and hydroxyproline content, while precluding analysis of cellular and extracellular proteins and RNA (**Table 1**).

Chondrocyte RNA expression in articular cartilage is rarely quantified in the same samples used for biochemical analysis of other components, owing partly to the low RNA yield obtained from this hypocellular tissue and partly to copurification of GAG, which interferes with RNA yield and purity *(8)*. Adjusting the RNA purification method *(8)* can minimize such proteoglycan interference. For small samples, mRNA expression can be studied using lysate RNase protection with radioactive probes *(9–11)* or quantitative or semiquantitative reverse transcriptase polymerase chain reaction (RT-PCR) *(12–14)*. Cartilage cellular protein expression can be analyzed by Western blot, from as little as a few milligrams of cartilage pulverized and extracted with detergent-based extraction buffers *(15)*. Alternatively, Western analysis can be performed from guanidine extracts of cartilage, provided that the guanidine salts that form precipitates with sodium dodecyl sulfate (SDS)-containing protein electrophoresis buffers are removed *(11,15)*. Most cartilage components, apart from type II collagen, may be solubilized from minced or pulverized cartilage with guanidine HCl (GuCl) and guanidine thiocyanate (GITC) *(11,16,17)*. Solubilized GAG, DNA, and RNA can be assayed directly from guanidine extracts *(4,11)*. The guanidine-insoluble pellet can be digested with papain for residual DNA and GAG quantification and further hydrolyzed for hydroxyproline determination (**Table 1**) *(11)*.

1.2. Biochemical Composition of Articular Cartilage

Some laboratories report GAG, collagen, and DNA content normalized to dry weight *(18–26)* and some to wet weight *(2,11,27–35)*. Cartilage water content is known to diminish with age and to increase in arthritic cartilage *(20,36–38)*. Although it is a highly relevant and even diagnostic parameter for cartilage, water content determination by lyophylization will degrade cellular RNA and labile proteins; therefore samples dedicated to molecular, as well as biochemical, analyses will necessarily be normalized to wet weight. Cartilage composition can be seen to vary for different anatomical locations, species, age, and load/nonload–bearing regions (**Tables 2A** and **2B**). Normal articular cartilage thus shows a range of 65–85% water, 12–24% collagen, 3–6% GAG, and 16,000–90,000 chondrocytes per mg tissue wet weight (**Table 2A**). A typi-

Table 1
Biochemical and Molecular Assays that Can Be Performed With Differently Prepared Cartilage Extracts

	Biochemical assays			Molecular assays	
Assay	DMB colorimetric (GAG)[a]	Hydroxyproline colorimetric (Hydroxyproline [collagen])[a]	Hoechst assay fluorimetric (DNA [cells])[a]	RNase protection (mRNA expression)[a]	Western blot (Protein expression)[a]
Sample lysate					
Direct papain digestion of wet or dry tissue samples	Yes	Yes	Yes	No	No
Multivalent extracts					
GuCl extract of pulverized sample	Yes	No[b]	Yes	Yes	Yes[d]
GITC extract of GuCl-insoluble pellet	No[b]	No[b]	(Yes)[c]	Yes[e]	Yes
Papain digest of GuCl/GITC-insoluble pellet	Yes	Yes[f]	Yes[g]	No	No

[a]Species detected.
[b]Extract incompatible with assay, unless guanidine salt is removed.
[c]Hoechst assay may be performed in the presence of guanidine thiocyanate (GITC); however, little DNA remains in this fraction. Also, GITC partly solubilizes chitosan, the presence of which is incompatible with the Hoechst assay.
[d]Contains most of the soluble cellular and extracellular proteins.
[e]Contains the major fraction of total RNA.
[f]Contains the major fraction of total hydroxyproline.
[g]Up to 10% of cellular DNA is trapped in the pulverized cartilage fragments.

cal articular cartilage sample of 1 mg wet mass is expected to harbor around 50 μg GAG, 150 μg collagen, and 0.2–0.6 μg DNA.

To interpret biochemical data further, some researchers have normalized their data to cell content or collagen content. Researchers have normalized tissue variables to collagen content *(18,35,37,38)*, based on its stability and extremely low turnover rate *(39)*. In contrast, GAG levels may fluctuate *in situ*, for instance increasing with short-term exercise *(26)*, or decreasing following brief cytokine-induced joint damage *(40)* or in "kissing" lesions, in which full-thickness defects are in direct contact on two articulating surfaces *(41)*. Cartilage cellularity will play a key role in the kinetics of reestablishing normal GAG content, the rebound of which has been observed in rabbit joints following depletion caused by interleukin-1β injection *(40)*. The amount of GAG per chondrocyte could serve as an instantaneous indication of GAG homeostasis, integrating its synthesis, deposition, and degradation, in any given cartilage sample. Between 0.4 and 3.5 ng GAG/chondrocyte can be calculated for articular cartilage from various species and anatomical locations, using data from six different studies *(11,24,27,30,32,33)* (**Tables 2A** and **2B**). An age-dependent increase in the quantity of GAG per chondrocyte has been seen *(11,24)*. Since GAG synthetic rates have been found to decline with age, for human articular chondrocytes of the femoral condyle *(42)*, and remain steady for bovine adult carpal chondrocytes *(43)*, an age-dependent increase in GAG per cell may reflect a loss in cell density, rather than greater synthetic output per cell.

1.3. Results Can Depend on Site of Harvest and Analytical Methods

Experimental bias may arise from random sample collection methods. For instance, sample biopsies simply skimmed from the cartilage surface will give relatively higher water content, higher cell density, higher collagen, and lower GAG content than full-thickness biopsies *(20)* (**Table 2B**). Samples taken from nonload–bearing regions will have higher cell density than load-bearing regions (*2,28*; **Table 2A**). Appreciable proximodistal gradients of GAG content can occur in the same joint surface *(25)*. The most representative biopsy for a biochemical assay must be therefore carefully selected.

Biochemical assay precision can be compromised by subtle differences in analytical methodology, including the choice of standards and the conversion factors. Standards should be of high purity and have uniform composition. In the hydroxyproline assay to estimate collagen content, standard L-hydroxyproline is routinely used. However, in converting hydroxyproline content to collagen type II content, there is little consensus on the appropriate factor. The hydroxyproline conversion factor (CF) for cartilage collagen content (μg

Table 2A
Reported Biochemical Composition of Articular Cartilage, Normalized to Wet Weight

A

Citation (ref)	species	age	joint area	sub-location	condition	% H20	CONTENT GAG	collagen	cell density	ng GAG per chondrocyte
Reported as Wet Weight							μg/mg	% wet wt	thousands/mg wet wt	
Kim 1988 (2)	Bovine	2 wks	FPG	Load-Bearing	normal				33.0	
Kim 1988 (2)	Bovine	2 wks	FPG	Non-Load Bearing	normal				59.0	
Eggli 1988 (28)	Lapine	Adult	MFC	Load-Bearing	normal				28.6 [a]	
Eggli 1988 (28)	Lapine	Adult	MFC	Non-Load Bearing	normal				40.6 [a]	
Hunziker 2002 (34)	Human	23-49 yrs	MFC	Load-Bearing	post mortem				23.7 ± 1.8 [a]	
Sah 1997 (29)	Lapine	Adult	MFC		Control	70 ± 4	28 ± 10 [b]			
Sah 1997 (29)	Lapine	Adult	MFC		ACL transected	75 ± 4	25 ± 9 [b]			
Treppo 2000 (31)	Human	14-45 yrs	Talus		normal	75	38 [b]	1.9% OH-Pro		
Treppo 2000 (31)	Human	14-45 yrs	distal femur	Pat + FPG + MFC	normal	78	27 [b]	1.8% OH-Pro		
Treppo 2000 (31)	Human	14-45 yrs	Tibial Plateau		normal	79	22 [b]	1.7% OH-Pro		
Lee 2000 (30)	Canine	> 2 yrs adult	Tibial Plateau	central medial	Control	81 [c]	55 [b]		16.3 [d]	**3.4**
Lee 2000 (30)	Canine	> 2 yrs adult	FPG	proximal	Control	71 [c]	54 [b]		28.6 [d]	**1.9**
Lee 2000 (30)	Canine	> 2 yrs adult	MFC	anterior	Control	73 [c]	47 [b]		28.0 [d]	**1.7**
Buschmann 1982 (27)	Bovine	2 wks	FPG		normal		57 ± 11 [b]		73 ± 17	**0.78**
Hoemann 2002 (11)	Bovine	2 week	Shoulder	Load-Bearing	normal		58 ± 4 [b]	16% ± 2% [e]	65 ± 4	**0.89**
Hoemann 2002 (11)	Bovine	Adult	Shoulder	Load-Bearing	normal		49 ± 15 [b]	18% ± 2% [e]	30 ± 4	**1.6**
Dumont 1999 (32)	Bovine	1-2 yr M	Shoulder	Load-Bearing	normal		31 [b]		38.3 ± 8.3	**0.81**
Ameer 2002 (33)	Porcine	4-6 months	FPG		normal	85	40 ± 7.6	7.2%	89 [d]	**0.44**
Lewis 1998 (35)	Bovine	adult	metacarpal	centromedial "#10"	normal	65 ± 4	40 [b]	23% [f]		

MFC, medial femoral condyle; FPG, femoral patellar groove, Pat, patella; OH-Pro, hydroxyproline (not converted to collagen content).
[a]By stereometry.
[b]Used chondroitin 6-sulfate C as the DMB standard.
[c]Based on converting published data given as (wet wt – dry wt)/dry wt.
[d]Assuming 7.7 pg DNA/cell *(2)*.
[e,f]Conversion factor from mg OH-Pro to mg collagen given as 8.3[e] or 7.1 [f].

Table 2B
Reported Biochemical Composition of Articular Cartilage, Normalized to Dry Weight

B

Citation (ref)	species	age	joint area	sub-location	condition	------- % H20	CONTENT GAG	------- collagen	cell density	ng GAG per chondrocyte
Reported as Dry Weight							µg/mg dry wt	% dry wt	thousands/mg dry wt	
Mankin 1970 (18)	Human	36-80yr M/F	femoral head		normal [a, m]		53.6 ± 21.5 [d]	6.8% OH-Pro	5.31 ng DNA/mg	
Mankin 1970 (18)	Human	61-88yr M/F	femoral head		OA [a]		43.1 ± 22.6 [d]	6.5% OH-Pro	6.16 ng DNA/mg	
Kempson 1970 (19)	Human	42 yr F	femoral head	averaged 12 sites	post mortem		8.5 ± 1.5 [d]	54% ± 7 [e]		
Venn 1977 (20)	Human	51-77 yrs	femoral head	superficial zone	post mortem	74	12 [d]	84% [f, h]		
Venn 1977 (20)	Human	51-77 yrs	femoral head	middle zone	post mortem	72	20 [d]	57% [f, h]		
Venn 1977 (20)	Human	51-77 yrs	femoral head	deep zone	post mortem	67	22 [d]	70% [f, h]		
Venn 1977 (20)	Human	51-77 yrs	femoral head	superficial zone	OA [a]	76	8 [d]	83% [f, h]		
Venn 1977 (20)	Human	51-77 yrs	femoral head	middle zone	OA [a]	78	16 [d]	55% [f, h]		
Venn 1977 (20)	Human	51-77 yrs	femoral head	deep zone	OA [a]	74	14 [d]	50% [f, h]		
Amiel 1988 (21)	Lapine	Adult M	MFC		normal		38 ± 3 [d]	60%		
Richardson 1990 (22)	Equine	Adult	radial carpal	distomedial	away from lesion		48 [d]		143 [k]	
Richardson 1990 (22)	Equine	Adult	radial carpal	distolateral	opposite lesion		13 [d]		155 [k]	
Vachon 1991 (23)	Equine	Adult	radial carpal	distal	control		73.2 ± 7.9 [d]	56% [g]		
Vachon 1991 (23)	Equine	Adult	radial carpal	distal	periosteal repair		11.3 ± 1.2 [d]	60% ± 4% [g]		
Vachon 1991 (23)	Equine	Adult	radial carpal	distal	nongraft repair		12.9 ± 5.1 [d]	82% ± 18% [g]		
Brama 1998 (24)	Equine	Neonatal	metacarpal	middle, load-bearing	normal	78	156 ± 33 [c]	45% [l]	167 [k]	0.93
Brama 1998 (24)	Equine	5 months	metacarpal	middle, load-bearing	normal	70	190 ± 19 [c]	52% [l]	111 [k]	1.71
Brama 1998 (24)	Equine	1 year	metacarpal	middle, load-bearing	normal	67	141 ± 16 [c]	58% [l]	72 [k]	1.95
Murray 2001 (26)	Equine	Adult	radial carpal	dorsal	high exercise	68 ± 5	280 [b]	54% [g]	31.2 [k]	8.9
Murray 2001 (26)	Equine	Adult	radial carpal	palmar	high exercise	67 ± 7	310 [b]	52% [g]	28.6 [k]	10.8
Murray 2001 (26)	Equine	Adult	radial carpal	dorsal	low exercise	68 ± 3	220 [b]	62% [g]	29.9 [k]	7.3
Murray 2001 (26)	Equine	Adult	radial carpal	palmar	low exercise	69 ± 4	330 [b]	57% [g]	29.9 [k]	11.0
Burkhardt 2001 (25)	Ovine	2-3 yrs	MFC	anterior	normal		118 ± 3 [b]			
Burkhardt 2001 (25)	Ovine	2-3 yrs	MFC	posterior	normal		244 ± 2 [b]			

MFC, medial femoral condyle; OH-Pro, hydroxyproline (not converted to collagen content).
[a]Obtained from hip surgery.
[b]Used chondroitin 4-sulfate A as the DMMB standard.
[c]Used chondroitin 6-sulfate C as the DMMB standard.
[d–g]Calculated from glucosamine and galactosamine (hexosamine) content. Conversion factor from mg OH-Pro to mg collagen given as 6.94[e], 7.6[f], or 7.83[g].
[h]Converted to dry weight according to given average percent hydration.
[k]Assuming 7.7 pg DNA/cell *(2)*.
[l]Assumed 100 hydroxyproline residues per triple-helical collagen type II chain (no conversion factor given).
[m]Patients suffered a femoral neck fracture.

collagen = CF × μg hydroxyproline) is highly variable according to different laboratories: CF = 6.94 ***(19)***, 7.1 ***(35)***, 7.6 ***(20)***, 8.3 ***(11)***, or 10 ***(44,45)***. Experimentally, CF = 6.6 for bovine tendon collagen type I ***(7)***. The maximal theoretical number of proline targets for prolyl-hydroxylase in human collagen type II (Gly-Pro sequence in helical domain, SwissProt accession no. P02458) is 114 residues out of a cleaved 1060 residue collagen type II chain, which, when adjusted for mass by primary sequence, yields 13.2% hydroxyproline (w/w), or CF = 7.6 (13.2 mg OH-Pro/100 mg collagen type II), as employed by Venn and Maroudas ***(20)***. Incomplete hydroxylation will lead to values greater than 7.6. Omission of ascorbate from culture media will result in the absence of hydroxyproline for chondrocytes cultured in hydrogels. In the DMB assay to quantify GAG, standard chondroitin sulfate is used; however, some laboratories employ bovine trachea chondroitin 4-sulfate A ***(25,26)*** and others shark chondroitin 6-sulfate C ***(11,24,27,29–32)*** (**Tables 2A** and **2B**). Although these two standards, when mixed with GuCl, give similar curves in the DMB assay ***(4)***, their extinction coefficients deviate under normal assay conditions ***(46)***. Of note, average GAG levels extrapolated from hexosamine content are appreciably lower than those estimated using the DMB assay (**Table 2B**). All of this said, one must observe with caution the apparent health of the joint, medical condition, age of the animal, and precise zone from which the sample is analyzed, as well as analytical standards and conversion factors, in order to maximize the validity of the conclusions drawn from resulting biochemical data.

1.4. Biochemical Composition of Tissue-Engineered Cartilage

A substantial effort has gone into evaluating the biochemical content arising from scaffolding materials seeded with chondrocytes and grown in cultures or bioreactors or as implants in nude mice. Adult bovine cartilage harbors around 30,000 cells/mg and newborn cartilage, 60,000 cells/mg, yet many experimental hydrogel constructs are seeded with cell concentrations ranging from 2500 to 125,000 cells/mg ***(11,27,33,47–61)*** (**Table 3**). This disparity in cell density is partly owing to scaffold seeding limitations, as when cells must migrate into a solid scaffold, or when a hydrogel must solidify in the presence of 20 million cells/mL, which occupy up to 10% of the total volume when collected in a loose cell pellet prior to casting (our own observations; ***49***). Nevertheless, the GAG content of in vitro cultured constructs appears to depend heavily on initial cell density. After 6 wk in static culture, 2% agarose cultures seeded with 10,000 primary calf chondrocytes cells per mL harbored 16 μg GAG/mg and 18,300 cells/mg ***(27)***. In comparison, a 6-wk static culture of 4% polyglycolic (PGA) scaffolds seeded with 62,500 primary calf chondrocytes cells per mL harbored 25 μg GAG/mg and 49,500 cells/mg ***(48)***. However, when the 6-wk agarose and PGA cultures are analyzed for GAG content per chondrocyte, the

Table 3A
Biochemical Content Expressed in ng GAG/Chondrocyte for Tissue-Engineered Cartilage Cultured In Vitro[a]

A

Citation	source cartilage	P(n)	seed density	scaffolding material	Source Cartilage	ng GAG/chondrocyte week 1 day 3	week 1 day 7	week 2 day 14	week 3 day 21	week 4 day 28	week 5 day 36	week 6 day 42	week 7 day 49	week 10 day 70
In vitro cultures			million cells/ml											
Buschmann 1992 (27) [a]	newborn calf FPG	P0	10	2% AGAROSE	0.78		0.51	0.85	0.92	0.92	0.85	0.82	0.79	1.09
Hoemann 2002 (11) [a]	newborn calf FPG	P0	10	2% AGAROSE	0.89			0.95	1.03					
Hoemann *submitted* (49) [a]	newborn calf FPG	P0	10	1.3% Chitosan				0.43	0.5					
Vunjak-Novakovic 1999 (48) [a]	newborn calf FPG	P0	62.5	4% PGA-STATIC		0.12						0.55		
	newborn calf FPG	P0	62.5	4% PGA-MIXED		0.12						0.22		
	newborn calf FPG	P0	62.5	4% PGA-ROTATING		0.12						0.72		
Obradovic 1999 (50) [a]	newborn calf FPG	P0	~50	PGA-Control O2 [c]		0.03					0.43			
	newborn calf FPG	P0	~50	PGA-Infrequent O2 [c]		0.03					0.51			
	newborn calf FPG	P0	~50	PGA- low O2 [c]		0.03					0.31			
	newborn calf FPG	P0	~50	PGA-Infrequent feed [c]		0.03					0.55			
Wu 1999 (51) [a]	4 mo ovine FPG	P0	~ 30	PGA in bioreactor	~0.70				0.5					
Ameer 2002 (33) [a]	4-6 month pig knees	P0	125	PGA	0.44		0.1			0.15				
	4-6 month pig knees	P0	125	PGA+50 mg/ml fibrin			0.2			0.39				
Grande 1997 (52) [a]	bovine ankle joint	P1-P2	2.5	PGA static							0.27 [d]			
	bovine ankle joint	P1-P2	2.5	PGA closed culture							0.47 [d]			
	bovine ankle joint	P1-P2	2.5	collagen (I) static							0.29 [d]			
	bovine ankle joint	P1-P2	2.5	collagen (I) closed culture							0.46 [d]			
Yu 1997 (53) [b]	calf carpal deep zone	P0	1.6 [e]	collagen-coated Millicell				0.09		0.08		0.08		0.09
Sun 2001 (54) [b]	sheep 9mo tail-NP	P0	3.3 [e]	collagen-coated Millicell				0.04		0.07		0.49		1.65
Nehrer 1997 (55) [b]	2-3 yr canine,Tib,Pat	P1	20	collagen(1)+GAG sponge			0.04 [f]	0.07 [f]						
	2-3 yr canine,Tib,Pat	P1	20	collagen (II) sponge			0.07 [f]	0.07 [f]						
Toolan 1996 (56) [b]	4 mo rabbit hip,SH	P1	4.25	1% collagen(1) sponge								0.005 [g]		
Bryant 2001 (57)	newborn calf FPG	P0	75	PEG-photocrosslinked				0.2		0.4				
Kisiday 2002 (58)	newborn calf FPG	P0	15	2% AGAROSE			0.15 [h]							
	newborn calf FPG	P0	15	self-assembling peptide			0.12 [h]							
Wong 2001 (59)	1-2 yr cow humerus	P0	4	2% Pronova ALGINATE			0.53 [i]		0.55 [i]		0.53 [i]		0.72 [i]	

[a]Abbreviations and footnotes: *see* **Table 3B**.

Table 3B
Biochemical Content Expressed in ng GAG/Chondrocyte for Tissue-Engineered Cartilage Developed as Nude Mouse Implants

B

						ng GAG/chondrocyte								
			seed		Source	week 1	week 1	week 2	week 3	week 4	week 5	week 6	week 7	week 12
Citation	source cartilage	P(n)	density	scaffolding material	Cartilage	day 3	day 7	day 14	day 21	day 28	day 36	day 42	day 49	day 84
Nude mouse implants														
Passaretti 2001 (60) [b]	3-6 mo swine	P0	40	PBS	0.22							0.07		
	3-6 mo swine	P0	40	80 mg/ml porcine fibrin								0.07		
	3-6 mo swine	P1 [k]	40	80 mg/ml porcine fibrin								0.02		
	3-6 mo swine	P2 [k]	40	80 mg/ml porcine fibrin								0.002		
Elisseeff 1999 (61) [b]	newborn calf FPG	P0	50	10% PEO-dimethacrylate				1.23		0.50			1.40	
	newborn calf FPG	P0	50	20% PEO-dimethacrylate				1.22		0.94			1.17	
	newborn calf FPG	P0	50	30% PEO-dimethacrylate				0.35		0.62			1.20	
	newborn calf FPG	P0	50	40% PEO-dimethacrylate				0.52		0.75			0.65	
Sims 1998 (44) [b]	calf shoulder	P0	12.5	40-60 mg/ml human fibrin	0.05 [m]							0.004 [m]		0.05 [m]

P(n), passage number; P0, primary chondrocytes; P1, first passage; P2, second passage; FPG, femoral patellar groove; NP, nucleus pulposus; Tib, tibia; Pat, patella; SH, shoulder; PEG, polyethylene glycol; PEO, polyethylene oxide.

[a]Conversion factor given as 7.7 pg DNA per cell *(2)*.

[b]Assuming 7.7 pg DNA/cell.

[c]Oxygen tension was 84 mm for control, 86 mm for infrequent O_2, 42 mm for low O_2, and 84 mm for infrequent feeding.

[d]Assuming cell density doubles from 2.5 million/mL d 0, to 5 million/mL d 35, assuming PGA constructs had 90% hydration ***(48)***.

[e]2D culture: million cells/cm^2.

[f]Based on background-subtracted levels for GAG and DNA/collagen sponge.

[g]Based on reported values of 0.05 μg GAG/μL, and 10 million cells/cm^2 construct at 6 wk for collagen sponges seeded and grown in serum-free media + growth factors.

[h]Assuming no change in 2% agarose or 0.5% self-assembling peptide hydrogel thickness (3-mm diameter, 1.6-mm-thick = 11.3 mg/construct), GAG values extrapolated from **Fig. 3** at d 7 *(58)*.

[k]P1 = 4 cell doublings; P2 = 8 cell doublings.

[l]Assuming cell construct volume invariant (5.5-mm diameter, 2-mm-thick = 47.5 mg/construct), that cell density was at 4 million/mL at d 7, and at 8 million/mL at wk 3, wk 5, and wk 7.

[m]Based on published values of 4.38, 1.91, or 3.75% GAG, and 6.84, 40.62, or 5.41 mg DNA/mL (cartilage), for bovine cartilage, 6-wk implants, or 12-wk implants, respectively, assuming construct density = 1.

agarose cultures contain 0.82 ng GAG/cell, and PGA static cultures show 0.55 ng GAG/chondrocyte (**Table 3A**).

For each tissue engineering system, the ng GAG/cell variable is affected by apparent scaffold-, nutrient-, and cell-dependent properties (**Table 3**). For instance, 2% agarose cultures with newborn primary calf chondrocytes show the highest and steadiest GAG/cell content, close to that of adult cartilage, during a 2–10-wk culture (***11,27***; **Tables 2** and **3**). Lower GAG/cell values, closer to that of newborn cartilage, are seen when the scaffold is biodegradable such as PGA ***(48,50)*** or polyglycolic acid (PGA)-fibrin ***(33)***, or erodable, such as chitosan ***(11)***. Lower values are obtained when cells are grown on top of scaffolds ***(53)***, perhaps owing to initially unrestrained diffusion of GAG into the media. Lower values are obtained when the scaffold is unable to maintain cells uniformly in a rounded shape, as with collagen sponges ***(55)***, perhaps owing to lower GAG secretion by flattened, dedifferentiated cells. The GAG per chondrocyte level is severely depressed by extensive in vitro cell passage ***(56,60)***. In contrast, the GAG/cell value can be boosted by increasing media exchange during perfusion culture, compared with static culture ***(48,52)***. If biochemical assays and gene expression profiles were routinely performed on tissue-engineered cartilage, additional structure-function relationships could be culled.

To summarize, biochemical assays of cartilage or tissue-engineered cartilage can yield important information. Data resulting from accurate measurements can lead to a broader understanding of the relationships among absolute matrix components, chondrocyte phenotype, and the development, maintenance, or loss of cartilage mechanical function.

2. Materials

1. Room temperature reagents: guanidine hydrochloride, GITC, Tris-HCl, disodium EDTA dihydrate, urea (molecular biology grade), NaCl, sodium phosphate monobasic (NaH_2PO_4), sodium phosphate dibasic (Na_2HPO_4), NaOH, L-cysteine hydrochloride (Sigma, St. Louis, MO cat. no. C1276), phenol red, NaCl, glycine, L-*trans*-hydroxyproline, citric acid monohydrate, *p*-dimethyl-aminobenzaldehyde (Ehrlich's reagent), dimethyl methylene blue (Polysciences, Warrington PA); AG-1X8 anion-exchange resin (Bio-Rad, Mississauga, ON, Canada).
2. Solvents: ethanol, HCl_{conc} (37%), ddH_2O, *n*-propanol, 70% perchloric acid.
3. 4°C Reagents: Papain Type III 2x Crystallized (Sigma cat. no. P3125), chloramine T, Hoechst 33258.
4. –20°C Reagents: chondroitin 6-sulfate C from shark cartilage (Sigma cat. no. C4384), calf thymus DNA type I (Sigma cat. no. D1501).
5. Plasticware: 2.0-mL cryovials (Corning), sterile DNase/RNase-free pipet tips for p1000, p200 (Ambion), sterile DNase/RNase-free screw-cap 2.0-mL flat-bot-

tomed Eppendorf tubes with rubber gaskets, 1.5-mL Eppendorf tubes, individual 200-μL PCR tubes (for small-scale papain digestion), syringes, disposable plastic 1.0-mL spectroscopy cuvettes, black 96-well Fluro-Nunc 96-well plates (Canadian Life Technologies, Burlington, ON, Canada), standard 96-well ELISA flat-bottomed plates, 5.0-mL Combitips.

6. Precut p1000 pipet tips: wear gloves, and work on a clean surface (clean glass Pyrex plate) with a clean scalpel blade. Cut off around 3 mm from the tip of a blue, p1000 pipet tip. Put into a specially marked pipet tip rack for use in transferring pulverized sample slurry.
7. Other: bottle cap 0.22-μm filters, wide-mouth pyrex media bottles, 0.22-μm syringe-filters, Whatman paper #4 grade, Kimwipes, latex gloves, –80°C freezer boxes, liquid nitrogen or dry ice. Target DP 2-mL vials (C4000-1W, National Scientific Company), and DP green caps with TST silicone septa (C4000-53G, National Scientific Company) for protein hydrolysis.
8. Micromettler balance, pH meter, water purification unit, room temperature vortex mixer (Vortex Genie, Fischer), 4°C vortex mixer with 40-hole Eppendorf tube styrofoam adaptor, room temperature microfuge, 4°C microfuge, water bath, speed vac (to lyophilize chondroitin sulfate standard).
9. Calibrated pipetmen p1000, p200, p20, repeat pipetor with Combitips, 8-channel pipetor and boats
10. Spectrophotometers: standard VIS-UV spectrophotometer (550 nm for hydroxyproline, 260/280 nm for DNA quantification), enzyme-linked immunosorbent assay (ELISA) plate reader (530- and 590-nm filters for DMB), fluorimeter plate reader (Hoechst excitation 360 nm, emission 460 nm, cutoff 420 nm).
11. Biopulverizor (10–100 mg chamber, Biospec Products, OK cat. no. 59012N), small thermos, hammer, ear protectors (Fischer Scientific), safety glasses (Fischer Scientific).
12. –80°C Freezer for long-term sample storage, temperature-controlled 60°C Pasteur oven for papain digestion.

2.1. Solutions for Sample Extraction

1. 50 mL 6 *N* HCl: 25 mL ddH_2O + 25 mL HCl_{conc} (37% HCl_{conc} = 12.5 *N*).
2. 50 mL 10 *N* NaOH: 20 g NaOH pellets in 50 mL ddH_2O (for pH adjustment).
3. 100 mL 1 *M* Tris-HCl, pH 7.5: add 12.1 g Tris-HCl to 70 mL ddH_2O, pH to 7.5, with 6 *N* HCl prior to completing to 100 mL. Autoclave sterilize.
4. 100 mL 500 m*M* $Na_2EDTA{\cdot}2H_2O$: add 18.6 g $Na_2EDTA{\cdot}2H_2O$ to 70 mL ddH_2O, pH to 8.0, with 10 *N* NaOH prior to completing to 100 mL. Autoclave sterilize.
5. 100 mL GuCl extraction buffer (4 *M* GuCl/50 m*M* Tris-HCl/1 m*M* EDTA): to 38.2 g guanidine HCl, add ddH_2O to 80 mL. Add 5 mL 1 *M* Tris-HCl, pH 7.5. Add 200 μL 500 m*M* EDTA. Stir until completely dissolved. Bring volume to 100 mL with ddH_2O. Filter through Whatman #4 paper. Store at 4°C.
6. 100 mL GITC extraction buffer: 4 *M* GITC, 50 m*M* Tris-HCl, 1 m*M* EDTA. To 47.3 g GITC, add ddH_2O to 80 mL. Add 5 mL 1 *M* Tris-HCl, pH 7.5. Add 200 μL 500 m*M* EDTA. Stir until completely dissolved. Bring volume to 100 mL with ddH_2O. Filter through Whatman #4 paper. Store at 4°C.

7. 1 L PBE buffer (100 m*M* sodium phosphate buffer/10 m*M* Na_2EDTA): Dissolve 6.53 g Na_2HPO_4, 6.48 g NaH_2PO_4, and 10 mL 500 m*M* EDTA in 900 mL ddH_2O. Adjust pH to either 6.5 (cartilage, agarose) or pH 7.5 (chitosan hydrogel). Bring volume to 1 L with ddH_2O. Sterilize and remove dust particles by filtering through 0.22-µm bottle cap filter into a sterile media bottle.
8. Papain digestion buffer (100 m*M* sodium phosphate buffer/10 m*M* Na_2EDTA/ 10 m*M* L-cysteine/0.125 mg/mL papain) *Prepare under laminar flow hood. Cysteine and papain enzyme are unstable; use fresh.*
   a. Prepare 40 mL PBE-10 m*M* cysteine: combine 40 mL PBE buffer with 63.0 mg L-cysteine hydrochloride. Filter sterilize with a 0.22-µm syringe filter.
   b. Prepare 20 mL papain digestion buffer: transfer 20 mL sterile PBE-cysteine to a fresh 50-mL conical tube. Add papain enzyme using sterile technique. Swipe rubber stopper of the papain enzyme vial with ethanol, swirl to resuspend, and remove papain solution with sterile 1-mL syringe and hypodermic needle to a sterile Eppendorf tube. Use a pipetman to add 2.5 mg papain enzyme to 20 mL PBE-cysteine (add 100 µL if papain is 25 mg/mL).
9. 75% Ethanol stored at –20°C.

2.2. Solution for Western Blot

1. 8 *M* Urea: 4.84 g urea to 10 mL total volume with ddH_2O.

2.3. Solutions for Hoechst Assay (see *Note 1*)

1. PBE buffer: 100 m*M* phosphate buffer, 10 m*M* EDTA, pH 6.5 or 7.5; *see* **Subheading 2.1.**).
2. 1 L TEN buffer: 10 m*M* Tris-HCl, 1 m*M* EDTA, 100 m*M* NaCl. Combine 1.21 g Tris-HCl, 5.84 g NaCl, and 2 mL 500 m*M* EDTA in 800 mL ddH_2O. Adjust pH to 7.5 before bringing volume to 1 L. Filter.
3. Hoechst 33258 stock: 2 mg Hoechst 33258/mL in ddH_2O = 10,000X stock. Store 4°C under foil up to 1 yr. Working solution: dilute 3 µL stock into 30 mL TEN (prepare fresh).

2.4. DMB Assay

1. 1 L DMB solution; mix 900 mL ddH_2O, 2.37 g NaCl, and 3.04 g glycine. Dissolve 16 mg DMB in 5 mL 100% ethanol in a clean, dry, capped glass scintillation vial wrapped in foil for 2–16 h with a magnetic stir bar. Add dissolved DMB to NaCl-glycine solution, and transfer residual DMB with a 200-µL ethanol rinse. Adjust pH to 3.00 with 1 *N* HCl (~9 mL). Complete to 1 L with ddH_2O. Filter with Whatman #4 paper, and store in foil-wrapped glass bottle at room temperature. The solution is stable for 3–6 mo. Discard if optical density $(OD)_{595}$ declines appreciably 0.9 *(47)*, or if precipitates are visible.

2.5. Solutions for Hydroxyproline Assay

1. 6 *N* HCl, or HCl_{conc}.
2. 50 mL 6 *N* NaOH: 12 g NaOH in 50 mL ddH_2O total volume.

3. 10 mL 0.2% Phenol red: 20 mg phenol red dissolved in 10 mL ddH_2O.
4. 500 mL citrate buffer: combine 300 mL ddH_2O with 25 g citric acid (monohydrate, 210 g/mol), 6 mL acetic acid, 35.75 g anhydrous sodium acetate (82 g/mol), 17 g NaOH (40 g/mol), adjust to pH 6.0 before bringing to 500 mL with ddH_2O. Filter with Whatman paper. Store at 4°C.
5. 17.5% Half-saturated NaCl: 17.5 g NaCl/100 mL ddH_2O. Autoclave sterilize. Store at room temperature.
6. 50 mL Oxidizing agent (for 100 reactions): prepare fresh. Dissolve 0.177 g chloramine T in 15 mL *n*-propanol (substitutes for methylcellulose) in a 50-mL conical tube. Add 10 mL ddH_2O and 25 mL citrate buffer.
7. 50 mL Colorimetric reagent with oxidative neutralizing solution (for 100 reactions): prepare fresh. Dissolve 1.25 g Ehrlich's reagent (*p*-dimethylaminobenzaldehyde) in 25 mL *n*-propanol (65°C for 10 min to dissolve). In a separate tube, mix 11.4 mL 70% perchloric acid with 13.6 mL ddH_2O to make 32% perchlorate. Add 25 mL Ehrlich's reagent to 25 mL 32% perchlorate.

3. Methods

3.1. Guanidine Salt Extraction (see Notes 2–5)

1. Collect sample: tare a labeled cryovial. Wick any liquid from the sample before weighing to obtain the precise weight of a fresh cultured or dissected sample. Immediately freeze the sample in liquid nitrogen, and store at –80°C until extraction.
2. Pulverize the sample.
   a. Place a clean and dry biopulverizer with a piston in a small thermos holding around 2 cm of liquid nitrogen. Allow to cool until the nitrogen stops boiling (a few minutes).
   b. Transfer a preweighed, frozen sample to the biopulverizer. Biopulverize by striking the steel piston with a hammer a few times. Pivot the piston and strike several more times. Repeat three more times. (**Caution:** *Wear ear protectors and safety glasses. Strike as hard as you can, as inadequate pulverization can drastically affect the percentage of DNA extracted*). Do not lift the piston up and down, as this action may cause an air flux that causes the sample powder to disperse out of the chamber.
3. Extract with GuCl.
   a. With one hand, carefully lift the piston (do not shake off any powder stuck to it) and add GuCl extraction buffer directly to the bottom of the open barrel with a p1000 pipetman. Add 1000 μL to either a 20-mg cartilage sample or 40-mg hydrogel culture, or a proportionate amount for any other sample weight (*see* **Note 5** and **Table 4**). The buffer will freeze instantly. Place the piston back into the biopulverizer while the GuCl buffer is still frozen, so that the sample powder on the piston thaws in the presence of GuCl.
   b. Allow the GuCl buffer to thaw completely; you can speed this up by carefully placing the biopulverizer in a shallow water bath. *The buffer once thawed may flood above the pulverizer hole; this is desirable, since any powder that escaped the hole will come in contact with the extraction buffer.*

Table 4
Example Assay Conditions for Quantitative Biochemical Assays of Cartilage Components

Assay	Species detected	Standard curve	Linear range	Suggested test sample volume	Total assay volume	Typical content per mg wet weight: Adult cartilage	Typical content per mg wet weight: Agarose culture[a]
Hoechst	Double-stranded DNA (cell density)[b]	Sheared calf thymus DNA	10–125 ng (0–800 FU)	GuCl or Papain extract 2–10 μL	250 μL (96-well plate)	300 ng	150 ng
DMB	Chondroitin sulfate, keratin sulfate sodium salt (GAG content)[c]	Chondroitin sulfate C sodium salt	0.125–1.25 μg (OD_{530} minus OD_{590}: 0–0.8)	GuCl or papain extract 2–0 μL (cartilage) 10–20 μL (in vitro culture)	250 μL (96-well plate)	30 μg	12 μg
OH-Pro	*L-trans*-hydroxyproline (collagen content)[d]	*L-trans*-hydroxy-proline	0.5–5.0 μg (OD_{550}: 0–0.9)	Neutralized acid hydrolyzate 2–10 μL (cartilage) 25–75 μL (in vitro culture)	1.5 mL (1.0-mL plastic cuvet)	2.0 μg (17 μg)	0.06 μg (0.5 μg)

GuCl, guanidine hydrochloride; DMB, dimethyl methylene blue; OH-Pro, hydroxyproline; FU, fluorescence intensity units.
[a]Optimal 3-wk agarose hydrogel culture seeded with 10 million primary newborn chondrocytes per mL.
[b]Conversion factor: 7.7 pg DNA per bovine chondrocyte ***(2)***; most mammalian cells harbor 6–8 pg DNA/cell ***(61)***.
[c]Polyanions, including hyaluronic acid, heparin, and SDS, will cause positive interference in this assay.
[d]As an indication of prolyl hydroxylase-modified helical collagen type II and/or type I content.

c. Transfer the extract containing sample particles and buffer to an Eppendorf screw-cap tube using a p1000 blue pipetman tip with the end cut off. As sample particles tend to adhere to plastic and metal surfaces, transfer small, 200-μL aliquots in the suggested manner. First, remove any solution floating on the top of the biopulverizer unit to a clean screw-cap microfuge tube. Then remove the piston, and rinse the piston with the clear extract removed from the top of the biopulverizer. Do not rinse the piston with extract from inside the biopulverizer, since this tends to deposit even more sample fragments on the piston. Using a swirling motion, remove the GuCl extract and the entire pulverized sample to the microfuge tube. Examine the barrel of the pulverizer for sample. If sample fragments are visible, pulse-spin the extract, and collect these remaining fragments by rinsing the barrel with the clear supernatant and transferring fragments and supernatant to the screw-cap microfuge tube.
d. Vortex the extract and dispersed sample crumbs continuously for 30 min at 4°C, using a vortex mixer styrofoam adapter for 40 Eppendorf tubes.
e. Microfuge the sample for 10 min at 21,000*g* at 4°C.
f. If the sample did not pellet correctly, that is, if there is a large, viscous DNA mass at the bottom of the tube (over 300 μL vol) this means that the sample contained many cells. More GuCl buffer must be added, to solubilize the genomic DNA fully. If this is the case, add an additional 1 mL GuCl buffer to the pellet, vortex, and recentrifuge for 15 min. Combine the supernatant with the first GuCl extract, and if necessary place in a larger tube (**GuClsup**). Store the **GuClsup** at –80°C until ready to analyze. Vortex well upon thawing.

4. Extract twice with GITC.
   a. This step solubilizes a major fraction of RNA, which is recalcitrant to GuCl extraction, as well as some GuCl-insoluble proteins. To the pellet, add an amount of GITC extraction buffer that equals 1/4 the volume of 4 *M* GuCl buffer used (250 mL GITC, if 1 mL GuCl was used).
   b. Disperse the pellet completely, using a pipet tip if necessary (especially for cells grown in hydrogels).
   c. Vortex continuously for 5 min at 4°C. Centrifuge the sample for 10 min at 21,000*g* at 4°C. Remove the supernatant to a fresh tube.
   d. To the pellet, add another 1/4 volume GITC buffer. Disperse the pellet and vortex for 5 min at 4°C. Centrifuge for 10 min at 21,000*g* at 4°C.
   e. Combine the second GITC supernatant with the first GITC supernatant (**GITCsup**), and mix well.
   f. Store the GITCsup at –80°C until ready to analyze. Vortex well upon thawing.

3.2. Papain Digestion (see *Note 6*)

1. Either the *guanidine-insoluble pellet, or an unextracted tissue sample* may be submitted to papain digestion.
2. Rinse the GITC-insoluble pellet extremely well with 75% ethanol before papain digestion to get rid of all trace GITC: add 500 μL –20°C, 75% ethanol to the pellet, vortex briefly, microfuge 5 min at 21,000*g*, and discard supernatant.

Table 5
Suggested Extraction Volumes for Cartilage and Hydrogel Samples[a]

Cartilage weight (mg)	Tube size (mL)	GuCl buffer volume (mL)	GITC buffer volume (mL × 2)	Papain buffer volume (mL)
1–2	0.2 PCR	—	—	0.1
2–4	0.2 PCR	—	—	0.2
5	1.5	0.25	0.065	0.125
20	2.0	1.0	0.25	0.5
Hydrogel weight				
40 mg gel (10^7 cells/mL)	2.0	1.0	0.5	0.5

[a]For optimal vortex mixing, do not exceed 1.5 mL extraction volume per 2-mL tube, or 1.0 mL extraction volume per 1.5-mL tube. Do not exceed 20 mg cartilage or 40 mg hydrogel sample per 2-mL tube.

Perform a second wash with 75% ethanol. After discarding supernatant, flash-spin, and remove all residual ethanol with a p200 pipet tip. Allow to air dry for 10–15 min at room temperature. *Incomplete washing will result in GITC contamination of the pellet, which negatively interferes with the hydroxyproline assay and may completely suppress the signal.*

3. To the rinsed guanidine-insoluble pellet, add a volume of papain digestion buffer, pH 6.5, for cartilage or agarose hydrogels, or pH 7.5 for chitosan hydrogels, equal to one-half the volume of GuCl buffer employed, according to guidelines given in **Table 5** (*see* **Note 5**).
4. In a cryovial, or rubber gasket-sealed screw-cap Eppendorf tube, digest between 18 and 24 h at 60°C, in a temperature-controlled incubator. Make sure the tube is screwed completely shut, but not so tight that the gasket cracks, to avoid evaporation. An oven is preferred to a water bath, because during long incubations in a water bath, liquid condenses on the inner lid, leading to altered sample salt concentrations.
5. Postdigestion hydrogel samples: agarose, polysaccharides, and artificial polymers are not substrates for papain. DNA must be further liberated from these hydrogels by melting (70°C water bath for 10 min, agarose) or crushing (Eppendorf pestle, chitosan). After melting agarose or crushing chitosan hydrogel, vortex briefly, and then microfuge for 5 min at 10,000*g* at room temperature to pellet any remaining debris. Do not heat agarose above 70°C, or DNA may denature and fail to bind with Hoechst dye.
6. Postdigestion cartilage/bone samples: no visible cartilage matrix should remain for cartilage-only samples. Bone or calcified cartilage will appear as white pre-

cipitates that do not digest in papain. Remove with centrifugation at room temperature, 10,000*g* for 5 min.

7. Proceed immediately to the Hoechst DNA assay without freezing the papain-digested sample. Up to 10% of cellular DNA in a pulverized sample is trapped in the guanidine-insoluble pellet. Sample freezing can reduce apparent DNA yield by as much as half, although GAG and hydroxyproline yield is unaffected. Analyze aliquots of cleared papain supernatant by DMB assay (for unextracted GAG), and hydroxyproline assay (for insoluble collagen).

3.3. RNase Protection Assay

1. For RNase protection assay, combine 10 μL **GuClsup** with 10 μL **GITCsup** for each RNase protection sample.
2. Add 25 μL Direct Protect Buffer from the Ambion Direct Protect RNase Protection kit.
3. Add radioactive antisense RNA probe(s) in 5 μL Direct Protect Buffer, for a total sample volume of 50 μL. Proceed as suggested by the kit instructions.

3.4. Western Blot Analysis of Guanidine-Soluble Proteins

1. For Western blot analyses, the **GuClsup** and **GITCsup** extracts can be analyzed separately, or combined.
2. Precipitate 100 μL guanidine extract (either **GuClsup**, or **GITCsup**, or 50 μL of each supernatant combined) with 500 μL of –20°C ethanol, at –80°C overnight for maximal precipitation.
3. Centrifuge at 21,000*g* for 15 min at 4°C. Carefully remove supernatant.
4. To wash residual guanidine salts away, add 250 μL –20°C 75% ethanol, vortex, and centrifuge for 5 min at 21,000*g*.
5. Remove supernatant, pulse-spin tube, and carefully remove the last traces of ethanol with a p200 pipet tip (don't disturb pellet). It is important to wash the guanidine salt from the pellet, or else the sodium dodecyl sulfate (SDS) in the protein gel loading buffer will precipitate. Allow ethanol to evaporate from the open tube for 15 min on the bench.
6. Resuspend the pellet in 50 μL 8 *M* urea with thorough pipeting (room temperature). Once the pellet is resuspended, place immediately on ice to avoid proteolysis. Partly denatured proteases can still exhibit protease activity.
7. For Western blot analysis of relatively abundant cellular or extracellular proteins, analyze 10 or 20 μL per minigel lane. Transfer a 20-μL aliquot to a fresh tube and mix with an equal volume of 2X Laemmli loading buffer. Ice at all times. Boil the samples for 3 min in a dry heat block, and ice until loading onto the SDS-polyacrylamide gel electrophoresis (PAGE) minigel.
8. Transfer to polyvinylidene difluoride (PVDF) membranes with a semi-dry transfer apparatus for immunodetection.

3.5. Hoechst Assay

1. DNA standard preparation (sheared, filtered calf thymus DNA). Keep sterile to prevent DNA degradation.
   a. Dissolve 5 mg calf thymus DNA overnight at 37°C in 5 mL sterile buffer (standard for papain digests) or TEN buffer (standard for guanidine extracts).
   b. Read OD_{260}/OD_{280} to make sure DNA is fully dissolved (the 280/260 ratio should be above 1.8).
   c. Pipet DNA around 40 times with a sterile glass pasteur pipet to shear the DNA, and then filter through 0.45-μm syringe filter.
   d. Determine the precise DNA stock concentration by the OD_{260} reading from a 1:20 dilution (a 50 μg/mL solution has an OD_{260} of 1.00).
   e. Based on the precise concentration, generate 10 mL each of diluted standards, 1, 2, 4, 6, 8, and 12.5 μg/mL in PBE (standards for papain lysates), as well as diluted standard solutions of 1, 2, 4, 6, 8, and 12.5 μg/mL in TEN (standards for guanidine extracts).
   f. Confirm the standard concentrations by OD_{260} before freezing aliquots.
   g. Store as frozen 100-μL aliquots.
   h. Vortex well upon thawing.
   i. Use 10 μL of each standard for a standard curve from 10 to 125 ng DNA.
2. DNA standard curve validation. Verify all diluted standard concentrations by OD_{260}. An inconsequential difference in standard curve slope occurs between DNA standards made in PBE pH 6.5 or pH 7.5. Verify a linear curve by Hoechst assay (*see* **Table 4**).
3. Hoechst assay procedure (*see* **Notes 7–10**).
   a. Set up file in Fluorimeter Plate Reader. First two columns: blank [A1,A2] and [H1,H2] and standards [B1,B2 to G1,G2]. Standard range = 10, 20, 40, 60, 80, and 125 ng DNA per well.
   b. Pipet standards and samples into a 96-well NuncFluor plate.
      i. Papain-digested samples: in duplicate in the first two columns, pipet 10 μL PBE buffer for blanks and 10 μL of each PBE-DNA standard. In sample wells, analyze duplicate samples at two distinct concentrations to guarantee linear readout (5 μL sample + 5 μL PBE) and (10 μL sample + 0 μL PBE).
      ii. GuCl-extracted samples: in duplicate in the first two columns, pipet 10 μL TEN buffer for blanks and 10 μL of each TEN-DNA standard. Add 10 μL GuCl buffer to blanks and standards. In sample wells, analyze duplicate samples at two distinct concentrations to guarantee linear readout (5 μL sample + 5 μL GuCl + 10 μL TEN) and (10 μL sample + 0 μL GuCl + 10 μL TEN).
   c. Using an eight-well, multichannel pipet, add 200 μL of freshly prepared 0.2 μg/mL Hoechst 33258 in TEN to all wells, and read fluorescence immediately (360 nm excitation, 460 nm emission, 420 nm cutoff).

d. Repeat assay with a new plate for samples that fall outside the standard curve, or for samples that do not have a linear relationship between two sample concentrations.
e. Determine cellularity: use a conversion factor of 7.7 pg DNA/cell for bovine chondrocytes, or determine DNA content for other species. Mammalian cells generally harbor from 5 to 8 pg DNA/cell *(62)*.

3.6. DMB Assay

1. DMB standard: chondroitin 6-sulfate C sodium salt standard (*see* **Note 11**). Speed vac dry 100 mg chondroitin sulfate C. In a 50-mL conical tube, weigh approx 10.0 mg chondroitin sulfate, and, according to the precise weight, add PBE buffer to generate a 0.5 mg/mL solution (~20 mL). Vortex for several minutes to dissolve fully. Generate serial dilutions in PBE, to constitute the standard curve, at 12.5, 25, 50, 75, 100, 125 μg/mL chondroitin sulfate, to give a standard curve range of 0.125–1.25 μg/well for 10 μL of standard per 96-well. Store as 100-μL frozen aliquots. Vortex well upon thawing.
2. Chondroitin sulfate C sodium salt standard validation. Generate a standard curve using fresh DMB assay solution. Using PBE and DMB dye as the blank, the OD_{530} of 1.25 μg chondroitin sulfate C, with subtraction of the OD_{590} negative peak, should be between 0.65 and 0.8.
3. DMB assay procedure (*see* **Notes 7** and **12**).
   a. Perform a pilot visual test with several samples and standards in a dummy plate, to determine the correct sample dilution to use, in order to fall within the linear range of the standard curve.
   b. Set up file in visible light Plate Reader: read the OD_{530} and the OD_{590}, with baseline subtraction of the negative peak at OD_{590} *(1)* from the reading at OD_{530} for increased assay sensitivity. First two columns: DMB dye blank [A1,A2], [H1,H1] and standards [B1,B2 to G1,G2]. Use 10 μL of each standard for a standard range of 0.125, 0.25, 0.5, 0.75, 1.0, and 1.25 μg sodium chondroitin sulfate C per well.
   c. Pipet standards and samples in a 96-well flat-bottomed ELISA plate.
      i. Papain-digested samples: in duplicate in the first two columns, pipet 10 μL PBE buffer for blanks, and 10 μL of each standard. In sample wells, analyze duplicate samples at two distinct concentrations to guarantee linear readout (2 μL sample + 8 μL PBE) and (10 μL sample + 0 μL PBE).
      ii. GuCl-extracted samples: In duplicate in the first two columns, pipet 10 μL PBE buffer for blanks, and 10 μL of each standard. Add 10 μL GuCl buffer to blanks and standards. In sample wells, analyze duplicate samples at two distinct concentrations to guarantee linear readout (2 μL sample + 8 μL GuCl + 10 μL PBE) and (10 μL sample + 0 μL GuCl + 10 μL PBE).
   d. Using an Eppendorf repeat pipetor with a 5.0-mL Combitip, dispense 250 μL of DMB assay solution rapidly into all wells.

e. Read plate immediately at OD_{530} and OD_{590}.
f. Repeat assay with a new plate for samples that fall outside of the standard curve, or for samples that do not have a linear relationship between two sample concentrations.

3.7. Hydroxyproline Assay

1. Hydroxyproline standard. Put 100 μg/mL hydroxyproline in 1 m*M* HCl (as a bacteriostatic *[6]*). This is stable at 4°C for 6 mo. Use 5 to 50 μL standard to generate a standard curve from 0.5 to 5.0 μg hydroxyproline.
2. Hydroxyproline assay sample preparation: includes hydrolysis in 6 *N* HCl, dilution with ddH_2O, neutralization with 6 *N* NaOH, and decolorization with resin.
   a. Combine 50–200 μL papain-digested sample with an equal volume of concentrated HCl (37%) in a fail-safe Target DP vial (National Scientific). Ordinary rubber gaskets will not seal properly at 110°C.
   b. If you suspect that the collagen content of your sample is less than 100 μg, Speed-Vac 200 μL of sample until dry in an Eppendorf tube, resuspend in 50 μL 6 *N* HCl, and transfer to hydrolysis vial. Beware of possible negative interference by protein in such concentrated samples.
   c. Make sure the tube is closed well, or else the sample may evaporate and generate erroneous results.
   d. Incubate for 18 h at 110°C in a Pasteur oven.
   e. After cooling, pulse spin and use a calibrated pipetman to determine the precise sample volume remaining. Complete to twice the original volume with ddH_2O (*see* **Notes 13** and **14**).
   f. To each sample, add 2–4 μL of a solution of 0.2% phenol red in water as a pH indicator.
   g. If the hydrolyzate was black (*see* **Note 15**), dilute the sample severalfold until the pale pink color is discernable.
   h. Add 6 *N* NaOH, start with 75% the volume of 6 *N* HCl added at first, and then add 10 μL 6 *N* NaOH aliquots until the solution turns pink.
   i. Decolorize phenol red from the sample by adding around 50 mg AG-1-X8 ion exchange resin. Vortex, and microfuge for 1 min at room temperature at 21,000*g*.
   j. If the resin does not pellet, filter the solution through a blue pipet tip containing a small volume of 500-μm-diameter glass beads at the tip, with a small layer of 100-μm-diameter glass beads above.
   k. If solution is still pink, add more resin and recentrifuge.
   l. Transfer the samples to fresh tubes. If necessary, store frozen until ready to perform the assay (*see* **Note 16**).
3. Hydroxyproline assay (*see* **Note 17**).
   a. 1.5-mL Assay volume in a standard 1.5-mL Eppendorf tube.
   b. Use nonoxidized sample as a reagent blank *(7)* or simply water.
   c. Use **Table 6** as a guide for setting up the standard curve and samples to be analyzed.

Table 6
Hydroxyproline Standards, Samples, and Reagent Volumes for 1.5-mL Sample Assay Volume

ddH_2O (µL)	Half-saturated NaCl (µL)	Hydroxyproline stock (µL)	Chloramine T 4 min room temperature (µL)	Ehrlich's reagent 12 min 60°C, then ice (µL)
Standards				
250	250	0	500	500
245	250	5 (0.5 µg)	500	500
240	250	10 (1.0 µg)	500	500
220	250	15 (1.5 µg)	500	500
225	250	25 (2.5 µg)	500	500
200	250	50 (5 µg)	500	500
Samples		Sample volume (µL)		
245	250	5 500	500	
200	250	50 500	500	

d. To each tube add sequentially: ddH_2O (to complete sample or standard to 250 µL), 250 µL half-saturated NaCl, and sample or standard.
e. Perform **steps f–h** under a chemical fume hood.
f. Use the Eppendorf repeat pipettor to add 0.5 mL chloramine T solution (*see* **Note 17**). Close all tubes and shake.
g. Incubate at room temperature for 4 min.
h. Use the Eppendorf repeat pipetor to dispense the 0.5 mL of Ehrlich's reagent. Close all tubes and shake.
i. Place all tubes in a floating rack, and place all at once at 60°C in a water bath, for better heat transfer than a heat block or incubator. Incubate at 60°C for 12 min. Place briefly on crushed ice to chill. Read OD_{550} in a visible spectrophotometer in 1.0-mL plastic disposable cuvettes.
j. Taking into account all hydrolyzate sample dilution factors, extrapolate data to determine original sample hydroxyproline content. Use a conversion factor of 7.6 to extrapolate theoretical collagen content.
k. Dispose of samples as hazardous liquid waste.

4. Notes

1. In the Hoechst fluorimetric assay, any particulate or dust will cause positive interference via light scattering. TEN and PBE solutions should be filtered with a 0.22-µm filter to remove dust particles. Glassware, plasticware, and bench spaces, should be dust-free.

2. For good experimental design, generate three to four samples for each condition, to obtain a statistically relevant number of samples. For cells cultured in hydrogels, generate several types of negative control sample, including hydrogel samples without cells, which are cultured in complete media for at least 1 d, and hydrogel with cells from d 1 culture for initial composition. The recorded mass of the cultured hydrogel samples at harvest can be used to determine shrinkage or swelling of the matrix. Negative control samples will show how many cells survive the initial seeding density, whether the cells proliferate during culture, whether the construct shrinks or swells, and whether the hydrogel or media causes positive or negative interference in the biochemical assays. Some biochemical assays may not be feasible, if the hydrogel is completely or partly composed of collagen, hyaluronic acid, or GAG. In this case, metabolic assays may be useful alternatives to estimate synthetic rates. Certain biochemical assays may need to be revalidated when performed in the presence of interfering hydrogel scaffolding that leaches into the extraction buffers. The lower the cell density, the greater the possible interference from hydrogel contaminants. It is for this reason that all samples should be solubilized according to their mass, and not simply in one convenient volume (for example, 1 mL) extraction buffer. Hydrogel components that partition into the extraction buffer can potentially interfere positively or negatively with biochemical assays. To judge the level of interference, compare a standard curve harboring the extraction buffer alone with a standard curve harboring the same volume of extract from hydrogel cultured without cells as that volume of extract needed to detect a particular biochemical component. If the curve is affected by more than 10%, it may be necessary to include hydrogel-only extracts in the standard curve.
3. Several special precautions should be taken before commencing sample extraction. Bench surfaces should be cleaned and fresh bench paper used. Gloves should be worn at all times, when procuring Eppendorf tubes from plastic bags and when handling pipet tips, to avoid contaminating samples with skin nucleases, proteases, and oils. Pipetmen barrels should be cleaned in soapy water before use. The thermos and biopulverizer should be cleaned and dried with a lint-free Kimwipe before use, to prevent sample contamination. Safety glasses should be worn while handling liquid nitrogen and guanidine solutions. Ear protection should be worn while pulverizing. Guanidine extraction buffers are highly corrosive. Wash inner pipetman barrels, and wipe the inside of the microfuge with a damp cloth after performing the assay, to avoid development of rust.
4. Samples should be weighed prior to frozen storage, since humidity can collect on frozen samples and falsify wet mass. Once calibrated, the Micromettler balance cannot be displaced, so samples must be harvested next to the balance. For very small samples, each numbered cryovial should be tared immediately before recording sample weight. If wet, wick off liquid from the sample with a clean Kimwipe prior to weighing. If water content must be established, sample tube weights must be recorded prior to sample weighing, lyophilization, and reweighing, for further papain digestion of GAG, DNA, and hydroxyproline analysis

only. Parallel empty plastic tubes should be weighed, lyophilized, and reweighed to determine any mass contribution by tube humidity. RNA analysis and protein analysis by Western blot can only be conducted on hydrated samples immediately frozen in liquid nitrogen. Store at –80°C, or proceed immediately to GuCl extraction. (If a –80°C freezer is not available, extracts can be kept a few months at –20°C in guanidine extraction buffer.) Samples should at no time be allowed to thaw before pulverizing. Have all reagents prepared for Hoechst DNA assay before proceeding to papain digestion of the insoluble pellet, as freeze-thaw leads to papain enzyme precipitation and loss of up to 50% DNA signal.

5. Extraction buffer volumes should be determined prior to sample extraction. Before beginning sample extraction, generate a table of all samples, sample weights, extraction volumes for GuCl, GITC, and papain digestion buffer, and paste into your lab notebook. The sample-to-buffer volume ratio plays a critical role in determining whether the test molecule is completely solubilized, falls within the detection limits of the assay (**Table 4**), and has minimal interference from other species present in the extract, including papain enzyme. The buffer-to-sample volume ratios suggested in **Table 5** permit satisfactory solubilization of the test molecules within the sensitivity ranges of the colorimetric assays for GAG and hydroxyproline, the fluorimetric Hoechst DNA assay, chemiluminescent detection of proteins by Western blot, and radioactive detection of RNAse protection products. A 20-mg cartilage sample and a 40-mg tissue-engineered hydrogel sample generate enough sample material to perform multiple biochemical assays in triplicate. Note that to be able to make a semiquantitative analysis of cellular proteins or mRNA expression levels, it may be preferable to adjust extraction volumes according to estimated cell densities.
6. Papain is active at pH 6.0 *(2)*, pH 6.5 *(27)*, pH 6.8 *(1)*, and pH 7.5 *(11)*. For cartilage samples, papain digestion can be routinely performed at pH 6.5. However, to analyze samples in the presence of chitosan, the pH of the digestion buffer must be altered to pH 7.5 to prevent chitosan association with nucleic acids and GAG. It is essential that the digestion buffer and tissue samples be kept sterile during the 60°C incubation, as microbial contaminants could introduce nucleases into the samples, resulting in DNA degradation. When placing milligram samples in papain digestion buffer, visually verify that the samples are immersed prior to the 60°C incubation.
7. For 96-well plate colorimetric or fluorimetric assays, make sure all wells contain the same volumes and buffer concentrations. When GuCl extracts are being analyzed, standards must harbor an equal amount of GuCl solution. Samples should comprise no more than 50 μL total volume. Test two different concentrations of each sample, to rule out positive/negative interference.
8. The presence of GuCl will depress the fluorescence reading proportionally to the amount of GuCl added.
9. GITC extracts of chitosan-cultured samples cannot be analyzed for DNA content, since GITC partly solubilizes the chitosan, which causes fluorescence light scattering. For cartilage GITC extracts, however, duplicate aliquots of 10 or 20 μL of

GITCsup can be tested against a standard curve containing the same amount of GITC extraction buffer.

10. Analysis of some hydrogel-cultured samples may further require the inclusion of negative control extracts in the DNA standard curve. The interference of hydrogel will be more pronounced for cultures with cell densities below 5 million cells/mL. To determine whether hydrogel present in GuCl extracts or papain digests causes positive or negative interference in the assay, compare the DNA standard curves with standard curves harboring 10 μL of GuCl-extracted or papain-digested hydrogel cultured without cells. If the slope is altered by more than 20%, extrapolate samples against a standard curve harboring hydrogel extracts.
11. The DMB assay standard in fact reflects the mg weight of the *salt* form of chondroitin sulfate C. The sodium content of a 100% salt from chondroitin sulfate powder is 8.76% (Na_2/Na_2CS = 44 g/mol/502 g/mol). Therefore, a 0.5 mg/mL standard prepared from a CS lot number carrying approx 7 to 9% Na^+ will represent 0.5 mg/mL CS-salt standard, provided the water content is negligible.
12. The use of visible light microplate readers and multiwell or automatic pipetors has significantly improved the DMB assay, which is highly sensitive to reagent precipitation. Have the plate reader ready to read the plate before dispensing the DMB reagent into the 96-well plate. GITC will cause an instant purple color of the DMB reagent; therefore GITC extracts cannot be used directly in the DMB assay.
13. The neutralized hydrolyzate contains 6 *N* NaCl. One volume of water is added to reduce salt concentration and sample buoyant density, so that during the decolorization step with ion exchange resin, the resin particles may be removed by centrifugation.
14. The precise volume of samples at all steps of the hydrolysis/dilution/neutralization procedure must be recorded, in order to calculate the original sample hydroxyproline content from diluted samples.
15. The presence of sugars, or GAG, in the 110°C hydrolysis step will result in caramelization, or blackening of the samples. Decoloring may be necessary for papain-digested cartilage prior to the hydroxyproline assay. Diluting the papain lysate before hydrolysis will proportionally reduce blackening. Samples that have been extracted with guanidine before papain digestion will not caramelize, as nearly all the sugars have been removed by the guanidine extraction.
16. For safe storage, transfer hydrolyzate to a cryovial prior to freezing.
17. In the hydroxyproline assay, when using the repeat pipetor, eject the initial few mL back into the original solution until liquid flow is steady. Stop ejecting before the end, as liquid velocity is higher, increasing the chance of sample spill. Start with a row of tubes, and always add reagents in the same order to keep similar incubation times. Chloramine T oxidizes the hydroxyproline. The perchloric acid in the Ehrlich's reagent solution destroys the chloramine T reagent, to arrest oxidation, whereas Erlich's reagent reacts colorimetrically with oxidized hydroxyproline. After adding Ehrlich's reagent, the samples can sit for a few minutes without harming the assay, before the 60°C incubation. For the best reproducibility, do not exceed the temperature, or the time of incubation. The standard curve

must be included with the samples, or else you cannot extrapolate your concentrations, as every curve differs slightly according to precise time of incubation and pause before reading. Place samples at room temperature when cool, to avoid condensation accumulating on chilled cuvettes. Chilling will slow the colorimetric reaction but not stop it entirely. Therefore, immediately read the samples in a visible light spectrophotometer in plastic disposable cuvettes. Blank with a negative control sample (i.e., papain digestion buffer sample), or with a nonoxidized sample *(7)*. The cuvettes can be rinsed afterward, for recycling. Use of plate readers is not recommended, owing to the highly corrosive perchlorate in the hydroxyproline sample.

Acknowledgments

The methods described are reprinted in greater detail from reference 11 (copyright 2002, with permission from Elsevier). The author would like to thank the Canadian Arthritis Network for financial support, as well as Dr. Michael Buschmann, Nicholas Tran-Khanh, and Jun Sun at Ecole Polytechnique for helpful discussions.

References

1. Farndale, R. W., Buttle, D. J., and Barrett, A. J. (1986) Improved quantitation and discrimination of sulphated glycosaminoglycans by use of dimethylmethylene blue. *Biochem. Biophys. Acta* **883,** 173–177.
2. Kim Y. J., Sah, R. L., Doong, J.-Y. H., and Grodzinsky, A. J. (1988) Fluorometric assay of DNA in cartilage explants using Hoechst 33258. *Anal. Biochem.* **174,** 168–176.
3. Farndale, R. W., Sayers, C. A., and Barrett, A. J. (1982) A direct spectrophotometric microassay for sulfated glycosaminoglycans in cartilage cultures. *Connect. Tissue Res.* **9,** 247–248.
4. Chandrasekhar, S., Esterman, M. A., and Hoffman, H. A. (1987) Microdetermination of proteoglycans and glycosaminoglycans in the presence of guanidine hydrochloride. *Anal. Biochem.* **161,** 103–108.
5. Stegemann, H. and Stalder, K. (1967) Determination of hydroxyproline. *Clin. Chim. Acta* **18,** 267–273.
6. Woessner, J. F. (1961) The determination of hydroxyproline in tissue and protein samples containing small proportions of this imino acid. *Arch. Biochem. Biophys.* **93,** 440–447.
7. Burleigh, M. C., Barrett, A. J., and Lazarus, G. S. (1974) A lysosomal enzyme that degrades native collagen. *Biochem. J.* **137,** 387–398.
8. Chomczynski, P. and Mackey, K. (1995) Modification of the tri reagent procedure for isolation of RNA from polysaccharide-and proteoglycan-rich sources. *Biotechniques* **19,** 942–945.
9. Haines, D. S. and Gillespie, D. H. (1992) RNA abundance measured by a lysate RNase protection assay. *Biotechniques* **12,** 736–741.

10. Binette, F., McQuaid, D. P., Haudenschild, D. R., Yaeger, P. C., McPherson, J. M., and Tubo, R. (1998) Expression of a stable articular cartilage phenotype without evidence of hypertrophy by adult human articular chondrocytes in vitro. *J. Orthop. Res.* **16L,** 207–216.
11. Hoemann, C. H., Sun, J., Chrzanowski, V., and Buschmann, M. D. (2002) A multivalent assay to detect DNA, RNA, glycosaminoglycan, protein, and collagen content of milligram samples of cartilage or chondrocytes grown in chitosan hydrogel. *Anal. Biochem.* **300,** 1–10.
12. Gehrsitz, A., McKenna, L. A., Soder S., Kirchner, T., and Aigner T. (2002) Isolation of RNA from small human articular cartilage specimens allows quantification of mRNA expression levels in local articular cartilage defects. *J. Orthop. Res.* **19,** 478–481.
13. Matyas, J. R., Huang, D., Chung, M., and Adams, M. E. (2002) Regional quantification of cartilage type II collagen and aggrecan mRNA in joints with early experimental osteoarthritis. *Arthritis Rheum.* **46,** 1536–1543.
14. Bluteau, G., Gouttenoire, J., Conrozier, T., et al. (2002) Differential gene expression analysis in a rabbit model of osteoarthritis induced by anterior cruciate ligament (ACL) section. *Biorheology* **39,** 247–258.
15. Langelier, A., Suetterlin, R., Hoemann, C. D., Aebi, U., and Buschmann, M. D. (2000) The chondrocyte cytoskeleton in mature articular cartilage: structure and distribution of actin, tubulin and vimentin filaments. *J. Histochem. Cytochem.* **48,** 1307–1320.
16. Sajdera, S. W. and Hascall, V. C. (1969) Proteinpolysaccharide complex from bovine nasal cartilage. *J. Biol. Chem.* **244,** 77–87.
17. Heinegard, D. and Sommarin, Y. (1987) Isolation and characterization of proteoglycans. *Methods Enzymol.* **144,** 319–372.
18. Mankin, H. J. and Lippiello, L. (1970) Biochemical and metabolic abnormalities in articular cartilage from osteo-arthritic human hips. J. *Bone Joint Surg. Am.* **52,** 424–434.
19. Kempson, G. E., Muir, H., Swanson, S. A. V., and Freeman, M. A. R. (1970) Correlations between stiffness and the chemical constituents of cartilage on the human femoral head. *Biochem. Biophys. Acta.* **215,** 70–77.
20. Venn, M. and Maroudas, A. (1977) Chemical composition and swelling of normal and osteoarthritic femoral head cartilage. *Ann. Rheum. Dis.* **36,** 121–129.
21. Amiel, D., Coutts, R. D., Harwood, F. L., Ishizue, K. K., and Kleiner, J. B. (1988) The chondrogenesis of rib perichondrial grafts for repair of full thickness articular cartilage defects in a rabbit model: a one year postoperative assessment. *Connect. Tissue Res.* **18,** 27–39.
22. Richardson, D. W. and Clark, C. C. (1990) Biochemical changes in articular cartilage opposing full- and partial-thickness cartilage lesions in horses. *Am. J. Vet. Res.* **51,** 118–122.
23. Vachon, A. M., McIlwraith, C. W., and Keeley, F. W. (1991) Biochemical study of repair of induced osteochondral defects of the distal portion of the radial carpal bone in horses by use of periosteal autografts. *Am. J. Vet. Res.* **52,** 328–332.

24. Brama, P. A., Tekoppele, J. M., Bank, R. A., Barneveld, A., and VanWeeren, P. R. (2000) Functional adaptation of equine articular cartilage: the formation of regional biochemical characteristics up to age one year. *Equine Vet. J.* **32,** 217–221.
25. Burkhardt, D., Hwa, S. Y., and Ghosh, P. (2001) A novel microassay for the quantitation of the sulfated glycosaminoglycan content of histological sections: its application to determine the effects of diacerhein on cartilage in an ovine model of osteoarthritis. *Osteoarthritis Cartilage* **9,** 238–247.
26. Murray, R. C., Birch, H. L., Lakhani, K., and Goodship, A. E. (2001) Subchondral bone thickness, hardness and remodelling are influenced by short-term exercise in a site-specific manner. *J. Orthop. Res.* **19,** 1035–1042.
27. Buschmann, M. D., Gluzband, Y. A., Grodzinsky, A. J., Kimura, J. H., and Hunziker, E. B. (1992) Chondrocytes in agarose culture synthesize a mechanically functional extracellular matrix. *J. Orthop. Res.* **10,** 745–758.
28. Eggli, P. S., Hunziker, E. B., and Schenk, R. K. (1988) Quantitation of structural features characterizing weight- and less-weight-bearing regions in articular cartilage: a stereological analysis of medial femoral condyles in young adult rabbits. *Anat. Rec.* **222,** 217–227.
29. Sah, R. L., Yang, A. S., Chen, A. C., et al. (1997) Physical properties of rabbit articular cartilage after transection of the anterior cruciate ligament. *J. Orthop. Res.* **15,** 197–203.
30. Lee, C. R., Grodzinsky, A. J., Hsu, H. P., Martin, S. D., and Spector, M. (2000) Effects of harvest and selected cartilage repair procedures on the physical and biochemical properties of articular cartilage in the canine knee. *J. Orthop. Res.* **18,** 790–799.
31. Treppo, S., Koepp, H., Quan, E. C., Cole, A. A., Kuettner, K. E., and Grodzinsky, A. J. (2000) Comparison of biomechanical and biochemical properties of cartilage from human knee and ankle pairs. *J. Orthop. Res.* **18,** 739–748.
32. Dumont, J., Ionescu, M, Reiner A., et al. (1999) Mature full-thickness articular cartilage explants attached to bone are physiologically stable over long-term culture in serum-free media. *Connect. Tissue Res.* **40,** 259–272.
33. Ameer, G. A., Mahmood, T. A., and Langer, R. (2002) A biodegradable composite scaffold for cell transplantation. *J. Orthop. Res.* **20,** 16–19.
34. Hunziker, E. B., Quinn, T. M., and Hauselmann, H. J. (2002) Quantitative structural organization of normal adult human articular cartilage. *Osteoarthritis Cartilage* **10,** 564–572.
35. Lewis, R. J., MacFarland, A. K., Anandavijayan, S., and Aspden, R. M. (1988) Material properties and biosynthetic activity of articular cartilage from the bovine carpo-metacarpal joint. *Osteoarthritis Cartilage* **6,** 383–392.
36. Mankin, H. J. (1974) The reaction of articular cartilage to injury and osteoarthritis (Second of Two Parts). *N. Engl. J. Med.* **291,** 1335–1340.
37. Mow, V. C., Ratcliffe, A., and Poole A. R. (1992) Cartilage and diarthrodial joints as paradigms for hierarchical materials and structures. *Biomaterials* **13,** 67–97.
38. Maroudas, A. (1990) Different ways of expressing concentration of cartilage constituents with special reference to the tissue's organization and functional proper-

ties, in *Methods in Cartilage Research* (Maroudas, A. and Kuettner, K. E., eds.), Academic, London, pp. 211–219.

39. Eyre, D. (2001) Collagen of articular cartilage. *Arthritis Res.* **4,** 30–35.
40. Page Thomas, D. P., King B., Stephens, T., and Dingle, J. T. (1991) In vivo studies of cartilage regeneration after damage induced by catabolin/interleukin-1. *Ann. Rheum. Dis.* **50,** 75–80.
41. Richardson, D. W. and Clark, C. C. (1990) Biochemical changes in articular cartilage opposing full- and partial-thickness cartilage lesions in horses. *Am. J. Vet. Res.* **51,** 118–122.
42. Verbruggen, G., Cornelissen, M., Almqvist, K. F., et al. (2000) Influence of aging on the synthesis and morphology of the aggrecans synthesized by differentiated human articular chondrocytes. *Osteoarthritis Cartilage* **8,** 170–179.
43. Front, P. Aprile, F., Mitrovic, D. R., and Swann, D. A. (1989) Age-related changes in the synthesis of matrix macromolecules by bovine articular cartilage. *Connect. Tissue Res.* **19,** 121–133.
44. Sims, C. D., Butler, P. E. M., Cao, Y. L., et al. (1998) Tissue engineered neocartilage using plasma derived polymer substrates and chondrocytes. *Plast. Reconst. Surg.* **101,** 1580–1585.
45. Riesle, J., Hollander, A. P., Langer, R., Freed, L. E., and Vunjak-Novakovic, G. (1998) Collagen in tissue-engineered cartilage: types, structure, and crosslinks *J. Cell. Biochem.* **71,** 313–327.
46. Hollander, A. P., Heathfield, T. F., Webber, C., et al. (1994) Increased damage to type II collagen in osteoarthritic articular cartilage detected by a new immunoassay. *J. Clin. Invest.* **93,** 1722–1732.
47. Stone, J., Akhtar, H., Botchway, S., and Pennock, C. A. (1994) Interaction of 1,9-dimethylmethylene blue with glycosaminoglycans. *Ann. Clin. Biochem.* **31,** 147–152.
48. Vunjak-Novakovic, G., Martin, I., Obradovic, B., et al. (1999) Bioreactor cultivation conditions modulate the composition and mechanical properties of tissue-engineered cartilage. *J. Orthop. Res.* **17,** 130–138.
49. Hoemann, C. D., Sun, J., Légaré, A., McKee, M. D., and Buschmann, M. D. Tissue engineering of cartilage using an injectable and adhesive chitosan-based cell-delivery vehicle. Submitted.
50. Obradovic, B., Carrier, R. L., Vunjak-Novakovic, G., and Freed, L. E. (1999) Gas exchange is essential for bioreactor cultivation of tissue engineered cartilage. *Biotechnol. Bioeng.* **63,** 197–205.
51. Wu, F., Dunkelman, N., Peterson, A., Davisson, T., De La Torre, R., and Jain, D. (1999) Bioreactor development for tissue-engineered cartilage. *Ann. NY Acad. Sci.* **875,** 405–411.
52. Grande, D. A., Halberstadt, C., Naughton, G., Schwartz, R., and Manji, R. (1997) Evaluation of matrix scaffolds for tissue engineering of articular cartilage grafts. *J. Biomed. Mater. Res.* **34,** 211–220.
53. Yu, H., Grynpas, M., and Kandel, R. A. (1997) Composition of cartilagenous tissue with mineralized and non-mineralized zones formed in vitro. *Biomaterials* **18,** 1425–1431.

54. Sun, Y., Hurtig, M., Pilliar, R. M., Grynpas, M., and Kandel, R. A. (2001) Characterization of nucleus pulposus-like tissue formed in vitro. *J. Orthop. Res.* **19,** 1078–1084.
55. Nehrer, S., Breinan, H. A., Ramappa, A., et al. (1997) Canine chondrocytes seeded in type I and type II collagen implants investigated in vitro. *J. Biomed. Mater. Res.* **38,** 95–104.
56. Toolan, B. C., Frenkel, S. R., Pachence, J. M., Yalowitz, L., and Alexander, H. (1996) Effects of growth-factor enhanced culture on a chondrocyte-collagen implant for cartilage repair. *J. Biomed. Mater. Res.* **31,** 273–280.
57. Bryant, S. J. and Anseth, K. S. (2001) Hydrogel properties influence ECM production by chondrocytes photoencapsulated in poly(ethylene glycol) hydrogels. *J. Biomed. Mater. Res.* **59,** 63–72.
58. Kisiday, J., Jin, M., Kurz, B., Hung, H., Semino, C., Zhang, S., and Grodzinsky, A. J. (2002) Self-assembling peptide hydrogel fosters chondrocyte extracellular matrix production and cell division: implications for cartilage tissue repair. *Proc. Natl. Acad. Sci. USA* **99,** 9996–10001.
59. Wong, M., Siegrist, M., Wang, X., and Hunziker, E. (2001) Development of mechanically stable alginate/chondrocyte constructs: effects of guluronic acid content and matrix synthesis. *J. Orthop. Res.* **19,** 493–499.
60. Passaretti, D., Silverman, R. P., Huang, W., et al. (2001) Cultured chondrocytes produce injectable tissue-engineered cartilage in hydrogel polymer. *Tissue Eng.* **7,** 805–815.
61. Elisseeff, J., Anseth, K., Sims, D., et al. (1999) Transdermal photopolymerization of poly(ethylene oxide)-based injectable hydrogels for tissue-engineered cartilage. *Plast. Reconstr. Surg.* **104,** 1014–1022.
62. Oegema, T. R., Carpenter, B. J., and Thompson, R. C. (1984) Fluorometric determination of DNA in cartilage of various species. *J. Orthop. Res.* **1,** 345–351.

9

Mechanical Characterization of Native and Tissue-Engineered Cartilage

Albert C. Chen, Stephen M. Klisch, Won C. Bae, Michele M. Temple, Kevin B. McGowan, Kenneth R. Gratz, Barbara L. Schumacher, and Robert L. Sah

Summary

Cartilage functions as a low-friction, wear-resistant, load-bearing tissue. During a normal gait cycle, one cartilage surface rolls and slides against another, all the while being loaded and unloaded. The durability of the tissue also makes for an impressive material to study. However, when cartilage is damaged or diseased, the tissue has little capacity to repair itself. The goal of cell-based repair strategies to replace damaged or diseased tissue requires that the functional biomechanical properties of normal (developing or mature), diseased, and repair cartilage be restored. This chapter addresses some of the major methods used to assess the biomechanical properties of native and tissue-engineered cartilage. First, the traditional methods of testing by compression, tension, shear, and indentation are reviewed. Next, additional methods to evaluate interfacial mechanics and lubrication are described. Thus, a variety of mechanical tests may be used to assess functional properties for normal, diseased, and tissue-engineered cartilage.

Key Words: Cartilage; biomechanics; tissue engineering; extracellular matrix; compression; tension; shear; stress; strain.

1. Introduction

Articular cartilage functions as a low-friction, wear-resistant, load-bearing tissue. Under normal circumstances, the composition and structure of cartilage confer remarkable mechanical properties on this tissue. The cartilage extracellular matrix is composed primarily of a proteoglycan gel and a collagen network. The proteoglycan gel has a high fixed-charge density and is compacted into a restricted volume relative to the free-swelling state, thereby imparting a large osmotic swelling pressure *(1)*. This swelling pressure is counteracted by tension developed in the collagen network, composed primarily of type II collagen *(2,3)*. The ability of cartilage to counterbalance the internal swelling pres-

From: *Methods in Molecular Medicine, Vol. 101: Cartilage and Osteoarthritis, Volume 2: Structure and In Vivo Analysis*
Edited by: F. De Ceuninck, M. Sabatini, and P. Pastoureau © Humana Press Inc., Totowa, NJ

sure and withstand compressive, tensile, and shear loads depends on the stiffness, resilience, and strength of the collagen network.

In physiological and pathophysiological circumstances, the mechanical properties of articular cartilage change. During development and prematuration growth, cartilage mechanical properties can evolve very rapidly (over ~8 wk from the late fetus to the young newborn), with a marked increase in compressive modulus (i.e., stiffening) ***(4)*** and also tensile modulus and strength ***(5)***. In contrast, with postmaturation aging and osteoarthritic degeneration, cartilage exhibits a decrease in compressive modulus (i.e., softening) ***(6)*** and tensile modulus and strength (i.e., integrity) ***(7,8)***. These changes appear to be related to alterations in the content and organization of the proteoglycan and collagen matrix components ***(9)***.

One approach to repairing damaged or diseased cartilage involves tissue engineering, in particular, the fabrication of cartilaginous tissue for implantation. The design and synthesis of tissue implants is directed toward variety of goals, ranging from endowing the tissue with the biomechanical properties of normal adult cartilage to those of the immature cartilage. Cartilaginous tissue with a range of biomechanical properties may be appropriate for therapeutic purposes, if it can be regulated to remodel appropriately under controlled postoperative rehabilitation regimes.

The mechanical properties of articular cartilage can be measured over a variety of length scales ***(10)***. Cartilage can be analyzed at length scales ranging from intact joints to full-thickness regions of cartilage over the joint surface, decreasing down to layers of cartilage tissue from different depths, to cellular and extracellular regions of cartilage tissue, to molecular constituents within these regions, and beyond. One set of biomechanical properties can be observed if articular cartilage is assumed to be homogeneous. Another set of very different properties can be observed if cartilage is analyzed at the finer length scale of tissue layers at varying depths from the articular surface ***(11,12)***. The length scale can be even finer, for example, to focus on the indwelling chondrocytes, which are relatively soft compared with the matrix ***(13)***, or the glycosaminoglycan component of the matrix ***(14)***. This chapter focuses on tissue-scale biomechanical properties of cartilage, as well as relationships between biomechanical properties at different length scales.

The mechanical properties of cartilage can be measured at structural or material levels. Structural properties reflect the body or joint as a whole and are influenced by cartilage material properties and sample geometry; material properties describe the characteristics of the cartilage material itself and are determined at a finer length scale than that for structural properties. The complex geometry of joints makes it challenging to assess cartilage biomechanical properties overall in a joint. To simplify experiments and the associated interpretation of results, experiments are often performed on parts of a joint or on excised tissue specimens. With appropriate boundary conditions and model assumptions (typically symmetry) so that variations occur in only one or two dimensions, material properties can be estimated from such tests. The biomechanical properties of tissue-engineered cartilage can also be analyzed prior to, or after, transplant.

The biomechanical methods range from in vitro benchtop tests to those that can be performed *in situ* or in vivo. Some biomechanical tests of cartilage that are traditionally performed in vitro are generally inappropriate for clinical implementation. Such tests may be destructive, requiring complete removal of tissue from the joint or testing to failure. Such tests may also require long durations that are impractical for clinical scenarios. Other biomechanical tests of cartilage may be performed *in situ* or in vivo. Such tests may be nondestructive and may be performed within a joint or on an intact section of tissue. Some mechanical tests of the articular cartilage may be difficult to perform. At early stages of osteoarthritis, it may be difficult to distinguish the subtle differences on the surface of the cartilage on a macroscopic level and hence difficult to discern differences between what may be considered normal and early degenerate tissue. Obviously, at the end stage, some regions of joints are devoid of cartilage, and it is not possible to perform any tests on cartilage.

A typical biomechanical test of articular cartilage requires mechanical test instrumentation, or a mechanical spectrometer, that applies displacement (or load) and measures the load (or displacement) response over time. In the displacement-controlled test, the deflection of the load-measuring component should be considered. Ideally, it will not deflect markedly relative to the displacement applied. However, if it does, the amount of deflection can often be corrected for if this quantity is small. A similar principle applies to a load-controlled test, wherein the load imparted by a displacement sensor should ideally be negligible.

Data should be stored for later reduction and analysis. Data storage typically consists of conversion of analog signals, such as voltages from a load cell or displacement transducer, to digital format by an analog-to-digital converter (A/D converter). During this process, the recorded signal may be erroneous if the sampling rate is not high enough. The Nyquist theorem gives the theoretical minimum sampling rate to prevent loss of information and states that an analog signal can be converted to a digital signal without loss of information as long as the sampling interval, T_s, satisfies $T_s < (1/2\ f_{max})$, where f_{max} is the highest frequency. In practice, sampling rates of two to five times the minimum sampling interval are used ***(15)***. The data must also be sampled at a resolution high enough to minimize errors in measurement. A data acquisition system typically has 16-bit resolution, resulting in the ability to measure up to 65,536 discrete levels over a voltage range.

Biomechanical measurements of cartilage should be conducted with the sample bathed in a defined solution. The water content of cartilage is approx 60–85% *(16)*, and that of engineered cartilaginous tissue at early stages of growth is typically even higher *(17)*. For measurements intended to reflect cartilage in its normal state, a physiological solution is typically used, and testing samples under conditions that cause evaporation and dehydration, or conversely, swelling, should be avoided. Phosphate-buffered saline (PBS) supplemented with proteinase inhibitors at physiological pH is typically used to hydrate samples *(18)*. Such inhibitors retard the breakdown of cell and matrix components by enzymes that may be active or become activated during the course of the testing procedure.

The reduction of test data and structural properties to material properties requires information about the sample geometry, such as sample diameter, thickness, width, and length, which provides a basis for normalization. Geometrical measurements can be determined with a contact-sensing dimension (thickness) gage *(12,19)*, although in principle, obtaining dimensions with any noncontact imaging device is appropriate *(20)*. Micrometers that sense electrical contact and microscopes have been used to measure the dimensions of the specimen accurately. When measuring sample dimensions, it is important to consider, especially with very delicate tissue, that mechanical perturbations may cause tissue deflection or even damage.

The poroelastic *(21)* or biphasic model *(11)* has been widely used to assess cartilage material properties. This model assumes the tissue to be composed of a solid and fluid phase. The solid phase consists of the collagen network and proteoglycan gel, and the fluid phase consists of water. Because articular cartilage is composed of interstitial fluid in addition to the extracellular matrix and a sparse population of cells, it exhibits viscoelastic behavior when tested in compression, tension, and shear. When a load is applied to cartilage, the flow of interstitial fluid, which is dependent on cartilage permeability (index of how easily fluid can flow within the tissue), can contribute to the resistance to that load (modulus).

This chapter reviews biomechanical test modalities that can be applied to assess the material properties of cartilage, at length scales ranging from mm down to μm. Cartilage has a number of material properties, some of which are elastic in nature; others involve specimen failure.

1.1. Compression Testing

A common method to assess the compressive properties of cartilage is the uniaxial confined compression test. In this test, typically, a cylindrical tissue

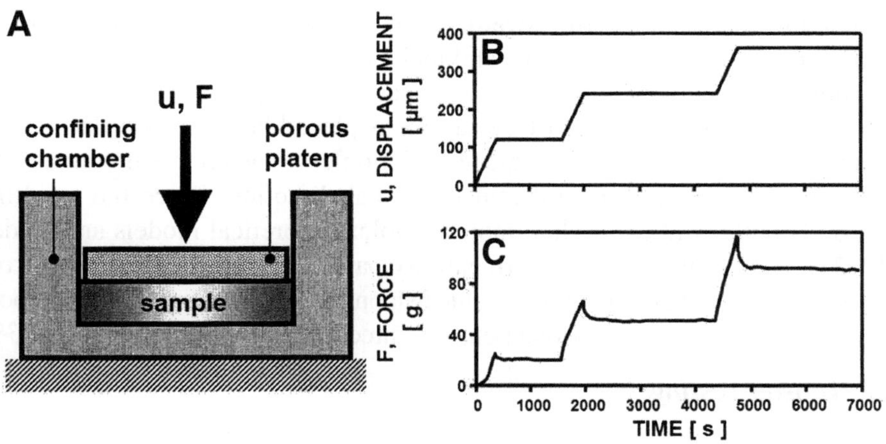

Fig. 1. Typical confined compression stress–relaxation test. **(A)** A cartilage disc is placed in a rigid confining chamber and a displacement, *u*, is applied to the cartilage disc via a porous platen, while measuring the resultant force, *F*. Typical **(B)** applied displacement and **(C)** measured loads from a test of articular cartilage.

sample is placed in a radially confining chamber, usually with an impermeable bottom surface and a porous platen covering the top surface. Relative motion between the platen and bottom surface causes fluid movement, ideally only through the porous platen, with resultant intratissue dynamics being in one dimension (**Fig. 1A**). Since the stiffness of the platen is high compared with the tissue, and the fluid is virtually incompressible, the major mechanism by which the tissue deforms is by exudation of the fluid through the surface that is in contact with the porous platen.

The compression test can be performed with control of either load or displacement. Under load control, the tissue undergoes creep displacement, gradually achieving an equilibrium. Under displacement control (**Fig. 1B**), the load dissipates over time (stress–relaxation), also leading to equilibrium (**Fig. 1C**). The modulus of the tissue can be computed from equilibrium values. From time-varying displacement and load, the permeability of the tissue can be determined by fitting the data to a theoretical model. There are certain advantages to performing a test in displacement control rather than load control. Displacement control allows testing a sample from a true "zero" displacement, which is straightforward to determine. In contrast, load control typically requires application of a nonzero load (and displacement) to initiate a test, and this alteration of sample thickness needs to be considered in reducing data to structural or material properties. Often in load control, only the change in sample thickness relative to an initial state is measured, with the initial state assumed to represent the free swelling state. However, tare loads can impart significant distortion to the tissue and make this assumption erroneous.

Another common method of assessing cartilage properties is the unconfined compression test. Here, a cartilage sample is placed between two flat, impermeable platens that are ideally rigid and frictionless. The sample is compressed and allowed to expand laterally in the radial direction. Since the resulting motion is both axial and radial, more complex theoretical models are needed *(22–27)*. Again, modulus and permeability parameters can be computed from the equilibrium *(22,28–36)* and dynamic responses *(37)*, although moduli in both the axial (compression) and radial (tension) directions may also be estimated *(38)*.

1.2. Tensile Testing

When performing a mechanical test in tension, a cartilage sample is typically extended at a constant dynamic rate of extension (**Fig. 2A**), or it can be extended sequentially by small displacements and allowed to relax to equilibrium states. Articular cartilage exhibits stress-relaxation behavior when tested in tension (**Fig. 2B**). This behavior has been described by quasi-linear viscoelastic theory *(39)*. When cartilage is loaded rapidly, the flow of interstitial fluid, which is dependent on cartilage permeability, can contribute to cartilage resistance to that load. Dynamic tensile experiments can yield stiffness values that are dependent on the interstitial fluid flow *(40)*, and use of these load values can lead to high estimates of intrinsic equilibrium tensile properties. Dynamic tensile experiments are convenient for assessing tissue strength and stiffness, whereas equilibrium tensile tests give measures allowing assessement of the elastic tensile material properties. Typically, human articular cartilage from the femoral condyles can exhibit a ramp modulus of 200 MPa and withstand a stress of 30 MPa before failing *(8)*. In contrast, at equilibrium, the same tissue exhibits an intrinsic tensile modulus of 5 MPa *(7)*. These values are site- and depth-dependent and can vary depending on the structure and content of collagen and glycosaminoglycans in the extracellular matrix *(7,41–43)*. However, for cases in which the cartilage has been eroded, with disruption of cartilage integrity or exposure of bone, a tensile test may not be suitable.

1.3. Shear Testing

An integral part of the function of cartilage is to withstand shear loading. The shear properties measured from simple and torsional tests are thought be measurements of fluid-independent properties of the solid matrix *(44–47)*. Furthermore, other types of shear testing (lap or adhesive shear and interfacial shear tests) may be important in determining properties of cartilage explants or cartilage repair at cartilage–cartilage interfaces.

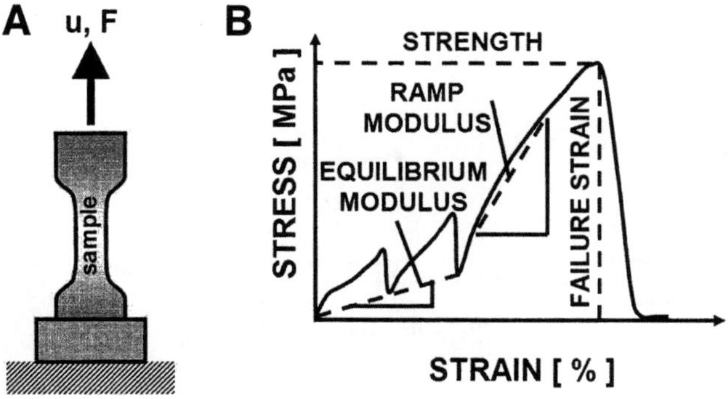

Fig. 2. **(A)** Dog-bone–shaped specimen used in a tensile test are extended at a constant rate while load is measured. **(B)** Equilibrium and dynamic tensile testing. Force and displacement are normalized to cross-sectional area and gage length at 0% strain, respectively, to give stress and strain. The strength, or failure stress, and failure strain is obtained from the dynamic stress–strain data. The ramp modulus is calculated as the slope of the best-fit line between 25 and 75% of the maximum stress. The equilibrium tensile modulus can be obtained from the best-fit line between the three equilibrium data points.

1.3.1. Simple and Torsional Shear

Shear testing of articular cartilage has been conducted in several configurations. Both simple and torsional shear configurations have been used to study static and dynamic shear moduli, or stiffness, properties that describe the ability of the tissue to withstand shear load (**Fig. 3A** and **3B**). Typically, incremental strains of 3–20% are used in these experiments. In dynamic shear measurements, some studies have used low-amplitude shear sinusoids at varying compressive strains ***(46)***, and others have used large-amplitude shear strains to measure the effects of fatigue ***(48)***. Alteration of specific matrix molecules has been shown to affect the dynamic shear modulus, with proteoglycan and collagen fragmentation decreasing the modulus and increased collagen crosslinking increasing the modulus ***(45)***. Shear testing has also been used to determine efficacy of repair tissue at different time points ***(49)***.

1.3.2. Cartilage Adhesion to Cartilage

Several types of testing have been used to assess the capacity of cartilage to repair both in vivo and in vitro. Specifically, direct-tensile, single lap-shear, and push-off tests have been used to test the quality of repair.

A measure of the adhesive strength is the direct-tensile test (American Society of Testing and Materials [ASTM] standard D 5179-98). In this test, samples

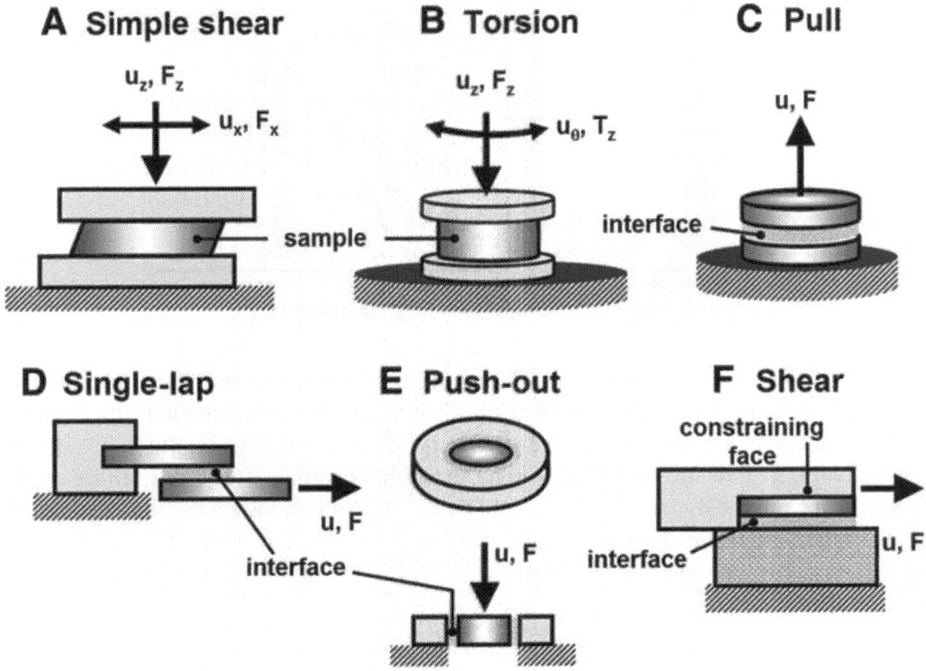

Fig. 3. Shear testing of articular cartilage. **(A)** Simple, **(B)** torsion, **(C)** pull, **(D)** single-lap, **(E)**, push-out, and **(F)** static shear tests. In (A) and (B), a displacement or force is applied to ensure the sample is securely held in place during the shear test. In (C), (D), and (E), the interface between two samples is analyzed by applying a constant rate displacement, *u*, to a sample, and measuring the resultant force, **F**, in the directions applied denoted by the arrows. In (F), the interface strength between the sample and underlying substrate is measured.

are placed in total apposition after addition of adhesive or start of culture. Prior to testing, portions of the cartilage are attached to test clamps. The test clamps are displaced at a low rate, and load is measured during displacement (**Fig. 3C**). The adhesive strength can be determined as the maximum force obtained prior to failure divided by the overlap area. Unlike the other tests of adhesive strength, samples undergoing this test will separate under a different failure mode than in the previous test, leading to possible differences in adhesive strength from samples tested in other manners ***(50)***. This method has been used to evaluate cartilage adhesion following laser soldering ***(51)*** and chondrocytes implanted in devitalized cartilage ***(52)***.

A single lap-shear shear test for cartilage integrative repair has been designed to mimic ASTM testing methods for adhesives (ASTM standard D

3983). In this configuration, cartilage blocks are placed in partial apposition in a specially designed chamber *(53,54)*. Following a period in culture, samples are tested by uniaxial extension (as described in **Subheading 1.2.**) at a low displacement rate (0.5 mm/min), while measuring both load and displacement to assess development of adhesive strength (**Fig. 3D**). The adhesive strength can be determined as the maximum force obtained prior to failure divided by the overlap area. Typically, samples tested in this manner failed at the overlap region and therefore lost the ability to sustain load. Using this type of testing, the effects on repair of collagen synthesis, deposition *(55)*, crosslinking *(56)*, developmental stage *(54)*, matrix properties *(57)*, and depth-dependent properties *(58)* have been elucidated in vitro. In addition, the interfacial strength of cartilage sample following photochemical welding *(59)* and following modulation of collagen crosslinking *(60)* were determined using the lap-shear test.

Push-out tests have been similarly used to assess the efficacy of cartilage repair. In these systems, a cylindrical core is removed from a disk of cartilage using a cylindrical punch. Following this "defect formation," the core and remaining annulus of tissue are placed together with or without adhesives and then cultured for a period of time. Upon testing of samples, the mechanical strength of the disc-annulus interface is tested by applying load on the inner disc while the outer ring is held fixed (**Fig. 3E**). Usually, plungers with a diameter equal in size to the central disc are used to ensure that the properties of the interface region are being tested. The plunger is displaced at a low displacement rate (0.5 mm/min) while measuring load. The adhesive strength is estimated as the maximum force divided by the area of interface. The configuration of this test is very similar to an allograft placed in a cartilage defect in vivo, creating the proper geometry for a clinical situation. However, a frictional force still remains, holding the disc inside the annulus after catastrophic failure of the interface region, perhaps recording higher values for adhesive strength as a result. Using this type of testing, interfacial strength of cartilage constructs *(61)* and enhancement of integration following enzymatic digestion *(62)* have been studied.

1.3.3. Cartilage-Bone Adherence

The osteochondral interface is a significant and still largely uninvestigated region. It is a clinically important region involved in growth and maturation of the joint. It demarcates one edge of the secondary center of ossification. It is also a site of fracture, primarily in the adolescent joint *(63–66)*. Properties of this interface are also relevant to tissue engineering. The osteochondral interface represents one boundary of mature articular cartilage. Normal values for interfacial biomechanical properties also provide a standard of comparison for engineered osteochondral constructs.

Investigation of the interfacial region requires an understanding of the structure of the interface and the properties of the tissues surrounding it. In the immature joint, the osteochondral interface is the junction of the deep cartilage and the subchondral bone, held together by interdigitating "fingers" of bone and cartilage ***(67,68)***. In the mature joint, however, the interfacial region has a different structure, complicated by the formation of a zone of calcified cartilage (ZCC) separating the uncalcified cartilage and bone. The ZCC is a transitional region that has a measured stiffness around 1/10 that of bone and 10–100 times that of cartilage ***(69)*** and is thought to help transmit loads efficiently from the cartilage to the underlying bone. It is bounded on one side by the osteochondral interface with the subchondral bone plate and on the other by the tidemark where the uncalcified cartilage begins. In samples from the mature joint, it is actually the latter of these two that is fractured in tests of the interfacial region ***(64,67,68,70)***.

The properties and dimensions of the tissues surrounding the interface greatly impact the test design for the region. Tests can be designed to avoid failure in the weaker surrounding regions. In the mature human joint, the shear strength of the osteochondral junction is 7.25 ± 1.35 MPa, whereas the full-thickness tensile strength of articular cartilage and the shear strength of the subchondral bone (beneath the subchondral bone plate) are only 3.75 ± 0.75 MPa and 2.45 ± 0.85 Mpa, respectively ***(70)***.

Despite the importance of the interfacial region and probably because of the constraints just discussed, few experiments aimed at determining its properties have been performed to date. Stress at the interface can be measured by a static shear strength apparatus such as that depicted in **Fig. 3F**. A dynamic fracture test created by Flachsmann et al. can be performed with either mixed-mode ***(64)*** or pure-mode II loading ***(67)***.

1.4. Indentation Testing

A typical indentation test is performed on cartilage tissue by compressing a surface (usually articular) of cartilage using a rigid (relative to cartilage) object of known size, shape, and boundary conditions (permeability and friction) (**Fig. 4A**), and then measuring load, displacement, and time (**Fig. 4B** and **C**). The indenter tip size (i.e., diameter) is typically smaller than the cartilage thickness in order to minimize the effect of the rigid underlying bone on the stiffness measurement. Indentation testing has been widely used ***(71–84)*** for characterizing the health and function of cartilage because of the relative ease of the experimental setup as well as the availability of classical ***(85,86)*** and more recent ***(78,87,88)*** mathematical solutions for estimating biomechanical properties of cartilage from indentation test results.

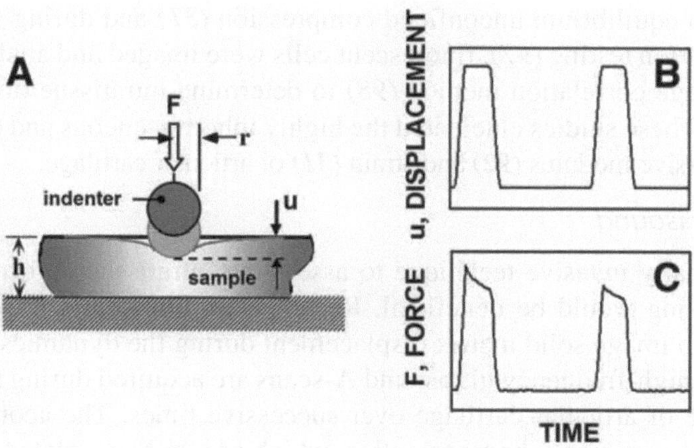

Fig. 4. **(A)** Cross-section schematic of indentation testing using a sphere-ended tip and a displacement-controlled protocol. **(B)** Applied displacement and **(C)** resultant load are illustrated.

1.5. Analysis of Intratissue Deformation

Most experimental studies used to evaluate the mechanical properties of cartilage have relied on controlling or measuring the surface displacement or load of tissue ***(11,89)***. However, these approaches do not allow direct measurement of spatially varying mechanical variables or properties. Theoretical models used to predict the spatial variations in equilibrium and nonequilibrium deformation and strain within a specimen of tissue based on observed spatial variations in composition and structure ***(11,90,91)*** have been difficult to verify because of the lack of a direct measurement method. The determination of intratissue deformation allows analysis of the spatial variation in tissue biomechanical properties.

1.5.1. Microscopy and Image Analysis

The spatial behavior of articular cartilage has been investigated by assessing the intratissue deformation with video microscopy in compression and tensile tests ***(12,20,31,92–94)***. For cartilage deformations that extend over length scales much larger than the size of an individual chondrocyte, the indwelling cells may be useful as intrinsic fiducial markers. The cells are essentially affixed to the extracellular matrix because the chondrocytes are three orders of magnitude greater than the effective pore size of the matrix (20–100 Å) ***(95,96)***. Cells can be localized with a fluorescent dye, visualized by fluorescent microscopy, digitally imaged, and tracked at equilibrium at different levels of compression. In equilibrium unconfined compression *(31)* and during short-duration indentation testing *(97)*, fluorescent cells were imaged and analyzed using a video image correlation method *(98)* to determine intratissue displacement and strain. These studies elucidated the highly inhomogeneous and depth-varying compressive modulus *(92)* and strain *(31)* of articular cartilage.

1.5.2. Ultrasound

A minimally invasive technique to assess the intratissue deformation in a clinical setting would be beneficial. Recently, an ultrasound transducer has been used to image solid matrix displacement during the dynamics of loading *(99)*. Here, high-frequency ultrasound A-scans are acquired during the loading of a sample of articular cartilage over successive times. The acoustic signal picks up the cartilage inhomogeneities, which are, in part, related to the collagen fibrils *(100)*. Using cross-correlation techniques, the displacement of the solid matrix of the tissue can be followed over the successive displacement profiles.

1.6. Friction Testing

There are a number of tissue surfaces in the body that are apposed and slide relative to one another with low friction and wear. In the joints, cartilage slides against cartilage, meniscus, synovium, and ligament. The rolling and sliding motion of articulating cartilage surfaces presents a challenging tribological system to test experimentally and model theoretically *(101)*. Lubrication plays a critical role in most bearing systems. In general, lubricants act at surfaces to reduce friction, heat, and wear. The molecular basis for the remarkable tribological behavior of tissue surfaces in the joint is unknown. Recent studies have focused on and implicated two main classes of molecules, lubricin/superficial zone protein *(102–108)* and surface-active phospholipids *(109–111)*. The exact role of these molecules in mediating boundary lubrication remains unclear.

A variety of in vitro mechanical test systems have been developed to determine friction coefficients, μ, and thus to characterize the effectiveness of lubrication as well as lubrication mechanisms. The tests typically involve application of a compressive force (W) to ensure contact between the opposing surfaces, application of a transverse or torsional displacement to one surface, and measurement of the resultant transverse force (F) or torque. For transverse motion, $\mu = F/W$. For torsional motion, torque is converted to an equivalent transverse force, with a correction factor for the effective radius that depends on the sample geometry *(112)*. Normal articular cartilage has a low μ, approx 0.001–0.05 *(112–114)*.

The test configurations for assessing friction have certain advantages and disadvantages. Typically, putative lubricants are in test solutions or applied to sample surfaces. Intact joints are tested with pendulum ("arthrotripsometer") instruments ***(113–119)*** (**Fig. 5A**). These have the advantage of retaining the most realistic, but also most complex, geometry; the large contact areas can make fluid exudation paths, and thus characteristic time constants, very long. Excised articular cartilage (in the form of osteochondral fragments) and noncartilage materials are tested in instruments that apply linear translation or rotation (**Fig. 5B** and **C**). Excised cartilage has often been tested in contact with glass ***(107,108,111,117,120–124)*** or metal ***(125)***, and lubricants have often been tested with latex against glass ***(104,126–129)*** (**Fig. 5D**). Only rarely have lubricants been examined with cartilage on cartilage ***(112)***. In linear translation, both fluid film and boundary lubrication are generally operative. On the other hand, in the rotational configuration ***(112)***, boundary lubrication predominates (since the same cartilage surfaces remain in contact), and putative lubricants can be examined in a realistic cartilage-on-cartilage scenario. The annular geometry results in the sliding velocity being approximately constant for the contacting cartilage surfaces.

The following sections describe methods that may be used to perform selected tests to assess the biomechanical properties of cartilage. Some materials are used for many tests, and some are specific to the test being described. The intent of this section is to provide a basis for testing, and the equipment is not limited to that listed here.

2. Materials

2.1. Tissue Harvest

1. Bovine knee.
2. Table vise.
3. Instruments: scalpel, forceps, squirt bottle, saw blade.
4. Autopsy saw.
5. PBS, pH 7.4 (Sigma).
6. Sledge microtome (Microm HM440E).
7. Contact-sensing micrometer (Mitutoyo) ***(12)***.

2.2. General Materials

1. Proteinase inhibitors (Sigma):
   a. 1 m*M* Phenylmethylsulfonyl fluoride.
   b. 2 m*M* Disodium ethylenediamine tetraacetate.
   c. 5 m*M* Benzamidine-HCl.
   d. 10 m*M* *N*-ethylmaleimide.

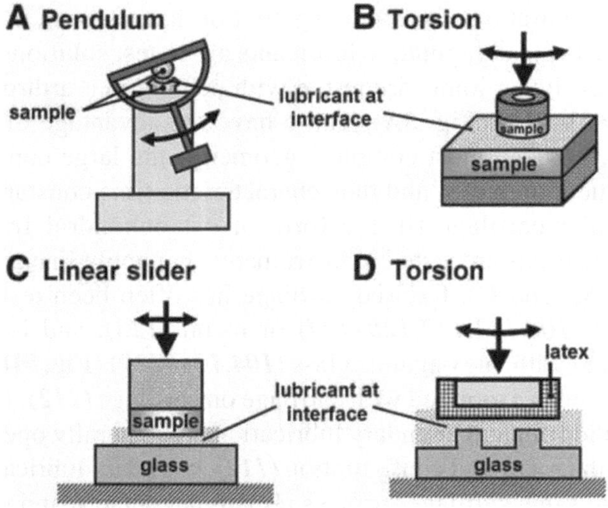

Fig. 5. Test modalities to assess lubrication function of cartilage and other materials. Cartilage can be tested in **(A)** pendulum **(B)** torsion, or **(C)** linear slider test scenarios. Alternatively, lubricants can be tested in a **(D)** torsion test between two nonbiological samples.

2. Mechanical spectrometer (e.g., from Biosyntech, Enduratec, IMASS, Instron, MTS).
3. Hydration system (pump).

2.3. Compression Specific Materials

1. Cylindrical punch.
2. Confining chambers.
3. Porous platen.
4. Loading plunger.

2.4. Tensile-Specific Materials

1. India ink.
2. Pin.
3. Custom dogbone-shaped punch.
4. Tensile clamps.

2.5. Shear-Specific Materials

1. Platens for holding tissue in place.
2. Horizontal actuator (e.g., from Newport).
3. Multiaxis load-cell (e.g., from Sensotec).
4. Tensile clamps.

2.6. Indentation Specific Materials

1. Indenter tip.
   a. material: solid or permeable stainless steel (pore size of ~1 μm).
   b. Plane-ended or hemisphere-ended cylinder.
   c. Approximately 1 mm diameter; aspect ratio (radius/cartilage thickness) must be tailored in order to avoid excessive "thickness effect."
2. 6 Degrees-of-freedom stage for sample positioning.
3. Displacement actuator/transducer: 1–2-mm range; 1-μm resolution.
4. Load cell: dependent on indenter diameter and the amount of load/displacement being applied. For a 1-mm-diameter plane-ended indenter tip displacing approx 300 μm from the tissue surface, approx 1 kg load can be expected as the upper range.
5. Time resolution: for short-time response, 1-ms resolution; for long-term responses, 1-s resolution should suffice.

2.7. Intratissue Deformation Analysis Specific

1. Fluorescent DNA dye Hoechst 33258 (Sigma).
2. Microcompression chamber.
3. Inverted microscope with mercury lamp for fluorescent microscopy, 4,6-diamino-2-phenylindole (DAPI) filter, and attached video camera.
4. Image acquisition program (NIH Image).

3. Methods

3.1. General Sample Preparation

1. Mount the knee joint in the table vise.
2. Using the autopsy saw, prepare osteochondral blocks approx 10 mm wide × 10 mm long × 10 mm tall, taking care to irrigate the tissue continuously during the cutting process.
3. Mount the osteochondral block into the clamp of the microtome and prepare cartilage of desired thickness, again keeping the tissue moist during the preparation process.

3.2. Generalized Confined Compression Stress–Relaxation Testing Procedures

3.2.1. Sample Preparation

1. From an osteochondral core or block, prepare a flat, plane-parallel section of tissue that is of desired thickness with a sledge microtome (*see* **Note 1**).
2. Prepare a cylindrical disk of desired diameter using a thin-walled cylindrical punch, taking care to enter the tissue perpendicular to the flat surface.
3. Measure the thickness of the test sample at locations along the circumference and at selected locations in the middle of the sample (*see* **Note 2**).

3.2.2. Stress–Relaxation Test

1. Set up the zero position of the actuator.
2. Place the sample in a radially confining chamber while submerged in the PBS solution and position the sample at the known thickness offset from the defined zero position.
3. Place a porous platen on top of the sample. The platen will apply the compression to the sample, while allowing fluid to flow freely out of the tissue (**Fig. 1A**).
4. From the known thickness, slowly bring the plunger into contact with the platen, relative to the zero position.
5. Apply a slow constant strain rate to compress the sample, and allow to relax for the appropriate time. Record data for the applied displacement and resultant load. Repeat as necessary to obtain a series of stress and strain points.
6. The duration of the test is governed by the characteristic time $[h^2/(4H_Ak_p)]$. In a test such as the uniaxial confined compression test, this is dictated by the thickness, h, of the sample. A doubling of the thickness will result in 4× the test time; decreases in the aggregate modulus (H_A) or permeability (k_p) will increase the relaxation time.

3.2.3. Parameter Estimation: Confined Compression Stress–Relaxation Experiments

Load should be normalized to the cross-sectional area of the disk, transforming it into stress. The displacement should be normalized to the height of the sample at 0% strain to transform it into strain. Two material constants that are commonly used to describe the mechanical properties of articular cartilage are the aggregate modulus, H_A, and the permeability, k_p. These parameters may be estimated from a confined compression stress–relaxation experiment. For a confined compression test, H_A describes the stiffness of the tissue such that, for a given applied strain, ε, the stress, σ, in the direction of the strain is equal to $H_A\varepsilon$. The permeability, k_p, represents the resistance to fluid flow through the solid matrix that may arise from frictional drag owing to solid-fluid interactions. A large value of k_p corresponds to a low resistance to fluid flow, whereas a small value of k_p corresponds to a high resistance to fluid flow. In a stress–relaxation experiment, smaller values of k_p lead to greater relaxation times to steady-state equilibrium. A direct measurement of k_p can be obtained from a 1D permeation experiment ***(130)***.

In one possible confined compression protocol, a cylindrical cartilage specimen is placed in a rigid confining chamber and is loaded via a rigid, permeable, porous platen that allows fluid to exude as the solid matrix is compressed. The other end of the specimen is placed against a rigid, impermeable platen. For stress–relaxation, displacement control is used so that a constant displacement rate, V_0, is applied during the loading phase ($0 \leq t \leq t_0$) followed by a fixed displacement ($u_0 = V_0 t_0$) during the relaxation phase ($t \geq t_0$). **Figure 1B** and **C** shows typical plots of applied displacement vs time and measured load vs time for three consecutive stress–relaxation cycles. At equilibrium, the total tissue compressive strain is $\varepsilon_{eq} = u_0/h$, where h is the specimen height. When the applied displacement rate and total displacement are small (e.g., a 10% total tissue strain applied over 1000 s), the linear biphasic model proposed ***(11)*** may be used to provide reasonable estimates of H_A and k_p. Although the mechanical properties of cartilage have been shown to be depth-dependent ***(12)***, it is common to assume that the tissue is homogeneous in order to obtain "depth-averaged" values.

Using the linear biphasic model, a governing partial differential equation for the solid matrix displacement can be derived and solved to obtain the displacement as a function of the depth coordinate and time ***(11)***. Letting z be the depth coordinate with z = 0 corresponding to the specimen's free-draining surface and $z = h$ corresponding to the specimen's impermeable surface, the solution for the solid matrix strain can be shown to equal ***(130)***:

$$\varepsilon(z,t) = \begin{cases} \dfrac{V_0 t_0}{h}\left[-\dfrac{t}{t_0} - \dfrac{1}{R^2}\left(\dfrac{z^2}{2h^2} - \dfrac{z}{h} + \dfrac{1}{3}\right) + \displaystyle\sum_{n=1}^{\infty} \dfrac{2}{n^2\pi^2R^2} e^{-(n\pi R)^2 t/t_0} \cos\left(\dfrac{n\pi z}{h}\right)\right], 0 \leq t \leq t_0 \\ \dfrac{V_0 t_0}{h}\left[-1 + \displaystyle\sum_{n=1}^{\infty} \dfrac{2}{n^2\pi^2R^2}\left(1 - e^{(n\pi R)^2}\right) e^{-(n\pi R)^2 t/t_0} \cos\left(\dfrac{n\pi z}{h}\right)\right], t \geq t_0 \end{cases} \quad (1)$$

during the ramp and relaxation phases, respectively, where $R^2 = H_A k t_0/h^2$ and $\varepsilon(z,t)$ signifies that the strain ε depends on both depth, z, and time, t. At steady-state equilibrium (i.e., as $t \rightarrow \infty$ in **Eq. 1**), the steady-state strain is recovered (i.e., $\varepsilon_{eq} = -u_0/h$, where the negative sign indicates compression).

The stress in the solid matrix at the free-draining surface (i.e., $z = 0$) can be obtained from the stress–strain relation

$$\sigma(0,t) = H_A \varepsilon(0,t). \quad (2)$$

At steady-state, the equilibrium stress is homogeneous and is determined from

$$\sigma_{eq} = H_A \varepsilon_{eq} = -H_A u_0/h. \quad (3)$$

Equations 1–3 can be used to estimate H_A and k as follows. For a single stress–relaxation cycle for which a total displacement u_0 is applied, the experimental solid surface stress is calculated as the load cell output, $F(t)$, divided by the cross-sectional area of the specimen, A:

$$\sigma(0,t) = F(t)/A. \quad (4)$$

This is used to calculate the equilibrium stress $\sigma_{eq} = F_{eq}/A$ where F_{eq} is the load cell value at equilibrium. Since this must equal **Eq. 3**, the aggregate modulus is calculated as:

$$H_A = (F_{eq}\, h)/(Au_0). \tag{5}$$

For cartilage, H_A is typically in the range 0.3–1.3 MPa (1 MPa = 1×10^6 N/m^2). For a series of consecutive stress–relaxation cycles, H_A can be determined from a best-fit linear regression of the equilibrium stress vs the equilibrium strain values using **Eq. 3**.

Once H_A has been determined, the permeability constant can be estimated from the experimental solid surface stress vs time data. A best-fit regression of the theoretical solid surface stress $\sigma(0,t)$ obtained from **Eqs. 1** and **2** and the experimental solid surface stress (**Eq. 4**) yields the optimal value of k. Various regression methods have been used to determine k in this manner. Perhaps the simplest method is to calculate the theoretical solution (**Eq. 2**) for different values of k and choose the value of k that results in the highest correlation coefficient (R^2) between the theoretical solution and the experimental data. Typical values of k for articular cartilage are in the range 1×10^{-15} to 1×10^{-16} m^2/(Pa·s).

Many refinements to the linear isotropic biphasic model have been proposed to provide a more accurate description of the mechanical properties of cartilage. For example, even for small applied displacements, the strains produced near the free-draining surface can be large enough to necessitate a large-deformation analysis. In that type of analysis, the solid matrix is modeled as a nonlinear elastic solid and the permeability is modeled as a nonlinear function of the solid matrix strain. Typically, two material constants are used to represent the stress–strain equation of the solid matrix, and two material constants are used to represent the strain-dependent permeability function. Recent papers have employed such nonlinear models for bovine articular cartilage and for human annulus fibrosus ***(131,132)***, both of which used consecutive stress–relaxation cycles. In an alternative approach, the strain-dependent permeability function was determined by superimposing small-strain oscillations on various static equilibrium offset strains ***(91)***.

Also, video microscopy has shown that the tissue strain field for full-thickness articular cartilage tested in confined compression is nonhomogeneous ***(12)***. Since the governing equations of the biphasic theory demand that the solid matrix stress be homogeneous, this observation reveals that the aggregate modulus H_A depends on depth from the articular surface. A nonhomogeneous biphasic model has been used to solve the confined compression stress-relaxation problem ***(133)*** to account for this tissue inhomogeneity. Other refinements include the modeling of the tissue's tension-compression nonlinearity ***(38)*** and the intrinsic viscoelasticity of the solid matrix ***(134)***.

3.3. Tensile Testing Procedures

3.3.1. Sample Preparation

1. Obtain cartilage on bone samples in the form of osteochondral cores or blocks.
2. Determine orientation of the splitline pattern at the regions near the edge of the sample (*see* **Note 3**).
3. Using a microtome, obtain a cartilage section approx 250 μm thick.
4. Prepare a dogbone-shaped specimen from the cartilage section. The taper allows the loads to be concentrated in the gage region, rather than at the clamps (**Fig. 2A**) (*see* **Note 4**).
5. Accurately measure the thickness and width of the specimen along the gage region (*see* **Note 5**).

3.3.2. Mounting Test Sample

1. Adjust the distance between the materials testing machine clamps to the proper gage distance (*see* **Note 6**).
2. Clamp the sample in the mechanical testing machine, ensuring that the sample is aligned parallel to the axis of tension and not twisted. Any slack in the sample will be removed later.
3. Hydrate the sample with PBS and proteinase inhibitors.
4. Adjust load transducer to zero reading.
5. Slowly extend the sample to desired preload (typically 2–5 g). This is to remove any slack in the sample. This should be considered the point of 0% strain.
6. Apply a prescribed tensile load/displacement protocol.

3.3.3. Specific Tensile Test Protocol

3.3.3.1. Dynamic Tensile Test

1. Apply a constant strain rate of approx 5 mm/min ***(8)***.
2. Obtain data for the load and displacement (assumed to be the clamp-to-clamp distance) of the specimen every second until the specimen fails. The load should increase with displacement approximately linearly, with the exception of the toe region, until failure when the load falls to zero.

3.3.3.2. Equilibrium Tensile Loading Protocol

1. Apply a constant strain rate until the specimen reaches 10% strain.
2. Allow the sample to relax until it reaches an equilibrium state of loading. The duration of the test is governed by the characteristic time ($h^2/E_t k_p$), where E_t is the equilibrium tensile modulus.
3. Apply a constant strain rate again until the specimen reaches 20% strain.

4. Allow the sample to relax until it reaches an equilibrium state of loading as defined in **step 2**. The load should increase with displacement approximately linearly up to each strain level and then decrease as the sample relaxes.

3.3.3.3. Combined Equilibrium and Dynamic Tensile Loading Protocol

The dynamic and equilibrium loading protocol can be combined. After the specimen has reached equilibrium after the 20% strain level, a constant strain rate of 5 mm/min can be applied until the specimen fails. The load should increase with displacement approximately linearly, then decrease as the sample relaxes at each equilibrium strain level, and then increase linearly until the sample fails (**Fig. 2B**).

3.3.4. Data Reduction

The data can be reduced to provide several indices of tensile properties. From the load-displacement curves, stress–strain plots can be obtained (**Fig. 2B**). Load is normalized to the cross-sectional area of the sample transforming it into stress. The displacement is normalized to the gage length of the sample at 0% strain to transform it into strain. From the dynamic stress–strain data, stress at failure, or strength, and strain at failure can be reported. The slope of the best-fit line between 0 and 100% of the maximum stress can be reported as the dynamic stiffness. From the equilibrium stress–strain data, the slope of the best-fit line between the equilibrium stress and strain data points can be reported as the tensile or equilibrium modulus.

3.4. Shear Testing Methods

3.4.1. Sample Preparation

1. Obtain cartilage on bone samples in the form of osteochondral cores or blocks.
2. Using a microtome, prepare a cartilage section of desired thickness.
3. For simple shear, a square or rectangular block of cartilage can be used. For torsional tests, a disc of cartilage should be prepared according to **Subheading 3.2.1.**
4. Measure thickness at multiple points and average.

3.4.2. Mounting Test Sample

1. Place the sample on a porous surface to ensure nonslip contact (*see* **Note 7**).
2. Apply a small compressive load or displacement to the cartilage sample, which is either made to adhere to the actuator or held in place with sandpaper to increase the frictional coefficient between the cartilage and actuator to prevent slippage.
3. Hydrate the sample with PBS and proteinase inhibitors.
4. Apply displacement perpendicular to the compressive load, either in a lateral shearing motion, or in a torsional motion (**Fig. 3A** and **B**).

3.4.3. Data Reduction

1. From load and displacement data, and tissue geometry, determine tissue stress and strain. Applied shear strain can be determined by dividing the displacement applied by the length of the sample over which it is displaced. This can be thought of as a percentage change. Tissue stress can be determined by resolving the forces into the tissue coordinate system (rectangular for simple shear, cylindrical for torsional shear) and dividing each force by the area perpendicular to that force.
2. Calculate a shear modulus for the given test using the stress and strain data. In general, the shear modulus can be determined by the stress divided by the strain at any given time point. Often, stress of the tissue at equilibrium (after stress relaxation has occurred) is used. In addition, the shear modulus can be determined as a slope of a regression line through points on a stress–strain plot at various shear strain levels.

3.5. Static Shear Strength Test

See **refs. *64*, *67***, and ***68***.

3.5.1. Sample Preparation

1. Obtain osteochondral blocks (>5 mm long and wide) with flat articular surfaces.
2. Make a pair of full-thickness cartilage cuts, spaced 2.5 mm apart, across the width of the block and centered along its length.
3. Perform a second pair of cuts, centered along block's width and perpendicular to the earlier cuts, marking a 2.5 × 2.5 mm cartilage square.
4. Remove the cartilage surrounding the square down to the level of the subchondral bone.

3.5.2. Shear Test

1. Secure the block in the load frame and fit an L-shaped bracket over the test square.
2. Load the sample by pulling the bracket parallel to the surface of the block at a rate of 0.5 mm/s until failure occurs. (**Fig. 3F**)
3. Record load vs displacement data during the test.

3.5.3. Data Reduction

Failure stress is determined as the maximum load divided by the area of the test square (*see* **Note 8**).

3.6. Indentation Methods

3.6.1. Sample Preparation

1. Obtain testing samples in the form of osteochondral blocks or explants, taking care to ensure that the obtained sample is satisfactory using the guidelines given in **Subheading 3.1.** (*see* **Note 9**).

3. Measure the thickness of the cartilage by optical (osteochondral block), contact-sensing (explant), or needle-penetration (both) methods (*see* **Note 10**).
4. Keep the sample hydrated throughout testing.

3.6.2. Sample Alignment and Preloading

1. Clamp the sample onto a stage, and position it such that the cartilage surface of the sample is orthogonal to the axis of loading by the indenter.
2. Lower the indenter until it is in contact with the cartilage surface while not applying excessive load.
3. It may be advisable to apply a small amount of load (preload) at this point, to make sure that a good contact is established between indenter and the sample.

3.6.3. Testing Samples in Indentation

1. Load control: a predefined load is applied at a specified loading rate (usually very fast), and resultant displacement, along with time, is measured.
2. Displacement control: a predefined displacement (**Fig. 4A**) is applied at a specified displacement rate, and the resultant load, along with time (**Fig. 4B** and **C**), is measured. Displacement control may be preferred when it is difficult to apply a predefined load (i.e., hand-held applications).
3. For a short-term test, typical loading duration is approx 1 s; a long-term test may utilize a loading duration of 15 min or more.

3.6.4. Specific Indentation Protocols

3.6.4.1. Short-Duration Load Control Protocol Example

1. Apply a preload equivalent to stress (load normalized to largest cross-sectional area of the indenter) of 25 kPa for 30 s. Each load will be applied in 0.4 s
2. Apply test loads, each of 1-s duration followed by 30 s of preload. The test loads are three sets of four load magnitudes, generating additional (to preload) 25, 50, 100, and 200 kPa of stress.

3.6.4.2. Short-Duration Displacement Control Protocol Example

1. Find contact by lowering the indenter until a small load (~1 g) is measured.
2. Apply test displacement (at 500 μm/s) ramps, each of 1 s duration followed by 30 s of displacement. The test displacements are three sets of four displacement magnitudes of 25, 50, 100, and 200 μm.

3.6.4.3. Long-Duration Load Control Protocol Example

1. Apply a preload equivalent to stress of 25 kPa for 30 s. Each load will be applied for 0.4 s.
2. Apply a test load equivalent to 100 kPa stress and allow sample to equilibrate for 1000 s, during which the displacement is measured.

3.6.5. Data Reduction

1. Short-duration tests: for load-controlled tests, the jumps in displacement at the onset and release of the test load can be measured and averaged for each load. For displacement-controlled tests, the peak loads during the on-ramp phase of each test displacement are measured and averaged for each displacement. These data may be reduced further: (1) displacement-load (or vice versa) can be linearly fit to obtain apparent stiffness; or (2) using a theoretical equation and assuming certain properties of cartilage *(87)*, intrinsic properties such as Young's modulus can be estimated.
2. Long-duration tests: from the applied load and time-dependent displacement behavior, biphasic properties of the sample can be determined *(78,88)*.

3.7. Video Microscopy

3.7.1. Sample Preparation

1. From an osteochondral block of tissue, prepare a section of full-thickness articular cartilage approx 10 mm long × 2 mm wide × 10 mm tall while under hydration with PBS and proteinase inhibitors.
2. Incubate tissue in PBS, proteinase inhibitors, and 1 μg/mL Hoechst 33258 dye for 3 h at room temperature to stain cellular DNA.

3.7.2. Mechanical Compression

1. Place the sample into the microcompression chamber *(12,92)*.
2. Acquire the fluorescent image in the uncompressed reference state.
3. Compress sample to desired offset compression level and allow to reach equilibrium.
4. Acquire the fluorescent image in compressed state. Repeat as necessary.

3.7.3. Image Processing

1. Create a binary (black and white) image of each fluorescent image.
2. Divide the tissue into discrete layers.
3. Locate centroids of 40–60 cell nuclei through the depth of the tissue that appear in each of the acquired images.
4. Track the displacement from the uncompressed reference state to each of the compressed states.

3.7.4. Data Analysis

1. The slope of the linear regression in each layer will yield an estimate of the strain, $\Delta u/\Delta z$, with the z-direction being from the articular surface to the subchondral bone.

4. Notes

1. Compression sample preparation.
   a. Thinner samples (<0.25 mm) are generally more difficult to test, as the stiffness and compliance of the test frame may affect outcome measurements.
   b. The walls of the cylindrical disk should be perpendicular to the two faces of the sample. This will help ensure complete confinement of the sample during loading.
2. Thickness measurements: For displacement control experiments, thickness measurements are critical. Errors in measurement will result in errors in applied displacement, since the reference point of the surface will not be in the proper location.
3. Tensile sample preparation.
   a. A splitline pattern can be observed in human articular cartilage ***(135)***, which is thought to follow the predominant direction of the collagen fibers at the surface ***(136,137)***. By assessing the splitline pattern at the edge, the region from which the tensile test strip will be obtained will not be damaged.
   b. The strength and stiffness of articular cartilage are greater when the axis of tension is parallel rather than perpendicular to the splitline direction or surface collagen ***(42,138)***. Specimens should be tested such that the axis of tension is parallel to the splitline direction in order to standardize sample preparation and optimize specimen loading. The determination of splitline direction in osteoarthritic samples may be more difficult as the surface zone may have eroded away.
   c. Sample dimensions can vary depending on the mechanical testing machine, clamping mechanism, and desired loads and displacements.
4. Thickness measurements should be made accurately. Load will be normalized to the thickness to obtain stress.
5. The dogbone or dumbell-shape is commonly used in engineering tests as established by the ASTM and allows the central "gage" region to experience uniform tensile stress, the magnitude of which is much greater than the stress at the enlarged ends, so that the sample fails in the gage region. Sample size can be as large as 32 mm long × 10 mm wide × 200 mm thick overall, with a central gage region of 6.35 mm long × 1.6 mm wide ***(42)*** or as small as was stated above. However, the sample width, thickness, and length (clamp-to-clamp distance) in this gage region should be accurately measured, as they are used later to normalize the load and displacement to stress and strain, respectively.
6. Specimen clamping.
   a. In the method described above, it is assumed that the clamp-to-clamp distance is the length the sample has extended plus the initial gap distance. However, should the sample slip during the test this might not be correct. Another method of measuring strain might be to mark points on the sample and monitor the change in distance of those points during the test using a camera ***(139)***.
   b. When clamping the sample, it is important to consider the amount of applied force on the sample ends. Although it is important that the sample does not

slip during the test, it is also important not to crush the sample in clamps or alter the mechanical properties of the tissue. Spring-loaded clamps offer variable clamping force. One could glue the sample to the clamps, but this may alter the mechanical properties of the tissue. The addition of sandpaper to the clamps could offer extra resistance to slippage.

7. Shear lap sample preparation.
   a. Gluing of the cartilage surfaces may affect the mechanical properties of the tissue by stiffening a portion of the cartilage at the surface.
   b. In addition, many shear testing protocols use full-thickness cartilage explants, which may have different shear properties from those from cartilage samples from varying depths, since cartilage has many depth-varying properties, including other mechanical properties such as compression ***(12)*** and tension ***(140)***.
8. There is some question as to whether pure shear is obtained using this test setup. Additionally, there is a possibility of a "peeling" effect of the sample accompanying shearing.
9. Indentation sample requirements and considerations.
   a. In-plane boundary condition: there should be enough tissue peripheral to the indentation site. With the indentation site at the center of the sample, the sample diameter should be at least three to four times the indenter tip diameter to avoid "edge effects" ***(141)***.
   b. Cartilage thickness significantly affects the measured stiffness of the sample ***(87)***. It should be measured whenever possible.
   c. Typically, cartilage is modeled as a layer of material bonded to a rigid bottom (useful for *in situ* conditions). For explants or tissue-engineered material, different (unbonded) boundary condition must be taken into account during analysis ***(142,143)***.
10. The load and displacement measurements can be normalized to thickness.

References

1. Maroudas, A. (1968) Physicochemical properties of cartilage in the light of ion exchange theory. *Biophys. J.* **8,** 575–595.
2. Maroudas, A. (1976) Balance between swelling pressure and collagen tension in normal and degenerate cartilage. *Nature* **260,** 808–809.
3. Basser, P. J., Schneiderman, R., Bank, R., Wachtel, E., and Maroudas, A. (1998) Mechanical properties of the collagen network in human articular cartilage as measured by osmotic stress technique. *Arch. Biochem. Biophys.* **351,** 207–219.
4. Williamson, A. K., Chen, A. C., and Sah, R. L. (2001) Compressive properties and function-composition relationships of developing bovine articular cartilage. *J. Orthop. Res.* **19,** 1113–1121.
5. Williamson, A. K., Masuda, K., Chen, A. C., Thonar, E. J.-M. A., and Sah, R. L. (2003) Tensile mechanical properties of bovine articular cartilage: variations with growth and relationships to collagen network components. *J. Orthop. Res.* **21,** 872–880.

6. Armstrong, C. G. and Mow, V. C. (1982) Variations in the intrinsic mechanical properties of human articular cartilage with age, degeneration, and water content. *J. Bone Joint Surg. Am.* **64,** 88–94.
7. Akizuki, S., Mow, V. C., Muller, F., Pita, J. C., Howell, D. S., and Manicourt, D. H. (1986) Tensile properties of human knee joint cartilage: I. influence of ionic conditions, weight bearing, and fibrillation on the tensile modulus. *J. Orthop. Res.* **4,** 379–392.
8. Kempson, G. E. (1982) Relationship between the tensile properties of articular cartilage from the human knee and age. *Ann. Rheum. Dis.* **41,** 508–511.
9. Maroudas, A., Katz, E. P., Wachtel, E. J., Mizrahi, J., and Soudry, M. (1986) Physico-chemical properties and functional behavior of normal and osteoarthritic human cartilage, in *Articular Cartilage Biochemistry* (Kuettner, K., Schleyerbach, R., and Hascall, V. C., eds.), Raven, New York, pp. 311–329.
10. Sah, R. L. (2002) The biomechanical faces of articular cartilage, in *The Many Faces of Osteoarthritis* (Kuettner, K. E. and Hascall, V. C., eds.), Raven, New York, pp. 409–422.
11. Mow, V. C., Kuei, S. C., Lai, W. M., and Armstrong, C. G. (1980) Biphasic creep and stress relaxation of articular cartilage in compression: theory and experiment. *J. Biomech. Eng.* **102,** 73–84.
12. Schinagl, R. M., Gurskis, D., Chen, A. C., and Sah, R. L. (1997) Depth-dependent confined compression modulus of full-thickness bovine articular cartilage. *J. Orthop. Res.* **15,** 499–506.
13. Jones, W. R., Ting-Beall, H. P., Lee, G. M., Kelley, S. S., Hochmuth, R. M., and Guilak, F. (1999) Alterations in the Young's modulus and volumetric properties of chondrocytes isolated from normal and osteoarthritic human cartilage. *J. Biomech.* **32,** 119–127.
14. Buschmann, M. D. and Grodzinsky, A. J. (1995) A molecular model of proteoglycan-associated electrostatic forces in cartilage mechanics. *J. Biomech. Eng.* **117,** 179–192.
15. Schwarz, S. E. and Oldham, W. G. (1993) *Electrical Engineering: An Introduction*, 2nd ed. Harcourt Brace Jovanovich, Fort Worth, TX.
16. Venn, M. F. and Maroudas, A. (1977) Chemical composition and swelling of normal and osteoarthritic femoral head cartilage I: chemical composition. *Ann. Rheum. Dis.* **36,** 121–129.
17. Waldman, S. D., Spiteri, C. G., Grynpas, M. D., Pilliar, R. M., and Kandel, R. A. (2003) Long-term intermittent shear deformation improves the quality of cartilaginous tissue formed in vitro. *J. Orthop. Res.* **21,** 590–596.
18. Frank, E. H., Grodzinsky, A. J., Koob, T. J., and Eyre, D. R. (1987) Streaming potentials: a sensitive index of enzymatic degradation in articular cartilage. *J. Orthop. Res.* **5,** 497–508.
19. Buschmann, M. D., Gluzband, Y. A., Grodzinsky, A. J., Kimura, J. H., and Hunziker, E. B. (1992) Chondrocytes in agarose culture synthesize a mechanically functional extracellular matrix. *J. Orthop. Res.* **10,** 745–758.

20. Schinagl, R. M., Ting, M. K., Price, J. H., and Sah, R. L. (1996) Video microscopy to quantitate the inhomogeneous equilibrium strain within articular cartilage during confined compression. *Ann. Biomed. Eng.* **24,** 500–512.
21. Frank, E. H. and Grodzinsky, A. J. (1987) Cartilage electromechanics-II. A continuum model of cartilage electrokinetics and correlation with experiments. *J. Biomech.* **20,** 629–639.
22. Kwan, M. K., Lai, W. M., and Mow, V. C. (1984) Fundamentals of fluid transport through cartilage in compression. *Ann. Biomed. Eng.* **12,** 537–558.
23. Li, L. P., Buschmann, M. D. and Shirazi-Adl, A. (2000) A fibril reinforced nonhomogeneous poroelastic model for articular cartilage: inhomogeneous response in unconfined compression. *J. Biomech.* **33,** 1533–1541.
24. DiSilvestro, M. R., Zhu, Q., and Suh, J. K. (2001) Biphasic poroviscoelastic simulation of the unconfined compression of articular cartilage: II—Effect of variable strain rates. *J. Biomech. Eng.* **123,** 198–200.
25. DiSilvestro, M. R., Zhu, Q., Wong, M., Jurvelin, J. S., and Suh, J. K. (2001). Biphasic poroviscoelastic simulation of the unconfined compression of articular cartilage: I—Simultaneous prediction of reaction force and lateral displacement. *J. Biomech. Eng.* **123,** 191–197.
26. Korhonen, R. K., Laasanen, M. S., Toyras, J., et al. (2002) Comparison of the equilibrium response of articular cartilage in unconfined compression, confined compression and indentation. *J. Biomech.* **35,** 903–909.
27. Li, L., Soulhat, J., Buschmann, M. D., and Shirazi-Adl, A. (1999) Nonlinear analysis of cartilage in unconfined ramp compression using a fibril reinforced poroelastic model. *Clin. Biomech.* **14,** 673–682.
28. Armstrong, C. G., Lai, W. M., and Mow, V. C. (1984) An analysis of the unconfined compression of articular cartilage. *J. Biomech. Eng.* **106,** 165–173.
29. Fortin, M., Soulhat, J., Shirazi-Adl, A., Hunziker, E. B., and Buschmann, M. D. (2000) Unconfined compression of articular cartilage. Nonlinear behavior and comparison with a fibril-reinforced biphasic model. *J. Biomech. Eng.* **122,** 189–195.
30. Bursac, P. M., Obitz, T. W., Eisenberg, S. R., and Stamenovic, D. (1999). Confined and unconfined stress relaxation of cartilage: appropriateness of a transversely isotropic analysis. *J. Biomech.* **32,** 1125–1130.
31. Wang, C. C., Deng, J. M., Ateshian, G. A., and Hung, C. T. (2002) An automated approach for direct measurement of two-dimensional strain distributions within articular cartilage under unconfined compression. *J. Biomech. Eng.* **124,** 557–567.
32. Wang, C. C., Chahine, N. O., Hung, C. T., and Ateshian, G. A. (2003) Optical determination of anisotropic material properties of bovine articular cartilage in compression. *J. Biomech.* **36,** 339–353.
33. Langelier, E. and Buschmann, M. D. (2003). Increasing strain and strain rate strengthen transient stiffness but weaken the response to subsequent compression for articular cartilage in unconfined compression. *J. Biomech.* **36,** 853–859.
34. Li, L. P., Buschmann, M. D., and Shirazi-Adl, A. (2003) Strain-rate dependent stiffness of articular cartilage in unconfined compression. *J. Biomech. Eng.* **125,** 161–168.

35. Wong, M., Ponticiello, M., Kovanen, V., and Jurvelin, J. S. (2000) Volumetric changes of articular cartilage during stress relaxation in unconfined compression. *J. Biomech.* **33,** 1049–1054.
36. Korhonen, R. K., Laasanen, M. S., Toyras, J., Lappalainen, R., Helminen, H. J., and Jurvelin, J. S. (2003) Fibril reinforced poroelastic model predicts specifically mechanical behavior of normal, proteoglycan depleted and collagen degraded articular cartilage. *J. Biomech.* **36,** 1373–1379.
37. Kim, Y. J., Bonassar, L. J., and Grodzinsky, A. J. (1995) The role of cartilage streaming potential, fluid flow and pressure in the stimulation of chondrocyte biosynthesis during dynamic compression. *J. Biomech.* **28,** 1055–1066.
38. Soltz, M. A. and Ateshian, G. A. (2000) A conewise linear elasticity mixture model for the analysis of tension-compression nonlinearity in articular cartilage. *J. Biomech. Eng.* **122,** 576–586.
39. Fung, Y. C. (1972). Stress-strain history relations of soft tissues in simple elongation, in *Biomechanics: Its Foundations and Objectives* (Fung, Y. C., Perrone, N., and Anliker, M., eds.), Prentice-Hall, Englewood Cliffs, NJ, pp. 181–208.
40. Li, J. T., Armstrong, C. G., and Mow, V. C. (1983) The effect of shtain rate on mechanical properties of articular cartilage in tension, in: *Proceedings Biomechanics Symposium Trans ASME*, AMD, vol. 56, p. 117, ASME, Houston, TX.
41. Akizuki, S., Mow, V. C., Muller, F., Pita, J. C., Howell, D. S., and Manicourt, D. H. (1987) Tensile properties of human knee joint cartilage: II. correlations between weight bearing and tissue pathology and the kinetics of swelling. *J. Orthop. Res.* **5,** 173–186.
42. Kempson, G. E., Muir, H., Pollard, C., and Tuke, M. (1973) The tensile properties of the cartilage of human femoral condyles related to the content of collagen and glycosaminoglycans. *Biochim. Biophys. Acta* **297,** 456–472.
43. Kempson, G. E. (1991) Age-related changes in the tensile properties of human articular cartilage: a comparative study between the femoral head of the hip joint and the talus of the ankle joint. *Biochim. Biophys. Acta* **1075,** 223–230.
44. Hayes, W. C. and Mockros, L. F. (1971) Viscoelastic properties of human articular cartilage. *J. Appl. Physiol.* **31,** 562–568.
45. Hayes, W. C. and Bodine, A. J. (1978) Flow-independent viscoelastic properties of articular cartilage matrix. *J. Biomech.* **11,** 407–419.
46. Zhu, W., Mow, V. C., Koob, T. J., and Eyre, D. R. (1993) Viscoelastic shear properties of articular cartilage and the effects of glycosidase treatment. *J. Orthop. Res.* **11,** 771–781.
47. Zhu, W., Chern, K. Y., and Mow, V. C. (1994). Anisotropic viscoelastic shear properties of bovine meniscus. *Clin. Orthop.* **306,** 34–45.
48. Simon, W. H., Mak, A., and Spirt, A. (1990) The effect of shear fatigue on bovine articular cartilage. *J. Orthop. Res.* **8,** 86–93.
49. Woo, S. L.-Y., Kwan, M. K., Lee, T. Q., Field, F. P., Kleiner, J. B., and Coutts, R. D. (1987) Perichondrial autograft for articular cartilage: shear modulus of neocartilage studied in rabbits. *Acta Orthop. Scand.* **58,** 510–515.

50. Ahsan, T. and Sah, R. L. (1999). Biomechanics of integrative cartilage repair. *Osteoarthritis Cartilage* **7,** 29–40.
51. Zuger, B. J., Ott, B., Mainil-Varlet, P., et al. (2001) Laser solder welding of articular cartilage: tensile strength and chondrocyte viability. Lasers Surg. Med. 28, 427—434.
52. Peretti, G. M., Zaporojan, V., Spangenberg, K. M., Randolph, M. A., Fellers, J., and Bonassar, L. J. (2003) Cell-based bonding of articular cartilage: An extended study. *J. Biomed. Mater. Res.* **64A,** 517–524.
53. Reindel, E. S., Ayroso, A. M., Chen, A. C., Chun, D. M., Schinagl, R. M., and Sah, R. L. (1995) Integrative repair of articular cartilage *in vitro*: adhesive strength of the interface region. *J. Orthop. Res.* **13,** 751–760.
54. DiMicco, M. A., Waters, S. N., Akeson, W. H., and Sah, R. L. (2002). Integrative articular cartilage repair: dependence on developmental stage and collagen metabolism. *Osteoarthritis Cartilage* **10,** 218–225.
55. DiMicco, M. A. and Sah, R. L. (2001) Integrative cartilage repair: adhesive strength correlates with collagen deposition. *J. Orthop. Res.* **19,** 1105–1112.
56. Ahsan, T., Lottman, L. M., Harwood, F. L., Amiel, D., and Sah, R. L. (1999) Integrative cartilage repair: inhibition by β-aminoproprionitrile. *J. Orthop. Res.* **17,** 850–857.
57. Giurea, A., DiMicco, M. A., Akeson, W. H., and Sah, R. L. (2002) Development-associated differences in integrative cartilage repair: roles of biosynthesis and matrix. *J. Orthop. Res.* **20,** 1274–1281.
58. Englert, C., McGowan, K. B., Klein, T. J., Giurea, A., Schumacher, B. L., and Sah, R. L. (2003) Inhibition of integrative cartilage repair by synovial fluid components. *Trans. Orthop. Res. Soc.* **28,** 189.
59. Jackson, R. W., Judy, M. M., Matthews, J. L., and Nosir, H. (1997) Photochemical tissue welding with 1,8 naphthalimide dyes: in vivo meniscal and cartilage welds. *Trans. Orthop. Res. Soc.* **22,** 650.
60. McGowan, K. B. and Sah, R. L. (2003) Pre-treatment with β-aminoproprionitrile accelerates integrative cartilage repair. *Trans. Orthop. Res. Soc.* **28,** 723.
61. Obradovic, B., Martin, I., Padera, R. F., Treppo, S., Freed, L. E., and Vunjak-Novakovic, G. (2001) Integration of engineered cartilage. *J. Orthop. Res.* **19,** 1089–1097.
62. van de Breevaart Bravenboer, J., In der Maur, C. D., Bos, P. K., et al. (2003). Increased interfacial strength of transplanted cartilage in vivo following enzymatic treatment of wound edges. *Trans. Orthop. Res. Soc.* **28,** 188.
63. Matthewson, M. H. and Dandy, D. J. (1978) Osteochondral fractures of the lateral femoral condyle. *J. Bone Joint Surg. Br.* **60,** 199–202.
64. Flachsmann, R., Broom, N. D., Hardy, A. E., and Moltschaniwskyj, G. (2000). Why Is the adolescent joint particularly susceptible to osteochondral shear fracture? *Clin. Orthop.* **381,** 212–221.
65. Kennedy, J. C., Grainger, R. W., and McGraw, R. W. (1966) Osteochondral fractures of the femoral condyles. *J. Bone Joint Surg. Br.* **48,** 436–440.

66. Rosenberg, N. J. (1964) Osteochondral fractures of the lateral femoral condyle. *J. Bone Joint Surg. Am.* **46,** 1013–1026.
67. Flachsmann, E. R., Broom, N. D., and Oloyede, A. (1995) A biomechanical investigation of unconstrained shear failure of the osteochondral region under impact loading. *Clin. Biomech.* **10,** 156–165.
68. Broom, N. D., Oloyede, A., Flachsmann, R., and Hows, M. (1996) Dynamic fracture characteristics of the osteochondral junction undergoing shear deformation. *Med. Eng. Phys.* **18,** 396–404.
69. Mente, P. L. and Lewis, J. L. (1994) Elastic modulus of calcified cartilage is an order of magnitude less than that of subchondral bone. *J. Orthop. Res.* **12,** 637–647.
70. Kumar, P., Oka, M., Nakamura, T., Yamamuro, T., and Delecrin, J. (1991) Mechanical strength of osteochondral junction. *Nippon Seikeigeka Gakkai Zasshi* **65,** 1070–1077.
71. Hirsch, C. (1944) A contribution to the pathogenesis of chondromalacia of the patella. *Acta Chir. Scand.* **90 (suppl),** 9.
72. Elmore, S. M., Sokoloff, L., Norris, G., and Carmeci, P. (1963) Nature of "imperfect" elasticity of articular cartilage. *J. Appl. Physiol.* **18,** 393–396.
73. Sokoloff, L. (1966) Elasticity of aging cartilage. *Proc. Fed. Am. Socs. Exp. Biol.* **25,** 1089–1095.
74. Kempson, G. E., Freeman, M. A. R., and Swanson, S. A. V. (1971) The determination of a creep modulus for articular cartilage by indentation tests of the human femoral head. *J. Biomech.* **4,** 239–250.
75. Coletti, J. M., Akeson, W. H., and Woo, S. L.-Y. (1972) A comparison of the physical behavior of normal articular cartilage and the arthroplasty surface. *J. Bone Joint Surg. Am.* **54,** 147–160.
76. Parsons, J. R. and Black, J. (1977) The viscoelastic shear behavior of normal rabbit articular cartilage. *J. Biomech.* **10,** 21–29.
77. Parsons, J. R. and Black, J. (1979) Mechanical behavior of articular cartilage: quantitative changes with alteration of ionic environment. *J. Biomech.* **12,** 765–773.
78. Mow, V. C., Gibbs, M. C., Lai, W. M., Zhu, W. B., and Athanasiou, K. A. (1989). Biphasic indentation of articular cartilage-II. A numerical algorithm and an experimental study. *J. Biomech.* **22,** 853–861.
79. Jurvelin, J., Kiviranta, I., Saamanen, A.-M., Tammi, M., and Helminen, H. J. (1990). Indentation stiffness of young canine knee articular cartilage—influence of strenuous joint loading. *J. Biomech.* **23,** 1239–1246.
80. Athanasiou, K. A., Rosenwasser, M. P., Buckwalter, J. A., Malinin, T. I., and Mow, V. C. (1991) Interspecies comparisons of in situ intrinsic mechanical properties of distal femoral cartilage. *J. Orthop. Res.* **9,** 330–340.
81. Athanasiou, K. A., Niederauer, G. G., and Schenck, R. C. (1995) Biomechanical topography of human ankle cartilage. *Ann. Biomed. Eng.* **23,** 697–704.
82. Lyyra, T., Jurvelin, J., Pitkänen, P., Väätäinen, U., and Kiviranta, I. (1995) Indentation instrument for the measurement of cartilage stiffness under arthroscopic control. *Med. Eng. Phys.* **17,** 395–399.

83. Lyyra, T., Kiviranta, I., Vaatainen, U., Helminen, H. J., and Jurvelin, J. S. (1999). In vivo characterization of indentation stiffness of articular cartilage in the normal human knee. *J. Biomed. Mater. Res.* **48,** 482–487.
84. Franz, T., Hasler, E. M., Hagg, R., Weiler, C., Jakob, R. P., and Mainil-Varlet, P. (2001) In situ compressive stiffness, biochemical composition, and structural integrity of articular cartilage of the human knee joint. *Osteoarthritis Cartilage* **9,** 582–592.
85. Hertz, H. (1881) On the contact of elastic solids. *J. Reine Angew. Math.* **92,** 156.
86. Love, A. (1944) *A Treatise on the Mathematical Theory of Elasticity*, 4th ed, Dover, New York.
87. Hayes, W. C., Keer, L. M., Herrmann, K. G., and Mockros, L. F. (1972) A mathematical analysis for indentation tests of articular cartilage. *J. Biomech.* **5,** 541–551.
88. Mak, A. F., Lai, W. M., and Mow, V. C. (1987) Biphasic indentation of articular cartilage-I. theoretical analysis. *J. Biomech.* **20,** 703–714.
89. Lee, R. C., Frank, E. H., Grodzinsky, A. J., and Roylance, D. K. (1981) Oscillatory compressional behavior of articular cartilage and its associated electromechanical properties. *J. Biomech. Eng.* **103,** 280–292.
90. Grodzinsky, A. J. and Frank, E. H. (1990) Electromechanical and physicochemical regulation of cartilage strength and metabolism, in *Connective Tissue Matrix: vol. II. Topics in Molecular and Structural Biology* (Hukins, D. W. L., ed.), CRC Press, Boca Raton, FL, pp. 91–126.
91. Chen, A. C., Bae, W. C., Schinagl, R. M., and Sah, R. L. (2001) Depth- and strain-dependent mechanical and electromechanical properties of full-thickness bovine articular cartilage in confined compression. *J. Biomech.* **34,** 1–12.
92. Chen, S. S., Falcovitz, Y. H., Schneiderman, R., Maroudas, A., and Sah, R. L. (2001) Depth-dependent compressive properties of normal aged human femoral head articular cartilage. *Osteoarthritis Cartilage* **9,** 561–569.
93. Chang, D. G., Lottman, L. M., Chen, A. C., et al. (1999) The depth-dependent, multi-axial properties of aged human patellar cartilage in tension. *Trans. Orthop. Res. Soc.* **24,** 644.
94. Elliot, D. M., Narmoneva, D. A., and Setton, L. A. (2002) Direct measurement of the Poisson's ratio of human patella cartilage in tension. *J. Biomech. Eng.* **124,** 223–228.
95. Hunziker, E. B. (1992) Articular cartilage structure in humans and experimental animals, in *Articular Cartilage and Osteoarthritis* (Kuettner, K. E., Schleyerbach, R., Peyron, J. G., and Hascall, V. C., eds.), Raven, New York, pp. 183–199.
96. Maroudas, A. (1979) Physico-chemical properties of articular cartilage, in *Adult Articular Cartilage*, 2nd. ed. (Freeman, M. A. R., ed.), Pitman Medical, Tunbridge Wells, England, pp. 215–290.
97. Bae, W. C., Lewis, C. W., and Sah, R. L. (2003) Intra-tissue strain distribution in normal human articular cartilage during clinical indentation testing. *Trans. Orthop. Res. Soc.* **28,** 254.

98. Sutton, M. A., McNeill, S. R., Helm, J. D., and Chao, Y. J. (2000) Advances in two-dimensional and three-dimensional computer vision, in *Photomechanics*, vol. 77 (Rastogi, P. K., ed.), Springer, New York, pp. 323–372.
99. Fortin, M., Buschmann, M. D., Bertrand, M. J., Foster, F. S., and Ophir, J. (2003) Dynamic measurement of internal solid displacement in articular cartilage using ultrasound backscatter. *J. Biomech.* **36,** 443–447.
100. Agemura, D. H., O'Brien, W. D., Jr., Olerud, J. E., Chun, L. E. & Eyre, D. E. (1990). Ultrasonic propagation properties of articular cartilage at 100 MHz. *J. Acoust. Soc. Am.* **87,** 1786–1791.
101. Mow, V. C. and Ateshian, G. A. (1997) Lubrication and wear of diarthrodial joints. In Basic Orthopaedic Biomechanics 2nd edit. (Mow, V. C. and Hayes, W. C., eds.), Raven, New York, pp. 275–315.
102. Schumacher, B. L., Block, J. A., Schmid, T. M., Aydelotte, M. B., and Kuettner, K. E. (1994). A novel proteoglycan synthesized and secreted by chondrocytes of the superficial zone of articular cartilage. *Arch. Biochem. Biophys.* **311,** 144–152.
103. Schumacher, B. L., Hughes, C. E., Kuettner, K. E., Caterson, B., and Aydelotte, M. B. (1999) Immunodetection and partial cDNA sequence of the proteoglycan, superficial zone protein, synthesized by cells lining synovial joints. *J. Orthop. Res.* **17,** 110–120.
104. Jay, G. D. (1992) Characterization of a bovine synovial fluid lubricating factor. I. Chemical, surface activity and lubricating properties. *Connect. Tissue Res.* **28,** 71–88.
105. Swann, D. A. and Radin, E. L. (1972) The molecular basis of articular lubrication. *J. Biol. Chem.* **247,** 8069–8073.
106. Swann, D. A., Sotman, S., Dixon, M., and Brooks, C. (1977) The isolation and partial characterization of the major glycoprotein (LGP-I) from the articular lubricating fraction of synovial fluid. *Biochem. J.* **161,** 473–485.
107. Swann, D. A., Hendren, R. B., Radin, E. L., Sotman, S. L., and Duda, E. A. (1981) The lubricating activity of synovial fluid glycoproteins. *Arthritis. Rheum.* **24,** 22–30.
108. Swann, D. A., Silver, F. H., Slayter, H. S., Stafford, W., and Shore, E. (1985). The molecular structure and lubricating activity of lubricin isolated from bovine and human synovial fluids. *Biochem. J.* **225,** 195–201.
109. Hills, B. A. (1989) Oligolamellar lubrication of joints by surface active phospholipid. *J. Rheumatol.* **16,** 82–91.
110. Hills, B. A. (1995) Remarkable anti-wear properties of joint surfactant. *Ann. Biomed. Eng.* **23,** 112–115.
111. Hills, B. A. and Monds, M. K. (1998). Enzymatic identification of the load-bearing boundary lubricant in the joint. *Br. J. Rheumatol.* **37,** 137–142.
112. Malcolm, L. L. (1976) An experimental investigation of the frictional and deformational responses of articular cartilage interfaces to static and dynamic loading. Ph.D. Thesis, University of California, San Diego.

113. Linn, F. C. (1967) Lubrication of animal joints. I. the arthrotripsometer. *J. Bone Joint Surg. Am.* **49,** 1079–1098.
114. Linn, F. C. (1968) Lubrication of animal joints. II. the mechanism. *J. Biomech.* **1,** 193–205.
115. Murakami, T., Higaki, H., Sawae, Y., Ohtsuki, N., Moriyama, S., and Nakanishi, Y. (1998) Adaptive and multimode lubrication in natural synovial joints and artificial joints. *Proc. Inst. Mech. Eng. [H]* **212,** 23–35.
116. Mori, S., Naito, M., and Moriyama, S. (2002) Highly viscous sodium hyaluronate and joint lubrication. *Int. Orthop.* **26,** 116–121.
117. Kumar, P., Oka, M., Toguchida, J., et al. (2001) Role of uppermost superficial surface layer of articular cartilage in the lubrication mechanism of joints. *J. Anat.* **199,** 241–250.
118. Unsworth, A., Dowson, D., and Wright, V. (1975) Some new evidence on human joint lubrication. *Ann. Rheum. Dis.* **27,** 512–520.
119. Unsworth, A., Dowson, D., and Wright, V. (1975) The frictional behavior of human synovial joints: I. Natural joints. *Trans. ASME F. J. Lubr. Technol.* **97,** 360–376.
120. McCutchen, C. W. (1959) Mechanism of animal joints: sponge-hydrostatic and weeping bearings. *Nature* **184,** 1284–1285.
121. Radin, E. L., Paul, I. L., Swann, D. A., and Schottstaedt, E. S. (1971) Lubrication of synovial membrane. *Ann. Rheum. Dis.* **30,** 322–325.
122. Davis, W. H. J., Lee, S. L., and Sokoloff, L. (1978) Boundary lubricating ability of synovial fluid in degenerative joint disease. *Arthritis Rheum.* **21,** 754–760.
123. Hills, B. A. and Monds, M. K. (1998) Deficiency of lubricating surfactant lining in the articular surfaces of replaced hips and knees. *Br. J. Rheumatol.* **37,** 143–147.
124. Schwarz, I. M. and Hills, B. A. (1998) Surface-active phospholipids as the lubricating component of lubricin. *Br. J. Rheumatol.* **37,** 21–26.
125. Forster, H. and Fisher, J. (1996). The influence of loading time and lubricant on the friction of articular cartilage. *Proc. Inst. Mech. Eng. [H]* **210,** 109–119.
126. Jay, G. D., Lane, B. P., and Sokoloff, L. (1992) Characterization of a bovine synovial fluid lubricating factor III. The interaction with hyaluronic acid. *Connect. Tissue Res.* **28,** 245–255.
127. Jay, G. D., Haberstroh, K., and Cha, C.-J. (1998) Comparison of the boundary-lubricating ability of bovine synovial fluid, lubricin, and Healon. *J. Biomed. Mater. Res.* **40,** 414–418.
128. Jay, G. D. and Cha, D.-J. (1999) The effect of phospholipase digestion upon the boundary lubricating activity of synovial fluid. *J. Rheumatol.* **26,** 2454–2457.
129. Jay, G. D., Tantravahi, U., Britt, D. E., Barrach, H. J., and Cha, C. J. (2001) Homology of lubricin and superficial zone protein (SZP): products of megakaryocyte stimulating factor (MSF) gene expression by human synovial fibroblasts and articular chondrocytes localized to chromosome 1q25. *J. Orthop. Res.* **19,** 677–687.

130. Lai, W. M. and Mow, V. C. (1980) Drag-induced compression of articular cartilage during a permeation experiment. *Biorheology* **17,** 111–123.
131. Ateshian, G. A., Warden, W. H., Kim, J. J., Grelsamer, R. P., and Mow, V. C. (1997) Finite deformation biphasic material properties of bovine articular cartilage from confined compression experiments. *J. Biomech.* **30,** 1157–1164.
132. Klisch, S. M. and Lotz, J. C. (2000) A special theory of biphasic mixtures and experimental results for human annulus fibrosus tested in confined compression. *J. Biomech. Eng.* **122,** 180–188.
133. Wang, C. C.-B., Hung, C. T., and Mow, V. C. (2001) An analysis of the effects of depth-dependent aggregate modulus on articular cartilage stress-relaxation behavior in compression. *J. Biomech.* **34,** 75–84.
134. Mak, A. F. (1986) The apparent viscoelastic behavior of articular cartilage—the contributions from the intrinsic matrix viscoelasticity and interstitial fluid flows. *J. Biomech. Eng.* **108,** 123–130.
135. Meachim, G. (1972) Light microscopy of Indian ink preparations of fibrillated cartilage. *Ann. Rheum. Dis.* **31,** 457–464.
136. Bullough, P. and Goodfellow, J. (1968) The significance of the fine structure of articular cartilage. *J. Bone Joint Surg. Br.* **50,** 852–857.
137. Clark, J. M. (1991) Variation of collagen fiber alignment in a joint surface: a scanning electron microscope study of the tibial plateau in dog, rabbit, and man. *J. Orthop. Res.* **9,** 246–257.
138. Kempson, G. E., Freeman, M. A. R., and Swanson, S. A. V. (1968) Tensile properties of articular cartilage. *Nature* **220,** 1127–1128.
139. Roth, V. and Mow, V. C. (1980) The intrinsic tensile behavior of the matrix of bovine articular cartilage and its variation with age. *J. Bone Joint Surg. Am.* **62,** 1102–1117.
140. Temple, M. M., Bae, W. C., Rivard, K. L., and Sah, R. L. (2002) Age- and site-associated biomechanical weakening of human articular cartilage of the femoral condyle: relationship to cellularity and wear. *Trans. Orthop. Res. Soc.* **27,** 84.
141. Bae, W. C., Law, A. W., Amiel, D., Sah, R. L. (2004) Sensitivity of indentation testing to step off edges and interface integrity in cartilage repair. *Ann. Biomed. Eng.* (in press).
142. Waters N. E. (1965) The indentation of thin rubber sheets by cylindrical indenters. *Br. J. Appl. Physiol.* **16,** 1387–1392.
143. Waters, N. E. (1965) The indentation of thin rubber sheets by spherical indenters. *Br. J. Appl. Physiol.* **16,** 557–563.

10

Noninvasive Study of Human Cartilage Structure by MRI

Felix Eckstein

Summary

Magnetic resonance (MR) imaging is a 3D imaging technique that has recently begun to permit direct delineation of cartilage structure. This chapter summarizes current methodology for the morphological (e.g., volume, thickness) and compositional imaging of cartilage using quantitative MR as well as for semiquantitative scoring of cartilage disease. The chapter explains the relevance of MR in identifying disease status, in monitoring disease progression, and in identifying risk factors of osteoarthritis, as well as in evaluating treatment response to so-called structure-modifying osteoarthritis drugs. The practical methodological procedures presented involve the description of how to acquire MR images for structural analysis and the semiquantitative scoring of articular cartilage. We also present a description of image-analysis techniques for cartilage segmentation and characterization of cartilage structure (quantitative outcome parameters, such as volume and thickness) and guidelines for how to test the validity (accuracy), precision (reproducibility), and sensitivity to change of such methodologies in osteoarthritis.

Key Words: Articular cartilage; MR imaging; joints; osteoarthritis; MR sequences; image analysis; validation; reproducibility; sensitivity to change.

1. Introduction

1.1. Articular Cartilage Function

Articular cartilage is responsible for providing an almost frictionless gliding surface for the articulating bodies of human joints, so that physical forces can be transmitted evenly between body segments during static and dynamic activity. The maintenance of articular cartilage integrity and prevention of tissue destruction are thought to be of critical importance in the maintenance of adequate joint function and patient well-being. The degeneration and loss of articular cartilage, in contrast, are believed to represent the crucial step in degenerative joint disease, namely, osteoarthritis (OA).

From: *Methods in Molecular Medicine, Vol. 101: Cartilage and Osteoarthritis, Volume 2: Structure and In Vivo Analysis*
Edited by: F. De Ceuninck, M. Sabatini, and P. Pastoureau © Humana Press Inc., Totowa, NJ

1.2. Role of Quantitative MRI for Drug Development Trials in OA

An important obstacle in testing the efficacy and in optimizing therapeutic approaches to OA has been the inability to evaluate cartilage status directly by noninvasive means *(1,2)*. The advent of magnetic resonance imaging (MRI), a 3D, noninvasive imaging technique with multiplanar capabilities and unparalleled soft tissue contrast, has created the opportunity to assess cartilage structure quantitatively, specifically its macromorphology (such as volume and thickness) and its biochemical composition (such as proteoglycan, collagen, and interstitial water content). Because of its thin and geometrically complex morphology, its relatively short transverse relaxation time (T2), its complex composition, and various potential sources of artifact, however, articular cartilage imaging presents a true challenge to quantitative MRI. In OA, MRI poses an even greater challenge, since the surface becomes more difficult to define owing to focal signal changes, fibrillation, and tissue thinning, and to the appearance of repair tissue and osteophytes. Nevertheless, significant advances in MR and digital image-analysis technology have revolutionized noninvasive assessment of cartilage structure and composition by noninvasive means.

1.3. MRI-Based Studies on Cartilage Morphology

These techniques have already provided a large number of new insights into the physiology of cartilage structure and have permitted us to assess systematically the impact of gender *(3–6)*, level of maturity and age *(5,7–9)*, anthropometric measures (body weight and height) *(3,5,8,10–12)*, bone size *(3,5,10–12)*, muscle morphology and strength *(9,13)*, limb dominance *(13)*, level of physical exercise *(5,14–16)*, use of estrogen replacement *(17)*, and genetics *(18)* on the morphology of cartilage and human joints in general.

Even more importantly, however, MRI offers a unique potential to characterize cartilage loss in OA quantitatively, and to evaluate potential effects of medical or surgical treatment on disease progression, which may help these new therapies to gain regulatory approval *(1,19)*. The ability to detect structural treatment response to these drugs in OA depends on certain requirements.

1.4. Requirements for MRI-Based Quantitative Endpoints

1. The technique employed must be able to measure a surrogate marker (a process-related feature) that is related to the clinical outcome of the disease (a feature that is directly related to how a patient feels, functions, or survives). The surrogate marker should lie directly on the disease pathway and should register the relevant beneficial and adverse effects of the drug ("surrogate" validity). Although it is difficult to prove surrogate validity in OA, there is high consensus that articular cartilage structure and composition represent the most important surrogate markers to be monitored in OA.

2. The technique should be able to measure the surrogate marker with high accuracy ("technical" validity), and measurements should correspond to a true value.
3. The technique should be able to measure the surrogate marker with high precision (reproducibility). Precision errors should be sufficiently low in relation to the magnitude of expected change for a given marker in OA.

1.5. Objectives of This Chapter

This chapter aims to describe practical procedures in MRI technology, as applied to the study of cartilage research and to OA. These procedures involve:

1. How to acquire MR images for morphological analysis, semiquantitative scoring, and compositional imaging of articular cartilage.
2. A description of image-analysis techniques for cartilage segmentation and characterization of cartilage structure (quantitative outcome parameters).
3. Some guidelines for how to test the validity (accuracy), precision (reproducibility), and sensitivity to change of these methodologies in OA.

2. Materials

1. Clinical MRI scanner of at least 1.5 T.
2. T1-weighted gradient echo (GE) sequences with either fat suppression or preferably with water excitation for determining cartilage morphology (**Fig. 1**) and other MR sequences for semiquantitative scoring and compositional imaging of cartilage.
3. CD-ROM, DVD, or other media to store digital image data in DICOM or other format.
4. Workstation or PC for digital image analysis.
5. Dedicated software for cartilage segmentation and computation of relevant quantitative outcome parameters from contiguous MR sequences.
6. Comparative techniques to test the technical validity of the measurements.

3. Methods

3.1. Overview and General Considerations

Appropriate MR sequences (*see* **Subheading 3.2.**) for morphological analysis of cartilage (e.g., volume and thickness) and the semiquantitative scoring of cartilage are now available on almost all clinical MRI scanners at 1.5 T (**Figs. 1** and **2**). Protocols will therefore be described in detail in **Subheadings 3.2.1.** to **3.2.6.** MR sequences for compositional imaging of cartilage, however, require either special equipment or particular procedures and will therefore be only briefly mentioned, in **Subheading 3.2.6.** Semiquantitative scoring of cartilage lesions (*see* **Subheading 3.2.5.**) requires profound diagnostic experience and must be performed by an experienced clinician who rates images on a day-to-day basis. Quantitative analysis of cartilage morphology should also be per-

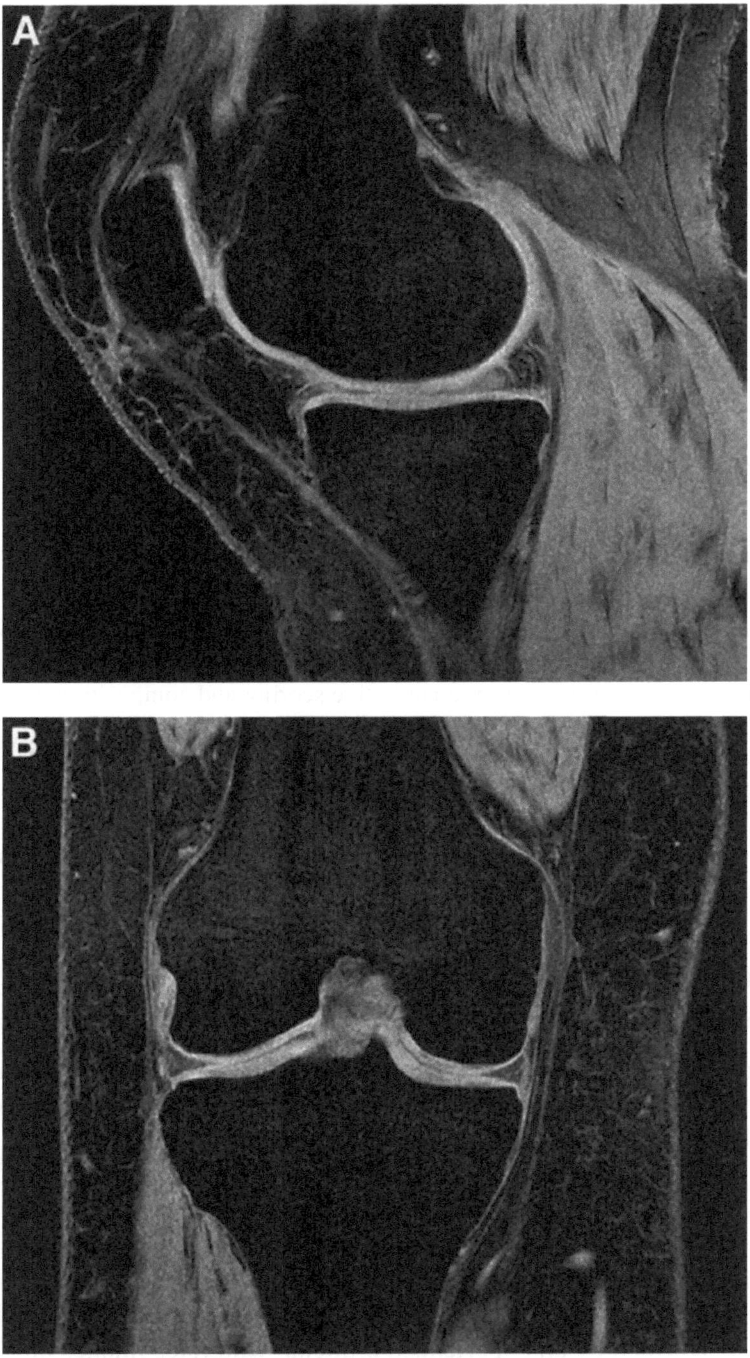
A
B

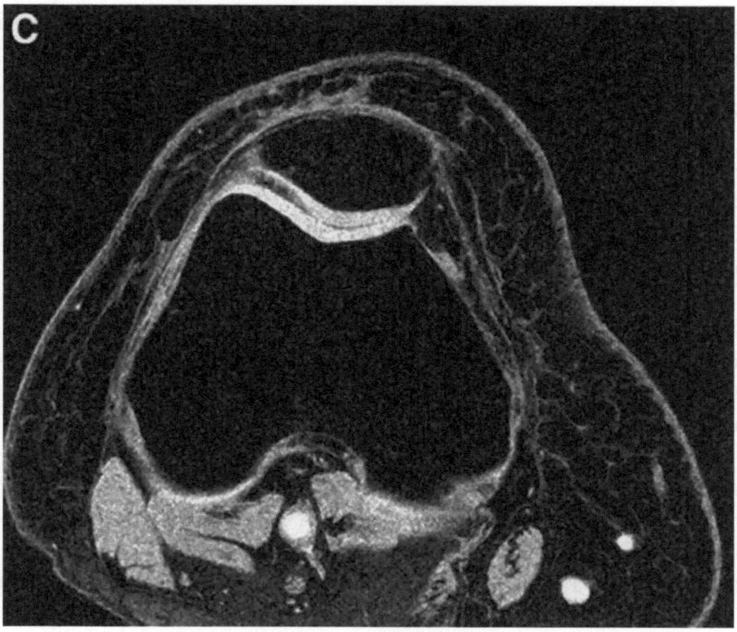

Fig. 1. Sagittal (**A**), coronal (**B**), and axial (**C**) MR image of a volunteer, acquired with a T1-weighted, fat-suppressed, water excitation gradient echo (GE) sequence. (Courtesy of Prof. David Felson, M.D., M.P.H., Arthritis and Musculoskeletal Disease Center, Boston University, Boston, MA.)

formed by trained and experienced personnel, to yield reliable results. Additionally, segmentation of cartilage and computation of quantitative cartilage outcome parameters (*see* **Subheading 3.3.**) require dedicated software that is currently available only at a few specialized centers and is not commercially available. Because no fully automated algorithms have been developed, these procedures require a high level of training, standardization, and quality control, in order to warrant a high level of consistency and reliability of the analyses. Owing to the digital nature of the data, however, images can be acquired at several clinical centers (e.g., within the context of multicenter studies) and may be centrally processed at specialized image-analysis centers, to which digital data are sent on CD-ROM or other media.

Subheading 3.3. will thus summarize some of the techniques that are currently used by these centers to derive quantitative parameters of cartilage morphology. **Subheading 3.4.** will eventually describe work and procedures that have been performed to evaluate the validity, reproducibility, and sensitivity to change of these quantitative parameters.

3.2. MR Sequence Description for Cartilage Imaging

3.2.1. General Considerations for Quantitative Imaging of Cartilage Morphology

To be suitable for quantitative assessment of cartilage status, MR sequences must fulfill the following requirements:

1. Sufficient signal (signal-to-noise ratio [SNR]) and contrast (contrast-to-noise ratio [CNR]) must be obtained for accurate delineation of the bone-cartilage interface and articular surface. No artifacts (geometric distortion or signal distortion should occur, particularly at the bone cartilage interface, where fat-bound and water-bound protons exist close together.
2. Measurements should be obtained at reasonable imaging times (6–15 min), to avoid movement artifact, to maintain patient comfort, and to keep the costs of the image acquisition within reasonable limits.
3. Because cartilage layers exhibit a thickness of typically 1–3 mm and even less in OA, sufficient spatial resolution is required so that a sufficient number of image points (pixels) is available to characterize the tissue thickness.
4. Note that SNR/CNR, acquisition time, and spatial resolution are interdependent and that optimization toward one of these parameters necessarily leads to sacrifices in the others. Increasing the resolution by a factor of two in all three dimensions, for instance, requires an increase in acquisition time by a factor of 64, when the SNR is to be kept constant. Therefore a delicate balance needs to be achieved between these parameters, for optimal delineation of a given joint or joint surface.

3.2.2. Type of MR Sequence for Quantitative Imaging of Cartilage Morphology

The MR sequences most commonly used for quantitative imaging of cartilage morphology over recent years have been T1-weighted spoiled GE sequences, e.g., fast low angle shot (FLASH) ***(20)*** or spoiled gradient recalled acquisition at steady state (SPGR). These have been implemented with either frequency selective spectral fat-suppression by a prepulse ***(21–24)*** or, more recently, by frequency selective water excitation ***(25–28)***, in order to provide a sufficient dynamic range of the image contrast, and to eliminate artifacts at the bone interface (**Fig. 1**):

1. The repetition time (TR) should be chosen below 60 ms with spectral fat suppression and below 20 ms with water excitation
2. The echo time (TE) should generally be as short as possible, preferably below 10 ms.

3. The optimal flip angle will depend on the choice of TR, TE, and bandwidth and may range from 10 to 30°; the optimal flip angle can be determined by parametric imaging of several patients with different flip angles.
4. The bandwidth of these sequences should be between 65 and 130 Hz/pixel, with higher values resulting in noisier images.
5. With regard to imaging at 3 T, *see* **Note 1**.
6. Acquisition times are usually shorter for water excitation protocols than for spectral fat suppression.

3.2.3. Spatial Resolution Required for Quantitative Imaging of Cartilage Morphology

The anisotropy of the spatial resolution of MR images is determined by the in-plane resolution and the slice thickness. The in-plane resolution is determined by the field of view (FOV) and the matrix (number of pixels by which the FOV is divided).

1. When imaging the knee, the FOV should be chosen at approx 160 mm, to accommodate the joints of large and of adipose subjects.
2. Using a 512-pixel matrix, a 160-mm FOV results in an in-plane resolution of 0.31 × 0.31 mm, which has frequently been used in quantitative cartilage imaging.
3. With regard to the use of an anisotropic in-plane resolution, *see* **Note 2**.

Hardy et al. ***(29)*** reported significantly higher precision errors for cartilage volume measurements at lower (0.55 × 0.55 mm) vs higher resolution (0.28 × 0.28 mm), despite considerably lower SNR and CNR and longer acquisition time (22 min) for the latter. When creating artificial cartilage lesions in rabbit joints, Link et al. ***(30)*** also showed that the ability to detect small lesions critically depends on the level of spatial resolution and that achieving a high resolution justifies sacrifices in SNR.

As images can be aligned roughly perpendicular to the joint surface; the slice thickness is less critical than the in-plane resolution. Marshall et al. ***(31)*** compared volume reconstructions from images with different section thickness with the actual volume of phantoms. They reported a mean difference of 1.7% for 1.0-mm section thickness, 3.5% for 1.5 mm, 6.4% for 2 mm, and 23% for 3 mm. They recommended use of a 1.5-mm section thickness, because of the long imaging time required with thinner slices. Hardy et al. ***(29)*** found no significant difference for inter-scan precision (reproducibility) of cartilage volume measurements in the human knee at 0.5-, 1-, and 2-mm section thickness and reported no significant difference in precision between these values.

1. We recommend using a 1.5-mm section thickness and an isotropic 0.3-mm in-plane resolution for the human knee, for which total coverage of the joint can be achieved at imaging times around 10–12 min.

2. The possibility of choosing a <100% slice resolution is discussed in **Note 3**.
3. Whether to use a sagittal, coronal, or transverse slice orientation at the knee depends on the specific research question and is discussed in **Note 4**.
4. For other joints with thinner cartilage, it may be necessary to use a higher in-plane resolution (e.g., 0.25 × 0.25 mm, interpolated to 0.125 × 0.125 mm) and lower section thickness (e.g., 1 mm) ***(27,32,33)***.

3.2.4. Other Settings for Quantitative Imaging of Cartilage Morphology

1. The number of sections to be acquired should be chosen in such a way that the entire region of interest is covered by the image dataset (anatomical coverage).
2. Acquiring excessive numbers of sections outside the region of interest will increase the imaging time. Acquiring too few sections will create problems in achieving anatomical coverage in subjects with large joints and can produce aliasing (folding) artifacts, in which anatomical structures from adjacent regions are projected into the peripheral images (beginning and end of the slab).
3. Aliasing artifacts can be avoided by either increasing the number of sections or by increasing slice oversampling (see below).

Recent MRI scanners offer a wide range of additional settings to modulate image contrast, resolution, and acquisition time:

1. If the image contrast is low with one acquisition (number of excitations [NEX] = 1), adding a second acquisition (NEX = 2) will double the imaging time and provide a 41% increase in SNR. In most cases, however, this will render imaging times too long for clinical practice.
2. Phase and slice oversampling permit one to increase SNR and imaging time in incremental steps; such oversampling is commonly used to reduce aliasing artifacts (*see* **Note 5**).
3. With regard to the use of phase partial Fourier, asymmetric echo, and elliptical scanning to reduce acquisition time, *see* **Note 6**.

3.2.5. Semiquantitative Scoring of Cartilage

3.2.5.1. Detection of Chondral Defects

Semiquantitative scoring of chondral defects includes features of cartilage signal alteration, cartilage surface irregularities, or cartilage thinning. A relatively high specificity and sensitivity in detecting chondral lesions has been demonstrated in cadaveric knee joints and in comparison with arthroscopy, both for the fat-suppressed GE sequences mentioned previously ***(21,34,35)*** and for fast spin echo (FSE) sequences (**Fig. 2**), which permit much shorter imaging times ***(36,37)***. Bredella et al. ***(38)*** have reported a sensitivity of 61% for detecting chondral lesions in the coronal plane (specificity 99%), 59% for the axial plane (specificity 99%), and 40% for the sagittal plane (specificity 100%) using fat-suppressed T2-weighted FSE sequences (**Fig. 2**). The authors con-

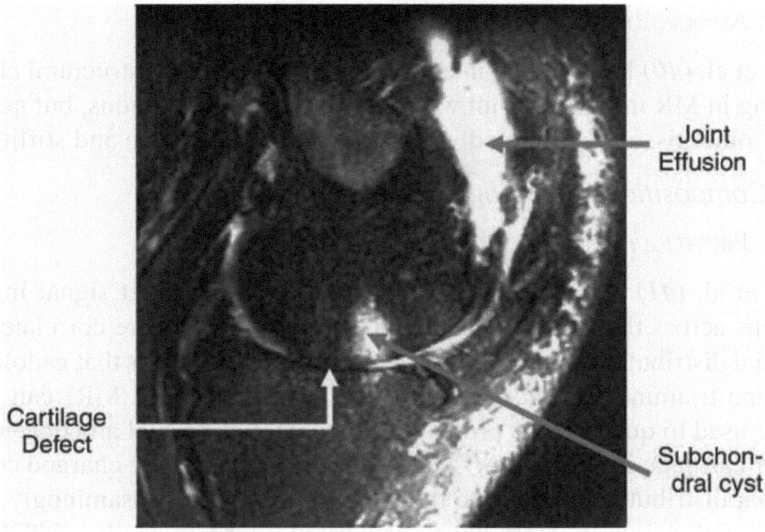

Fig. 2. Sagittal MR image of a patient with severe osteoarthritis of the knee, obtained with T2-weighted, fat-suppressed spin echo (SE) sequence. (Kindly provided by Prof. Thomas Link, Institute of Diagnostic Radiology, Klinikum rechts der Isar, München, Germany.)

cluded that combined axial and coronal planes offered sufficient coverage of articular surfaces and provided a high sensitivity and specificity for detecting chondral defects.

3.2.5.2. Current Efforts in the Detection of Chondral Defects

Current efforts aim at standardizing the scoring of cartilage lesions according to depth (size perpendicular to the surface), extension (size parallel to the surface), and anatomical location (joint compartment). However, to date there exists no single accepted grading system of cartilage lesions with MRI. The same MR sequence also permits analysis of structural abnormalities of other joint tissues (**Fig. 2**).

3.2.5.3. Grade 1 Lesions (Signal Heterogeneity)

Although the structural basis of grade 1 lesions (signal heterogeneity) is unknown, a recent paper ***(39)*** has shown that a relevant proportion of these lesions progresses toward morphological abnormality. Nevertheless, a relevant percentage of grade 1 lesions disappeared during the study period, and it remained unclear whether this was because of technical inability to reconfirm lesions in a follow-up examination or actual healing or repair.

3.2.5.4. Association With Clinical Symptoms

Link et al. ***(40)*** have shown in a recent paper that among structural changes occurring in MR images of joint with OA, only cartilage lesions, but not findings for other tissues, correlated with symptoms such as pain and stiffness.

3.2.6. Compositional Imaging of Articular Cartilage

3.2.6.1. Proteoglycans

Paul et al. ***(41)*** was some of the first to hypothesize that signal intensity variations across the cartilage (in a spin echo sequence) were correlated with the spatial distribution of the PGs. More recent work indicates that gadolinium-diethylene triamine pentaacetic acid (Gd-DTPA)-enhanced MRI can potentially be used to quantify the proteoglycan content of normal and degenerated articular cartilage in vivo ***(42–47)***. Gd-DTPA is a negatively charged contrast agent that distributes inversely to the concentration of glycosaminoglycans in cartilage. Other investigators have propagated T1rho relaxation ***(48,49)*** and sodium imaging for measuring proteoglycans ***(50–52)***, but these techniques require specific hardware, not yet available with clinical MRI scanners.

3.2.6.2. Collagen

Wolff et al. ***(53)*** employed magnetization transfer (MT) to evaluate cartilage macromolecules. This technique uses a low-power, off-resonance radiofrequency field, resulting in a decreased signal intensity in regions with tight magnetic coupling between fluid and macromolecules. Some authors suggested that MT is almost exclusively caused by collagen ***(54–56)***, whereas others have found a relevant contribution from the PGs ***(57,58)***. Clinically, it may be feasible to gain specific information on macromolecules (collagen) by obtaining MR images with and without an MT prepulse ***(59,60)***. Transverse relaxation times (T2) have also been used to derive specific information on spatial collagen architecture ***(61)***.

3.2.6.3. Interstitial Water Content

Attempts to evaluate the interstitial water content in cartilage have also been based on the measurement of T2 ***(62–65)*** and on proton density ***(66)*** but are awaiting further validation.

3.3. Image-Analysis Techniques for Cartilage Segmentation and Characterization of Structure (Quantitative Outcome Parameters)

3.3.1. Segmentation of OA Cartilage

1. To derive quantitative data from contiguous MR images, a first step requires labeling (segmentation) of the anatomical structure of interest (the articular cartilage) vs its neighborhood.
2. Owing to the relatively low contrast in some areas of the joint surface (e.g., joint contact areas, vicinity synovial folds, tendons and ligaments, repair tissue, and so on), reliable, fully automated segmentation of cartilage has not yet been achieved from MR images.
3. Various semiautomated segmentation techniques have been developed to date that require different levels of user interaction (*see*, e.g., **ref. *67***), but verification and manual editing by an experienced user is necessary on a section-by-section basis. For these reasons, cartilage segmentation is time-consuming and requires one to several hours per patient.
4. Cartilage volume is dependent on bone size and needs to be normalized to individual bone size for producing meaningful results in cross-sectional studies ***(68)***. Moreover, cartilage volume loss in longitudinal studies may represent either cartilage thinning or an increase in denuded surface areas. We therefore recommend treating the "original" bone cartilage interface (bone cartilage interface before the onset of disease) and the "current" cartilage surface (at the time of investigation) as two separate entities (**Fig. 3**).
5. In practice this means that in OA patients the bone cartilage interface is segmented as a whole (excluding peripheral osteophyte surfaces), whether or not it is covered by cartilage. This procedure requires particular diagnostic training and quality control, to achieve consistency between users. In case of segmentation of large denuded joint areas ("original" bone cartilage interface area), an even higher level of *a priori* knowledge and training is required by the user, because image contrast is relatively low in these areas and because differentiation from bone areas with no cartilage cover before the onset of disease requires thorough experience with joint anatomy. After the segmentation of the "original" bone cartilage interface, the cartilage or several cartilage fragments are then segmented in all non-denuded cartilage areas.

3.3.2. Computation of Quantitative Outcome Parameters

3.3.2.1. General Considerations

In the context of understanding cartilage physiology and pathophysiology, and for evaluating response to treatment in OA, there exists a great demand for fully quantitative parameters of cartilage macromorphology and cartilage loss.

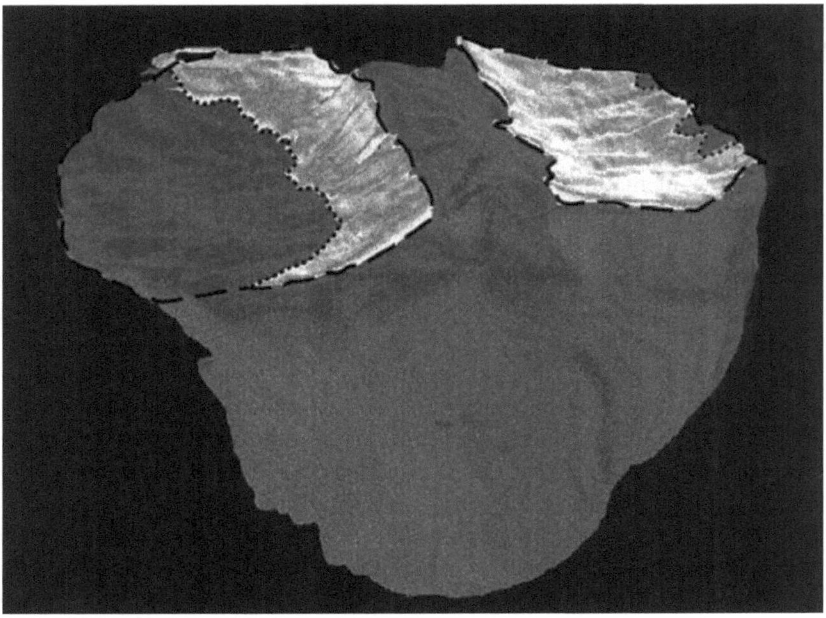

Fig. 3. Three-dimensional reconstruction of cartilage volume on tibial bone in a patient with severe knee osteoarthritis, after segmentation of tibial cartilage (white) on the tibial bone. The medial tibial plateau is on the left and the lateral one on the right. The broken line depicts the total "original" bone cartilage interface (before onset of the disease), and the dotted line depicts the cartilaginous joint surface area.

3.3.2.2. Cartilage Volume

After segmentation, computation of cartilage volume is achieved by numerical integration of the number of voxels attributed to the cartilage during the segmentation process (**Fig. 3**). If joints with relatively thin cartilage are imaged and if the in-plane resolution is relatively low, one can make use of the effect of "subpixel resolution" by interpolating the data to a higher in-plane resolution prior to segmentation ***(27,33)***.

3.3.2.3. Cartilage Thickness and Surface Areas

Cartilage volume, however, only provides a first step in the analysis of cartilage morphology. This can be pursued further by separating the cartilage volume into its two derivatives, namely, the cartilage thickness and the size of the cartilaginous joint surface or bone interface area ***(4,14)***. Computations of these parameters must, however, account for out-of-plane deviations of distances or areas; these must be performed in 3D and must be independent of the original section orientation ***(69,70)***.

3.3.2.4. Surface Geometry and Incongruity

Extraction of cartilage surface also permits determination of the geometric topography and curvature characteristics of diarthrodial joints ***(71)***. A mathematical representation of the surface can be achieved, for example, by fitting a continuous B-splines surface through the discretely segmented surface points ***(69,72,73)***. The principal curvatures can then be calculated from the B-spline surface and are identical to the eigenvalues of the Weingarten matrix ***(69)***. By computing an equivalent surface from two contacting cartilage layers, one can derive quantitative values of incongruity along the least and most congruent directions ***(69,74)***.

3.3.2.5. Fragmented Cartilage Morphology

When dealing with fragmented cartilage, as frequently present in OA, computational software should additionally be able to identify the number of cartilage fragments, the percentage of "original" bone interface currently covered by articular cartilage (or the % denuded/eroded areas), and the normalized cartilage volume (volume divided by the "original" bone-cartilage interface area) ***(68)***. This, however, requires separate segmentation of the "original" bone-cartilage interface (before disease onset) and the current cartilage cover (**Fig. 3**).

3.3.2.6. Cartilage Signal Intensity

To evaluate cartilage signal intensity quantitatively as a surrogate marker of cartilage composition (*see* **Subheading 3.1.6.**), Hohe et al. ***(75,76)*** have provided algorithms that permit one to map these signal intensities quantitatively across the cartilage, in both a layer- and region-specific manner.

3.4. Guidelines for How to Test the Validity (Accuracy), Precision (Reproducibility), and Sensitivity to Change of These Methodologies in OA

3.4.1. Validity (Accuracy) of Quantitative Cartilage Measurements

3.4.1.1. General Considerations on Validation Studies

Because the algorithms mentioned just above may be subject to error, validation vs independent, established methods is required. This should be performed not only in phantoms, but with the actual biological structure of interest, because most artifacts in MRI occur only when the actual tissue is placed in the magnetic field.

3.4.1.2. "Material" for Validation Studies

The technical validity of MRI-based measurements has been addressed by comparative analyses in unselected cadaver joints ***(23,73,77–81)***, in amputated joints *(3,22)*, and in knee joints of patients prior to total knee arthroplasty (TKA) *(3,22,28)*. The latter provides a unique opportunity for validating measurements, since patients can be imaged prior to surgery in vivo, and the tissue can be removed and analyzed after the operation.

3.4.1.3. Methods for Validation Studies

Various reference methods have been used as gold standards for comparative measurements, namely, water displacement of surgically retrieved tissue (either direct or by employing Archimedes' principle) *(3,22,28,32,78)*, anatomical sections obtained with high-precision bandsaws *(23,79)*, computed tomography (CT) arthrography *(27,80,81)*, A-mode ultrasound (not to be confused with clinical B-mode ultrasound) *(27,79)*, and stereophotogrammetry *(73)*.

3.4.1.4. Results of Important Validation Studies

Most of these validation studies have reported high agreement between methods, with random errors (absolute amount of pairwise over- or underestimation) around 5–10%. No consistent over- or underestimation has been revealed for MRI in comparison with reference methods across studies, and the degree of accuracy of MRI-based measurements has been similar for most cartilage surfaces throughout the human knee and other joints. Graichen et al. *(81a)* have recently demonstrated that, in patients with severe OA (prior to TKA), accurate data can also be obtained on the percentage of joint surface covered with cartilage (or on the percentage of denuded joint area) and on the thickness of the remaining cartilage layer. Validation studies have also been performed in smaller joints with thinner cartilage, for instance in the metacarpophalangeal joint *(32)* and in the elbow joint *(27)*.

3.4.2. Precision (Reproducibility) of Quantitative Cartilage Measurements

3.4.2.1. General Considerations on Measurement Precision and OA Progression

Measurement precision is of critical importance in clinical OA trials, because changes in cartilage status occur at a very slow rate. Highly reproducible techniques are therefore required to resolve these changes with statistical confidence, and in particular to resolve drug effects on these changes. Note that the level of technical precision is of major importance regarding the number of patients to be included in a trial and the study duration. It is evident that these factors have tremendous impact on the costs of clinical trials, because the examinations involved are costly and because there will be great financial benefits from reaching the market sooner with a novel agent *(82)*. Also, it may be critical from ethical point of view to expose large numbers of patients to a long study with an investigational new agent; equivalent information may be obtained using MRI in a shorter study with fewer patients.

3.4.2.2. Factors Affecting Precision

Precision on quantitative cartilage measurements from MRI depends (1) on the process of image acquisition, and (2) on the process of image analysis. In contrast to radiography, differences in joint positioning are less critical, because the technique is 3D and the relevant quantitative measures are obtained from reconstructions of serial images rather than from projection onto one image plane. This represents a potential advantage for multicenter clinical trials, which require robust acquisition techniques, whereas image analysis can be performed at specialized centers.

3.4.2.3. Statistical Measures of Precision

The way in which precision errors have most commonly been expressed is the standard deviation (SD) of repeated measurements, or the coefficient of variation (CV%; SD related to the mean value). When examining patients with OA, the CV% will necessarily be larger than that in healthy volunteers, even if the absolute error (SD) is similar. This is because patients display a lower value of cartilage volume, and the error is thus divided by a lower denominator, resulting in higher coefficients. The confidence limits of the SD and CV% reported in a precision study depend both on the number of subjects that have been examined and on the number of repeated scans, from which the SD or CV% have been calculated ***(83)***. Glüer et al. ***(83)*** have recommended to at least three or four repeated scans in at least 14 representative subjects; under these conditions, the "true" precision error in the population is not underestimated by more than 30%.

Note that there also exist different ways to report the average SD or CV% across several individuals in which repeated measurements have been taken. One way is to compute the median SD or CV% in the cohort. This, however, eliminates the impact of large precision errors and therefore involves underestimation of the "true" precision error in the population. Reporting the mean value of SD or CV% across subjects also underestimates the precision error in the population, because the measured variance (SD^2) and not the measured SD is considered an unbiased estimate of the parameter σ^2 of the gaussian normal distribution ***(83)***. For this reason, SDs or CV%s in each subject should be squared (giving more weight to large precision errors), and the analysis should report the square root of the mean of these values in the total sample (RMS SD or CV%) ***(83)***.

3.4.2.4. Results of Important Precision Studies for Cartilage Volume

Most studies have examined the precision of specific MRI acquisition protocols in conjunction with specific image-analysis tools under short-term acquisition conditions (images obtained within one imaging session, but with repositioning of the joint in between acquisitions—also termed immediate test-retest reproducibility). Results for important studies on the reproducibility of cartilage volume measurements are summarized in **Table 1** and may serve as benchmarks for new imaging protocols and image-analysis algorithms. The long-term and resegmentation precision of quantitative cartilage analysis has also been assessed in a recent paper ***(84)***.

3.4.2.5. Specific Results of Different Compartments and Section Orientations

When comparing results for different joint compartments and section orientations, the lowest precision errors (CV% ~ 1%) have been observed for axial protocols of the patella ***(85)***. Relatively large precision errors, in contrast, have been reported for analyses of the femoral condyles in sagittal scans ***(84)***, but this can be overcome by analyzing a selected region of interest (anterior femoral condyles) from coronal scans, using defined anatomical landmarks ***(85a)***.

3.4.2.6. Precision of Cartilage Thickness and Surface Areas

Precision errors of computation of the mean cartilage thickness throughout joint surfaces have been reported to be very similar to those of cartilage volume ***(28,70,86,87)*** as have been those for quantification of joint surface areas ***(68,69,87)***. These image-analysis steps thus do not involve a loss in precision vs the numerical integration of segmented voxels but may substantially broaden the information on specific structure-related disease processes in OA.

3.4.3. Sensitivity to Change of Quantitative Cartilage Measurements

3.4.3.1. Cross-Sectional Data

Estimates of cartilage thinning during normal aging (in the absence of OA) have been derived from cross-sectional data obtained in elderly healthy subjects without a history of knee joint symptoms, trauma, or surgery (50–78 yr) in relation to a cohort of young, healthy subjects that met the same conditions (20–30 yr). The authors ***(8)*** reported an estimated 0.3–0.5% reduction of cartilage thickness per annum for all knee compartments. In the patella, women displayed a higher estimated loss than men, but no gender difference was found for other compartments of the knee ***(8)***.

3.4.3.2. Longitudinal Data

Recently, the first data on changes in cartilage volume have become available from longitudinal studies. No significant changes in cartilage volume have been observed in healthy volunteers over periods of approx 2 yr ***(88)***, but significant cartilage loss was detected in a group of patients that had undergone partial meniscectomy ***(88)***. Despite differences in patient cohorts, the rate of cartilage loss observed in OA by different groups (~5% per annum) has been relatively similar across studies ***(89–91)***, with only one exception ***(92)***.

4. Notes

1. In terms of imaging at 3 T, similar T1-weighted 3D fat-suppressed GE sequences will soon become available. These permit a slight reduction in TR and TE, and a potential gain in SNR of up to 40% vs imaging at 1.5 T.
2. Note that the in-plane resolution can be chosen asymmetrically ***(24,31)***, with larger dimensions in the phase-encoding direction (phase resolution < 100%). This permits a substantial reduction in the acquisition time, but the effect on accuracy and precision of quantitative cartilage measurements has not yet been determined in comparative studies. Since a high resolution is generally required in both dimensions of the MR images, we recommend using an isotropic in-plane resolution.
3. An effective way to save imaging time and gain more signal is to reduce the slice resolution. This means that images are acquired with a larger section thickness but are interpolated to a smaller section thickness. Selecting a 75% slice resolution in combination with a 1.5-mm section thickness, for instance, implies that sections are acquired with a 2.0-mm section thickness but are interpolated to slices with a 1.5-mm geometric dimension. This approach has recently been validated in TKA patients ***(81a)***.
4. No relevant difference in precision errors has been identified for coronal and sagittal scans in the tibia of healthy volunteers. In our experience, however, coronal scans have advantages over sagittal images in OA, because of the partial volume effects that can occur at the internal aspects of the articular surfaces (adjacent to the intercondylar area) with sagittal images, and because of the pattern of cartilage loss in femorotibial OA, which frequently occurs in a mediolateral fashion ***(28)***. Because the cartilage is initially lost in the central aspects of the surface (but remains intact at the external and in particular at the internal aspects of the surface), transition from cartilaginous to denuded joint surface areas generally occurs from section to section with sagittal image data in OA, but within sectional images in coronal image data ***(28)***. Some current controversy exists between groups over which protocol (sagittal or a combination of axial and coronal scans) is favorable. To data, no face-to-face comparison of precision or longitudinal change between a sagittal vs a coronal (tibia) or axial (patella) protocol has been provided in the same cohort of OA patients. One of the reasons for this is the long imaging time that would be required on each patient for performing such a study.
5. If aliasing artifacts occur in the most peripheral images, one needs to increase slice oversampling; if they occur at peripheral parts of some images (in the in-plane phase-encoding direction), one needs to increase phase oversampling.

Table 1
In Vivo Short-Term Reproducibility for Cartilage Volume Measurements With MRI in the Knee to Serve as a Benchmark

Author	Surface	Orientation	Resolution	No. of subjects (type)	No. of repetitions	CV% (SD) RMS[a]	Upper 95% conf. limit; CV% (SD)[b]
Peterfy et al. ***(22)***	Patella	Sag	2.0/0.6 × 0.6	8 patients (3 amputated/5 TKA)	2–3	6.4 (210)	9.7 (319)
	Tot Fem	Sag		2		4.4 (580)	13 (1694)
	Tot Tib	Sag		2		3.6 (250)	11 (730)
Stammberger et al. ***(70)***	Patella	Sag	2.0/0.3 × 0.3	8 healthy vol.	6	1.5 (57)	1.8 (70)
	Med Tib	Sag				3.2 (75)	3.9 (92)
	Lat Tib	Sag				3.8 (106)	4.7 (130)
Cicuttini et al. ***(3)***	Patella	Sag	1.5/0.3 × 0.3	12 volunteers	2	3.0 (68)	4.6 (103)
	Tot Fem	Sag		(knee pain		2.0 (202)	3.0 (307)
	tot tib	sag		but no OA)		5.0 (152)	7.6 (231)
Cicuttini et al. ***(24)***	Patella	Sag	1.5/0.3 × 0.6	10 healthy vol.	4	2.4 (58)	3.0 (74)
	Tot Fem	Sag				2.6 (352)	3.3 (447)
	Total Tib	Sag				2.6 (68)	3.3 (86)
	Tot Fem	Sag		8 OA patients		2.9 (325)	4.2 (429)
	Tot Tib	Sag		(KLG 3)		3.2 (98)	4.2 (129)
Eckstein et al. ***(93)***	Patella	Axial	1.5/0.3 × 0.3	12 healthy vol.	4	1.0 (34)	1.2 (42)
Hyhlik-Dürr et al. ***(86)***	Med Tib	Cor	1.2/0.3 × 0.3	8 healthy vol.	6	2.3 (48)	2.8 (59)
	Lat Tib	Cor				2.6 (66)	3.2 (81)
Burgkart et al. ***(28)***	Med Tib	Cor	1.2/0.3 × 0.3	8 OA patients	2–4	5.5 (56)	7.8 (80)
	Lat Tib	Cor		(TKA)		3.8 (59)	5.4 (84)
Cicuttini et al. ***(94)***	Med FC	cor[c]	1.3/0.4 × 0.4	10 OA patients	4	2.6 (126)	3.3 (160)
	Lat FC	cor[c]				2.8 (114)	3.6 (145)
Eckstein et al. ***(84)***	Patella	Sag	1.5/0.3 × 0.3	14 healthy vol.	4	2.0 (79)	2.4 (96)
	Tot Fem	Sag				2.3 (303)	2.8 (370)
	Fem Tro	Sag				3.4 (180)	4.1 (220)

	Med FC	Sag				4.9 (211)	6.0 (257)
	Lat FC	Sag				5.3 (212)	6.5 (259)
	Med Tib	Sag				2.5 (56)	3.1 (68)
	Lat Tib	Sag				2.3 (77)	2.8 (94)
Glaser et al., submitted	Med FC	Cor	1.2/0.3 × 0.3	8 healthy vol.	4	3.2 (26)	4.2 (34)
	Lat FC	Cor				3.0 (25)	4.0 (33)
	Med FC	Cor		7 OA patients	2–4	6.2 (34)	8.9 (49)
	Lat FC	Cor		(TKA)		4.5 (37)	6.5 (53)

CV, coefficient of variation of repeated measurements; SD, standard deviation of repeated measurements; RMS, root mean square; upper 95% conf. limit., 95% (one-sided) upper confidence limit; Sag, Sagittal; cor, conronal; tot, total; med, medial; lat, lateral; tib, tibia; tot fem, total femur, including the trochlea and both condyles; FC, femoral condyle; fem tro, femoral trochlea; vol., volunteers; pat., patients; OA, osteoarthritis; KLG, Kellgren Lawrence grade.

[a]Data in parentheses are in μL.

[b]Data in parentheses are in μL.

[c]Analyzed from reformatted coronal scans (reformatted from sagittal plane).

6. There are several ways to decrease imaging time that do not affect the spatial resolution of the images. These include selection of phase partial Fourier (e.g., 7/8 or 6/8), elliptical scanning, or choice of a slightly asymmetric echo. However, these procedures may potentially cause ringing (replication of edges) or blurring (edges not sharp). As delineation of sharp edges at the bone-cartilage interface and articular surface is critical in quantitative cartilage imaging, these measures should be used with reservation and care.

Acknowledgments

The author would like to thank Wilhelm Horger (Siemens Medical Solutions, MR-Application Development, Erlangen Germany) for critical discussion of the manuscript. Thanks are also due to Maximilian Reiser and Christian Glaser (Institute of Diagnostic Radiology, LMU München), Karl-Hans Englmeier (Medis Institute, GSF National Research Center Neuherberg), Rainer Burgkart (Department of Orthopedics, TU München), Heiko Graichen (Department of Orthopedics, Frankfurt University), and David Felson (Arthritis and Musculoskeletal Disease Center, Boston University) for their excellent cooperation.

References

1. Peterfy, C. G. (2001) Role of MR imaging in clinical research studies. *Semin. Musculoskel. Radiol.* **5,** 365–378.
2. Beary, J. F., III (2001) Joint structure modification in osteoarthritis: development of SMOAD drugs. *Curr. Rheumatol. Rep.* **3,** 506–512.
3. Cicuttini, F., Forbes, A., Morris, K., Darling, S., Bailey, M., and Stuckey, S. (1999) Gender differences in knee cartilage volume as measured by magnetic resonance imaging. *Osteoarthritis Cartilage* **7,** 265–271.
4. Faber, S. C., Eckstein, F., Lukasz, S., et al. (2001) Gender differences in knee joint cartilage thickness, volume and articular surface areas: assessment with quantitative three-dimensional MR imaging. *Skeletal Radiol.* **30,** 144–150.
5. Jones, G., Glisson, M., Hynes, K., and Cicuttini, F. (2000) Sex and site differences in cartilage development: a possible explanation for variations in knee osteoarthritis in later life. *Arthritis Rheum.* **43,** 2543–2549.
6. Cicuttini, F. M., Wluka, A. E., Wang, Y., Davis, S. R., Hankin, J., and Ebeling, P. (2002). Compartment differences in knee cartilage volume in healthy adults. *J. Rheumatol.* **29,** 554–556.
7. Karvonen, R. L., Negendank, W. G., Teitge, R. A., Reed, A. H., Miller, P. R., and Fernandez-Madrid, F. (1994) Factors affecting articular cartilage thickness in osteoarthritis and aging. *J. Rheumatol.* **21,** 1310–1318.
8. Hudelmaier, M., Glaser, C., Hohe, J., et al. (2001) Age-related changes in the morphology and deformational behavior of knee joint cartilage. *Arthritis Rheum.* **44,** 2556–2561.

9. Hudelmaier, M., Glaser, C., Englmeier, K. H., Reiser, M., Putz, R., and Eckstein, F. (2003) Correlation of knee-joint cartilage morphology with muscle cross-sectional areas vs. anthropometric variables. *Anat. Rec.* **270A,** 175–184.
10. Eckstein, F., Winzheimer, M., Westhoff, J., et al. (1998) Quantitative relationships of normal cartilage volumes of the human knee joint—assessment by magnetic resonance imaging. *Anat. Embryol. (Berl.)* **197,** 383–390.
11. Eckstein, F., Winzheimer, M., Hohe, J., Englmeier, K. H., and Reiser, M. (2001) Interindividual variability and correlation among morphological parameters of knee joint cartilage plates: analysis with three-dimensional MR imaging. *Osteoarthritis Cartilage* **9,** 101–111.
12. Eckstein, F., Reiser, M., Englmeier, K. H., and Putz, R. (2001). In vivo morphometry and functional analysis of human articular cartilage with quantitative magnetic resonance imaging—from image to data, from data to theory. *Anat. Embryol. (Berl.)* **203,** 147–173.
13. Eckstein, F., Muller, S., Faber, S. C., Englmeier, K. H., Reiser, M., and Putz, R. (2002). Side differences of knee joint cartilage volume, thickness, and surface area, and correlation with lower limb dominance—an MRI-based study. *Osteoarthritis Cartilage* **10,** 914–921.
14. Eckstein, F., Faber, S., Muhlbauer, R., et al. (2002) Functional adaptation of human joints to mechanical stimuli. *Osteoarthritis Cartilage* **10,** 44–50.
15. Vanwanseele, B., Eckstein, F., Knecht, H., Stussi, E., and Spaepen, A. (2002) Knee cartilage of spinal cord-injured patients displays progressive thinning in the absence of normal joint loading and movement. *Arthritis Rheum.* **46,** 2073–2078.
16. Gratzke, C., Glaser, C., Englmeier, K. H., Reiser, M., and Eckstein, F. (2002) Comparison of cartilage morphology in professional weight-lifters and sprinters with normal volunteers suggests that human articular cartilage cannot adapt to functional stimulation. *Osteoarthritis Cartilage* **10 (suppl A),** S11 (abstract).
17. Wluka, A. E., Davis, S. R., Bailey, M., Stuckey, S. L., and Cicuttini, F. M. (2001) Users of oestrogen replacement therapy have more knee cartilage than non-users. *Ann. Rheum. Dis.* **60,** 332–336.
18. Siedek, V., Glaser, C., Englmeier, K. H., Reiser, M., and Eckstein, F. (2002) MRI-based analysis of knee and ankle cartilage in monocygotic twins suggests that its morphology is strongly determined by genetics. *Osteoarthritis Cartilage* **10 (suppl. A),** S56 (PS 110) (abstract).
19. Peterfy, C. G. (2002). Imaging of the disease process. *Curr. Opin. Rheumatol.* **14,** 590–596.
20. Frahm, J., Haase, A., and Matthaei, D. (1986) Rapid three-dimensional MR imaging using the FLASH technique. *J. Comput. Assist. Tomogr.* **10,** 363–368.
21. Recht, M. P., Kramer, J., Marcelis, S., et al. (1993). Abnormalities of articular cartilage in the knee: analysis of available MR techniques. *Radiology* **187,** 473–478.
22. Peterfy, C. G., van Dijke, C. F., Janzen, D. L., et al. (1994) Quantification of articular cartilage in the knee with pulsed saturation transfer subtraction and fat-suppressed MR imaging: optimization and validation. *Radiology* **192,** 485–491.

23. Eckstein, F., Gavazzeni, A., Sittek, H., et al. (1996) Determination of knee joint cartilage thickness using three-dimensional magnetic resonance chondrocrassometry (3D MR-CCM). *Magn. Reson. Med.* **36,** 256–265.
24. Cicuttini, F., Forbes, A., Asbeutah, A., Morris, K., and Stuckey, S. (2000) Comparison and reproducibility of fast and conventional spoiled gradient-echo magnetic resonance sequences in the determination of knee cartilage volume. *J. Orthop. Res.* **18,** 580–584.
25. Hardy, P. A., Recht, M. P., and Piraino, D. W. (1998) Fat suppressed MRI of articular cartilage with a spatial-spectral excitation pulse. *J. Magn. Reson. Imaging* **8,** 1279–1287.
26. Glaser, C., Faber, S., Eckstein, F., et al. (2001) Optimization and validation of a rapid high-resolution T1-w 3D FLASH water excitation MRI sequence for the quantitative assessment of articular cartilage volume and thickness. *Magn. Reson. Imaging* **19,** 177–185.
27. Graichen, H., Springer, V., Flaman, T., et al. (2000) Validation of high-resolution water-excitation magnetic resonance imaging for quantitative assessment of thin cartilage layers. *Osteoarthritis Cartilage* **8,** 106–114.
28. Burgkart, R., Glaser, C., Hyhlik-Durr, A., Englmeier, K. H., Reiser, M., and Eckstein, F. (2001) Magnetic resonance imaging-based assessment of cartilage loss in severe osteoarthritis: accuracy, precision, and diagnostic value. *Arthritis Rheum.* **44,** 2072–2077.
29. Hardy, P. A., Newmark, R., Liu, Y. M., et al. (2000) The influence of the resolution and contrast on measuring the articular cartilage volume in magnetic resonance images. *Magn. Reson. Imaging* **18,** 965–972.
30. Link, T. M., Majumdar, S., Peterfy, C., et al. (1998). High resolution MRI of small joints: impact of spatial resolution on diagnostic performance and SNR. *Magn. Reson. Imaging* **16,** 147–155.
31. Marshall, K. W., Guthrie, B. T., and Mikulis, D. J. (1995) Quantitative cartilage imaging. *Br. J. Rheumatol.* **34 (Suppl 1),** 29–31.
32. Peterfy, C. G., van Dijke, C. F., Lu, Y., et al. (1995) Quantification of the volume of articular cartilage in the metacarpophalangeal joints of the hand: accuracy and precision of three-dimensional MR imaging. *AJR Am. J. Roentgenol.* **165,** 371–375.
33. Al Ali, D., Graichen, H., Faber, S., Englmeier, K. H., Reiser, M., and Eckstein, F. (2002). Quantitative cartilage imaging of the human hind foot: precision and inter-subject variability. *J. Orthop. Res.* **20,** 249–256.
34. Recht, M. P., Piraino, D. W., Paletta, G. A., Schils, J. P., and Belhobek, G. H. (1996). Accuracy of fat-suppressed three-dimensional spoiled gradient-echo FLASH MR imaging in the detection of patellofemoral articular cartilage abnormalities. *Radiology* **198,** 209–212.
35. Disler, D. G., McCauley, T. R., Kelman, C. G., et al. (1996) Fat-suppressed three-dimensional spoiled gradient-echo MR imaging of hyaline cartilage defects in the knee: comparison with standard MR imaging and arthroscopy. *Am. J Roentgenol.* **167,** 127–132.
36. Broderick, L. S., Turner, D. A., Renfrew, D. L., Schnitzer, T. J., Huff, J. P., and Harris, C. (1994) Severity of articular cartilage abnormality in patients with

osteoarthritis: evaluation with fast spin-echo MR vs arthroscopy. *AJR Am. J. Roentgenol.* **162,** 99–103.
37. Kawahara, Y., Uetani, M., Nakahara, N., et al. (1998) Fast spin-echo MR of the articular cartilage in the osteoarthrotic knee. Correlation of MR and arthroscopic findings. *Acta Radiol.* **39,** 120–125.
38. Bredella, M. A., Tirman, P. F., Peterfy, C. G., et al. (1999) Accuracy of T2-weighted fast spin-echo MR imaging with fat saturation in detecting cartilage defects in the knee: comparison with arthroscopy in 130 patients. *AJR Am. J. Roentgenol.* **172,** 1073–1080.
39. Biswal, S., Hastie, T., Andriacchi, T. P., Bergman, G. A., Dillingham, M. F., and Lang, P. (2002). Risk factors for progressive cartilage loss in the knee: a longitudinal magnetic resonance imaging study in forty-three patients. *Arthritis Rheum.* **46,** 2884–2892.
40. Link, T. M., Steinbach, L. S., Ghosh, S., et al. (2003) Osteoarthritis: MR imaging findings in different stages of disease and correlation with clinical findings. *Radiology* **226,** 373–381.
41. Paul, P. K., Jasani, M. K., Sebok, D., et al. (1993) Variation in MR signal intensity across normal human knee cartilage. *J. Magn. Reson. Imaging* **3,** 569–574.
42. Trattnig, S., Mlynarik, V., Breitenseher, M., et al. (1999) MRI visualization of proteoglycan depletion in articular cartilage via intravenous administration of Gd-DTPA. *Magn. Reson. Imaging* **17,** 577–583.
43. Bashir, A., Gray, M. L., Boutin, R. D., and Burstein, D. (1997) Glycosaminoglycan in articular cartilage: in vivo assessment with delayed Gd(DTPA)(2-)-enhanced MR imaging. *Radiology* **205,** 551–558.
44. Allen, R. G., Burstein, D., and Gray, M. L. (1999) Monitoring glycosaminoglycan replenishment in cartilage explants with gadolinium-enhanced magnetic resonance imaging. *J. Orthop. Res.* **17,** 430–436.
45. Bashir, A., Gray, M. L., Hartke, J., and Burstein, D. (1999) Nondestructive imaging of human cartilage glycosaminoglycan concentration by MRI. *Magn. Reson. Med.* **41,** 857–865.
46. Burstein, D., Bashir, A., and Gray, M. L. (2000) MRI techniques in early stages of cartilage disease. *Invest. Radiol.* **35,** 622–638.
47. Gray, M. L., Burstein, D., and Xia, Y. (2001) Biochemical (and functional) imaging of articular cartilage. *Semin. Musculoskel. Radiol.* **5,** 329–343.
48. Duvvuri, U., Reddy, R., Patel, S. D., Kaufman, J. H., Kneeland, J. B., and Leigh, J. S. (1997). T1rho-relaxation in articular cartilage: effects of enzymatic degradation. *Magn. Reson. Med.* **38,** 863–867.
49. Duvvuri, U., Charagundla, S. R., Kudchodkar, S. B., et al. (2001). Human knee: in vivo T1(rho)-weighted MR imaging at 1.5 T—preliminary experience. *Radiology* **220,** 822–826.
50. Reddy, R., Insko, E. K., Noyszewski, E. A., Dandora, R., Kneeland, J. B., and Leigh, J. S. (1998) Sodium MRI of human articular cartilage in vivo. *Magn. Reson. Med.* **39,** 697–701.
51. Insko, E. K., Kaufman, J. H., Leigh, J. S., and Reddy, R. (1999) Sodium NMR evaluation of articular cartilage degradation. *Magn. Reson. Med.* **41,** 30–34.

52. Regatte, R. R., Kaufman, J. H., Noyszewski, E. A., and Reddy, R. (1999) Sodium and proton MR properties of cartilage during compression. *J. Magn. Reson. Imaging* **10,** 961–967.
53. Wolff, S. D., Chesnick, S., Frank, J. A., Lim, K. O., and Balaban, R. S. (1991) Magnetization transfer contrast: MR imaging of the knee. *Radiology* **179,** 623–628.
54. Kim, D. K., Ceckler, T. L., Hascall, V. C., Calabro, A., and Balaban, R. S. (1993). Analysis of water-macromolecule proton magnetization transfer in articular cartilage. *Magn. Reson. Med.* **29,** 211–215.
55. Aoki, J., Hiraki, Y., Seo, G. S., et al. (1996) [Effect of collagen on magnetization transfer contrast assessed in cultured cartilage]. *Nippon Igaku Hoshasen Gakkai Zasshi* **56,** 877–879.
56. Seo, G. S., Aoki, J., Moriya, H., et al. (1996) Hyaline cartilage: in vivo and in vitro assessment with magnetization transfer imaging. *Radiology* **201,** 525–530.
57. Gray, M. L., Burstein, D., Lesperance, L. M., and Gehrke, L. (1995) Magnetization transfer in cartilage and its constituent macromolecules. *Magn. Reson. Med.* **34,** 319–325.
58. Wachsmuth, L., Juretschke, H. P., and Raiss, R. X. (1997) Can magnetization transfer magnetic resonance imaging follow proteoglycan depletion in articular cartilage? *MAGMA* **5,** 71–78.
59. Vahlensieck, M., Dombrowski, F., Leutner, C., Wagner, U., and Reiser, M. (1994). Magnetization transfer contrast (MTC) and MTC-subtraction: enhancement of cartilage lesions and intracartilaginous degeneration in vitro. *Skeletal Radiol.* **23,** 535–539.
60. Vahlensieck, M., Gieseke, J., Traber, F., and Schild, H. (1998) [Magnetization transfer contrast (MTC)—which is the most MTC-sensitive MRI sequence?]. *Rofo Fortschr. Geb. Rontgenstr. Neuen Bildgeb. Verfahr.* **169,** 195–197.
61. Nieminen, M. T., Rieppo, J., Toyras, J., et al. (2001) T2 relaxation reveals spatial collagen architecture in articular cartilage: a comparative quantitative MRI and polarized light microscopic study. *Magn. Reson. Med.* **46,** 487–493.
62. Dardzinski, B. J., Mosher, T. J., Li, S., Van Slyke, M. A., and Smith, M. B. (1997) Spatial variation of T2 in human articular cartilage. *Radiology* **205,** 546–550.
63. Frank, L. R., Wong, E. C., Luh, W. M., Ahn, J. M., and Resnick, D. (1999). Articular cartilage in the knee: mapping of the physiologic parameters at MR imaging with a local gradient coil—preliminary results. *Radiology* **210,** 241–246.
64. Lusse, S., Claassen, H., Gehrke, T., et al. (2000) Evaluation of water content by spatially resolved transverse relaxation times of human articular cartilage. *Magn. Reson. Imaging* **18,** 423–430.
65. Liess, C., Lüsse, S., Karger, N., Heller, M., and Glüer, C. C. (2002) Detection of changes in cartilage water content using MRI T2-mapping in vivo. *Osteoarthritis Cartilage* **10,** 907–913.
66. Shapiro, E. M., Borthakur, A., Kaufman, J. H., Leigh, J. S., and Reddy, R. (2001) Water distribution patterns inside bovine articular cartilage as visualized by 1H magnetic resonance imaging. *Osteoarthritis Cartilage* **9,** 533–538.

67. Stammberger, T., Eckstein, F., Michaelis, M., Englmeier, K. H., and Reiser, M. (1999) Interobserver reproducibility of quantitative cartilage measurements: comparison of B-spline snakes and manual segmentation. *Magn. Reson. Imaging* **17,** 1033–1042.
68. Burgkart, R., Glaser, C., Hinterwimmer, S., et al. (2003) Feasibility of T- and Z-scores from MR image data for quantifying cartilage loss in osteoarthritis. *Arthritis Rheum.* **48,** 2829–2835.
69. Hohe, J., Ateshian, G., Reiser, M., Englmeier, K. H., and Eckstein, F. (2002) Surface size, curvature analysis, and assessment of knee joint incongruity with MRI in vivo. *Magn. Reson. Med.* **47,** 554–561.
70. Stammberger, T., Eckstein, F., Englmeier, K. H., and Reiser, M. (1999) Determination of 3D cartilage thickness data from MR imaging: computational method and reproducibility in the living. *Magn. Reson. Med.* **41,** 529–536.
71. Ateshian, G. A., Soslowsky, L. J., and Mow, V. C. (1991) Quantitation of articular surface topography and cartilage thickness in knee joints using stereophotogrammetry. *J. Biomech.* **24,** 761–776.
72. Ateshian, G. A. (1993) A B-spline least-squares surface-fitting method for articular surfaces of diarthrodial joints. *J. Biomech. Eng.* **115,** 366–373.
73. Cohen, Z. A., McCarthy, D. M., Kwak, S. D., etal. (1999) Knee cartilage topography, thickness, and contact areas from MRI: in-vitro calibration and in-vivo measurements. *Osteoarthritis Cartilage* **7,** 95–109.
74. Ateshian, G. A., Rosenwasser, M. P., and Mow, V. C. (1992) Curvature characteristics and congruence of the thumb carpometacarpal joint: differences between female and male joints. *J. Biomech.* **25,** 591–607.
75. Hohe, J., Faber, S., Stammberger, T., Reiser, M., Englmeier, K. H., and Eckstein, F. (2000) A technique for 3D in vivo quantification of proton density and magnetization transfer coefficients of knee joint cartilage. *Osteoarthritis Cartilage* **8,** 426–433.
76. Hohe, J., Faber, S., Muehlbauer, R., Reiser, M., Englmeier, K. H., and Eckstein, F. (2002) Three-dimensional analysis and visualization of regional MR signal intensity distribution of articular cartilage. *Med. Eng Phys.* **24,** 219–227.
77. Sittek, H., Eckstein, F., Gavazzeni, A., et al. (1996) Assessment of normal patellar cartilage volume and thickness using MRI: an analysis of currently available pulse sequences. *Skeletal Radiol.* **25,** 55–62.
78. Piplani, M. A., Disler, D. G., McCauley, T. R., Holmes, T. J., and Cousins, J. P. (1996) Articular cartilage volume in the knee: semiautomated determination from three-dimensional reformations of MR images. *Radiology* **198,** 855–859.
79. Eckstein, F., Adam, C., Sittek, H., et al. (1997) Non-invasive determination of cartilage thickness throughout joint surfaces using magnetic resonance imaging. *J. Biomech.* **30,** 285–289.
80. Eckstein, F., Schnier, M., Haubner, M., et al. (1998) Accuracy of cartilage volume and thickness measurements with magnetic resonance imaging. *Clin. Orthop.*, July, (352), 137–148.
81. Eckstein, F., Stammberger, T., Priebsch, J., Englmeier, K. H., and Reiser, M. (2000). Effect of gradient and section orientation on quantitative analysis of knee joint cartilage. *J. Magn. Reson. Imaging* **11,** 161–167.

81a. Graichen, H., Eisenhart-Rothe, R., Vogl, T., Englmeier, K. H., and Eckstein, F. (2004) Quantitative assessment of cartilage status in osteoarthritis by quantitative magnetic resonance imaging: technical validation for use in analysis of cartilage volume and further morphologic parameters. *Arthritis Rheum.* **50,** 811–816.
82. Peterfy, C. G. (2000) Scratching the surface: articular cartilage disorders in the knee. *Magn. Reson. Imaging Clin. N. Am.* **8,** 409–430.
83. Glüer, C. C., Blake, G., Lu, Y., Blunt, B. A., Jergas, M., and Genant, H. K. (1995) Accurate assessment of precision errors: how to measure the reproducibility of bone densitometry techniques. *Osteoporos. Int.* **5,** 262–270.
84. Eckstein, F., Heudorfer, L., Faber, S. C., Burgkart, R., Englmeier, K. H., and Reiser, M. (2002). Long-term and resegmentation precision of quantitative cartilage MR imaging (qMRI). *Osteoarthritis Cartilage* **10,** 922–928.
85. Eckstein, F., Lemberger, B., Stammberger, T., Englmeier, K. H., and Reiser, M. (2000). Patellar cartilage deformation in vivo after static versus dynamic loading. *J. Biomech.* **33,** 819–825.
85a. Glaser, C., Burgkart, R., Kutschera, A., Englmeier, K. H., Reiser, M., and Eckstein, F. (2003) Femoro-tibial cartilage metrics from coronal MR image data: technique, test-retest reproducibility, and findings in osteoarthritis. *Magn. Reson. Med.* **50,** 1229–1236.
86. Hyhlik-Dürr, A., Faber, S., Burgkart, R., et al. (2000) Precision of tibial cartilage morphometry with a coronal water-excitation MR sequence. *Eur. Radiol.* **10,** 297–303.
87. Eckstein, F., Heudorfer, L., Faber, S., Burgkart, R., Englmeier, K. H., and Reiser, M. (2002). Long-term and resegmentation precision of quantitative cartilage MR imaging (qMRI). *Osteoarthritis Cartilage* **10,** 922–928.
88. Cicuttini, F. M., Forbes, A., Yuanyuan, W., Rush, G., and Stuckey, S. L. (2002) Rate of knee cartilage loss after partial meniscectomy. *J. Rheumatol.* **29,** 1954–1956.
89. Wluka, A. E., Stuckey, S., Snaddon, J., and Cicuttini, F. M. (2002) The determinants of change in tibial cartilage volume in osteoarthritic knees. *Arthritis Rheum.* **46,** 2065–2072.
90. Cicuttini, F., Wluka, A., Wang, Y., and Stuckey, S. (2002) The determinants of change in patella cartilage volume in osteoarthritic knees. *J. Rheumatol.* **29,** 2615–2619.
91. Raynauld, J.-P., Pelletier, J.-P., Beaudoin, G., et al. (2002) A two-year study in osteoarthritis patients following the progression of the disease by magnetic resonance imaging using a novel quantification imaging system. *Arthritis Rheum.* **46,** S150 (abstract).
92. Gandy, S. J., Dieppe, P. A., Keen, M. C., Maciewicz, R. A., Watt, I., and Waterton, J. C. (2002). No loss of cartilage volume over three years in patients with knee osteoarthritis as assessed by magnetic resonance imaging. *Osteoarthritis Cartilage* **10,** 929–937.

93. Eckstein, F., Lemberger, B., Stammberger, T., Englmeier, K. H., and Reiser, M. (2000) Patellar cartilage deformation in vivo after static versus dynamic loading. *J. Biomech.* **33,** 819–825.
94. Cicuttini, F. M., Wluka, A. E., and Stuckey, S. L. (2001) Tibial and femoral cartilage changes in knee osteoarthritis. *Ann. Rheum. Dis.* **60,** 977–980.

11

High-Resolution MRI Techniques for Studies in Small-Animal Models

Olivier Beuf

Summary

High-field magnetic resonance (MR), which allows high-resolution imaging, is a powerful research tool to examine and visualize hyaline cartilage of small joints noninvasively. Recent studies have shown that qualitative assessment of degenerative joint disease, derived from MR images, was reliable. The ability to show pathologic changes throughout the time-course of the disease from 3D datasets has also been demonstrated. Quantitative imaging for accurate determination of cartilage volume and thickness are still to be confirmed. This chapter presents a MR protocol for in vivo imaging of small-animal knee joints on a 7-T imager. Technical aspects and specifics of modality and field strength are discussed, as well as future developments and expected evolutions of techniques.

Key Words: Osteoarthritis; articular cartilage; magnetic resonance imaging; high-resolution; small animals.

1. Introduction

Articular cartilage is a soft tissue that covers the load-bearing or articular surfaces of the ends of most bones at the movable joints. The major components are water (70%), collagen (10–20%), proteoglycans, and chondrocytes. When healthy, it is a smooth, lubricating, and load-bearing material, capable of withstanding a variety of mechanical forces. Depending on the acuteness of the disease, swelling, softening, and erosion of the cartilage predominate. Progressive thinning can result in an eventual loss of the entire articular cartilage. It is also characterized by the development of altered joint congruency, subchondral sclerosis, intraosseous cysts, and osteophytes.

In vivo high-resolution magnetic resonance imaging (HR-MRI) has significant potential as a tool to probe morphometric changes in articular cartilage. It is nonionizing, offers multiplanar capabilities and high spatial resolution, and

From: *Methods in Molecular Medicine, Vol. 101: Cartilage and Osteoarthritis, Volume 2: Structure and In Vivo Analysis*
Edited by: F. De Ceuninck, M. Sabatini, and P. Pastoureau © Humana Press Inc., Totowa, NJ

provides superior depiction of soft tissue detail *(1)*. Unlike other imaging modalities, MRI is capable of directly visualizing all components of the joint simultaneously, a necessity for accurate morphometric evaluation of articular cartilage *(2)*.

Magnetic resonance (MR) techniques have been proposed for assessing cartilage volume and thickness as well as structural degeneration in several human studies *(3)*. Recently, technological advances (*see* **Note 1**) have made MR a powerful research tool for the investigation of cartilage pathologies in small animal joints. Because of the limited size of joints, the technique is challenging *(4,5)* but HR-MRI could be a noninvasive method allowing the detection of osteoarthritic lesions as well as monitoring of disease progression and treatment response in joint disease *(6,7)*.

This chapter presents methods for assessing articular cartilage morphology using HR-MRI on small animals. MR acquisition protocols can be used on rat or guinea pig joints for diagnosis as well as for longitudinal studies using animal models.

2. Materials

1. Biospec system 70/20 (Bruker, Ettlingen, Germany) composed of a 7-T horizontal-bore magnet and equipped with 400 mT/m maximum gradient amplitude and 160 μs minimum rise time. The clear bore diameter is 120 mm.
2. A cylindrical birdcage body coil (72-mm inner diameter and 112-mm outer diameter) for transmission.
3. A 25-mm-diameter radiofrequency (RF) surface coil for signal reception only, operating at 300 MHz (corresponding to proton frequency at 7 T).
4. A home-made dedicated animal holder.
5. Gas anesthesia system for isoflurane (Minerve, Esternay, France) with a dedicated cone mask.
6. 2% Xylazine (Rompun, Bayer, France) and ketamine (Imalgène 1000, Merial, France).

3. Methods

Experiments must be constructed in accordance with the rules and regulations of the Ethics Committee on animal experimentation of the institution.

3.1. Anesthesia

Two possibilities can be considered for anesthesia depending on the available material and examination duration. Anesthesia can be induced with an intraperitoneal injection of 1 mg/kg using a cocktail composed of 50% vol of 2% xylazine and 50% vol of ketamine. For longer experiments and to avoid removal of the animal from the center of the magnet for additional injection, gaseous anesthesia is preferred. First the animal is introduced into an induction chamber for anesthesia using isoflurane gas at 4–5% and up to 4 L/min air flow for about 1 min. Hence, anesthesia is maintained with isoflurane gas at 1.5–2.5% and 1 L/min flow. Gas is administered with an approved system machine (Minerve, Esternay, France) and provided to the animal with a cone mask over the nose.

3.2. Animal Setup

The animal is laid out prone on a plastic bed. To ensure accuracy in animal positioning as well as to prevent motion artifacts, the leg is extended and the knee to be imaged is placed on a home-made dedicated holder just below the surface coil (as close as possible). The foot is fixed with surgical tape. The bed is introduced in the transmit body coil, and the knee joint is placed centrally within the body coil. Finally, the whole setup is centered precisely in the magnet. At this point, the knee to be imaged should be at the center of the surface coil, transmit coil and magnet. Animal setup and coil positioning is critical to maximize the signal-to-noise ratio (SNR) and image quality.

Note that for optimum SNR, the normal direction of the surface coil should be orthogonal to the main magnetic field direction. Note also that because of coupling between the surface and body RF coil, the B1 direction indicated on the body coil should be horizontal, and the B1 direction of the surface coil should be vertical, to minimize cross-coupling and be able to tune to 300 MHz and match both coils to 50 Ω.

3.3. Imaging Protocol

A gradient-echo localizer with three orthogonal orientations and reasonable (8 cm) field of view (FOV) is first used to identify the region of interest and allows graphical prescriptions of the scans to follow.

A series of two-dimensional (2D) sequences showing different tissue contrasts is performed to qualitatively assess peripheral joint tissues for such factors as edema, subchondral cysts, joint effusion, ligaments, and menisci. Using high-field strength, compared with clinical field strength (1.5 T), results in altered relaxation time and mainly in reduced longitudinal relaxation time (T1) contrast. Only proton density (PD) and transverse relaxation time (T2) contrast are proposed.

Sagittal multislice, multiecho 2D PD-weighted and T2-weighted images are performed with a rapid acquisition with relaxation enhancement (RARE) sequence *(8)* and the following parameters: repetition time (TR) 3000 ms; echo time (TE1/TE2) 19.2/50 ms; RARE factor 4; FOV 4 cm; 1-mm slice thickness; and reconstructed matrix 256 × 256.

Then a coronal 2D PD-weighted RARE sequence with fat suppression (FS) is performed with TR 3000 ms; TE 19.2 ms; RARE factor 4; FOV 4 cm; 1-mm slice thickness; and reconstructed matrix 256 × 256. Additionally, an axial 2D T2-weighted RARE sequence with FS is performed with TR 3000 ms; TE 40 ms; RARE factor 8; FOV 4 cm; 1-mm slice thickness; and reconstructed matrix 256 × 256. Representative images of 2D acquisitions are shown in **Fig. 1**. Again, because longitudinal relaxation time (T1) of tissues is longer at 7 T than at clinical field strength (1.5 T), the flip-back option is selected for all the above RARE sequences to improve image contrast with reasonable TR. The last spin echo pulse is followed by an additional flip-back pulse. This scheme realigns the longitudinal magnetization with the direction of the main magnetic field to restore it more rapidly.

More quantitative assessment of cartilage morphology is obtained from HR-MR images with a FS 3D gradient echo (GEFI) sequence (*see* **Notes 2** and **3**). Sixty-four partitions (312 μm thick) are acquired with an FOV of 40 mm and an acquisition matrix size of 512 × 384 (reconstructed to 512 × 512), leading to an in-plane spatial resolution of 78 × 78 mm^2. A flip angle (α) of 10°, TR of 30 ms, and TE of 4.8 ms TE with a 42-kHz receiver bandwidth (rbw) are used. The scan time is 24:34 min. Representative images obtained in sagittal and coronal planes are shown in **Fig. 2** (*see* **Note 4**).

A detailed list of acquisition parameters used for each sequence is reported in **Table 1**. The total measurement time per animal to perform the above MR protocol, including anesthesia and positioning in the magnet, is about 1 h. With this protocol, the anatomy (proximal tibia, distal femur, meniscus, synovial fluid, cruciate ligaments) and the pathology of the joint can be clearly seen.

For studies in which thickness assessment is required, spatial resolution can be increased but at the cost of scan time. For example, a 59-μm in-plane pixel size can be obtained with sufficient SNR in about a 45-min scan time (*see* **Note 5**). A representative image showing cartilage with higher spatial resolution is presented in **Fig. 3A**.

3.4. Intensity Correction

Since the images are acquired with a surface coil, the reception profile is nonuniform, leading to an intensity inhomogeneity depending on volume orientation with respect to coil orientation. Two correction schemes can be used, a phantom-based and a low-pass-filter (LPF)-based correction scheme. For phantom-based correction, data from uniform phantoms must be acquired to obtain the sensitivity profile of the coil. Cartilage images are corrected compared with this reference measurement. Alternatively, a 3D gaussian filter can be applied to the volume image *(9)*. The bandwidth of the gaussian filter is adjusted to achieve a compromise between the accurate location of true edges and noise reduction. An increase in filter bandwidth decreases noise, at the

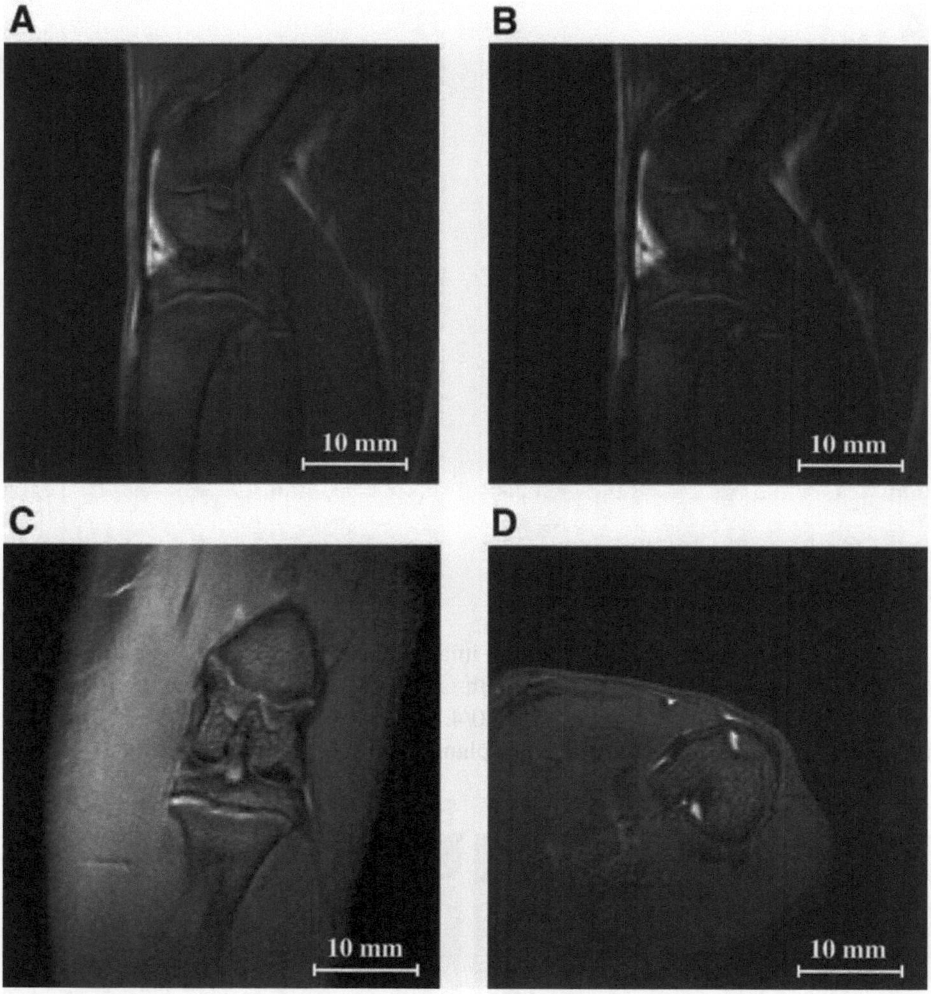

Fig. 1. Representative 2D images for qualitative assessment of peripheral joint tissues. **(A, B)** Sagittal proton density (PD)- and relaxation time T2-weighted image. **(C)** Coronal fat-suppressed PD-weighted image. **(D)** Axial fat-suppressed T2-weighted image.

cost of edge accuracy. Coil intensity correction improving the signal homogeneity of the image is shown in **Fig. 3B**.

3.5. 3D Analysis

Analysis of 3D volume can be done using multiplanar reconstruction (MPR) tools. With such software, images can be reformatted and viewed at the same

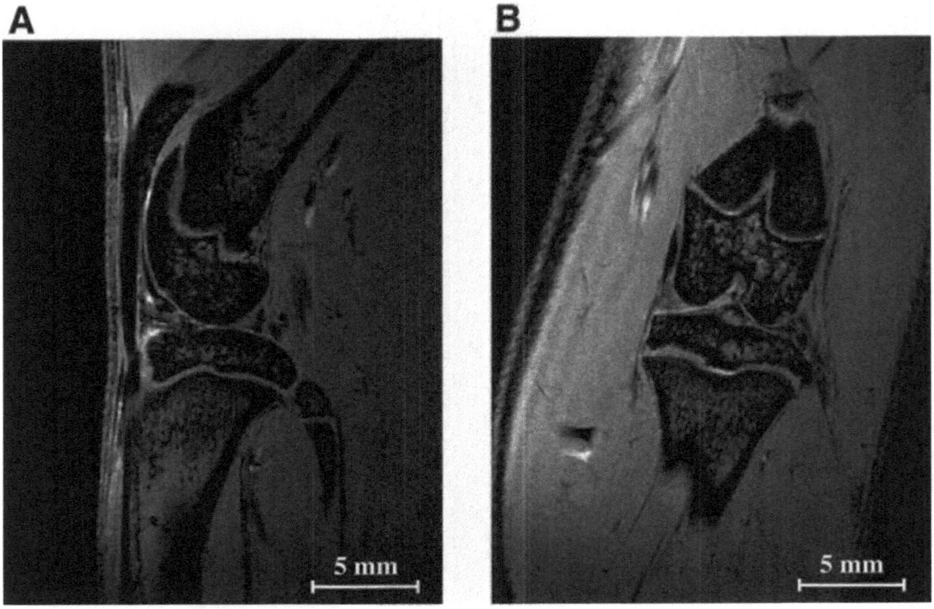

Fig. 2. Representative high-resolution images of a 9-wk-old rat knee in (**A**) sagittal and (**B**) coronal planes obtained at 7 T with fat-suppressed 3D gradient echo sequence with the following parameters: TR/TE: 30/4.8 ms; α 10°; FOV 40 mm; 312-µm slice thickness; 78×78 µm^2 reconstructed in-plane pixel size; 24 min scan time.

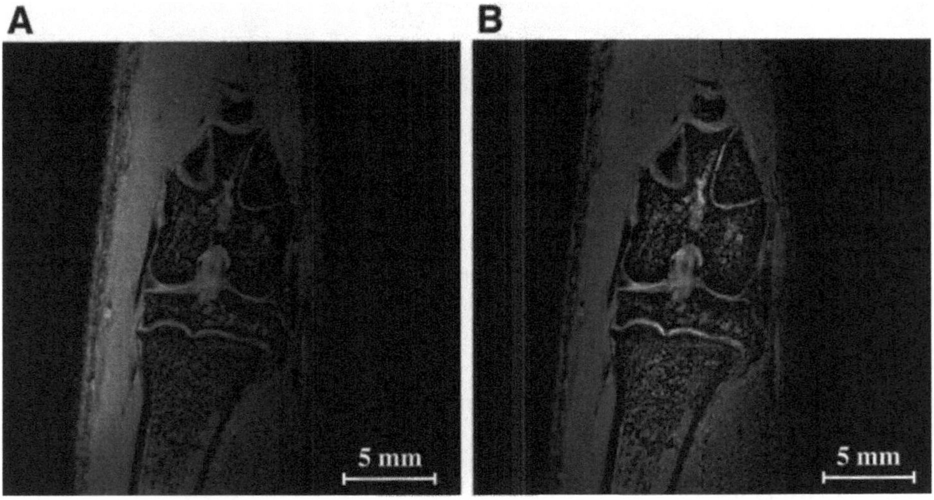

Fig. 3. (**A**) Representative very high-resolution coronal image of cartilage knee obtained on a 11-wk-old rat. In-plane resolution is 59×59 µm^2 and scan time is about 45 min. Image clearly depicts the femur and tibia cartilage boundaries. (**B**) Same image after low-pass filter-based correction.

Table 1
Proposed List of Sequences With Imaging Parameters Used on Small Animals for Knee Study at 7 T

Sequence description	FOV (cm)	Slice/slab thickness (mm)	No. of slices/ partitions	TR/TE (ms)	α (°)	Acq. matrix	Rec. pixel (μm)	Phase over-sampling	No. of excitations (NEX)	No. of echoes	RARE factor	rbw (kHz)	TA (min:sec)
3-Plane localizer	8.0	3	3	100/4	30	128 × 128	624	No	1	1	—	25	0:12
PD + T2 RARE 2D	4.0	1	11	3000/19.2/50	90	256 × 192	156	Yes	1	2	4	62	4:48
PD RARE 2D FS	4.0	1	11	3000/19.2	90	256 × 192	156	Yes	1	1	4	62	4:48
T2 RARE 2D FS	4.0	1	19	3000/40	90	256 × 192	156	Yes	2	1	8	62	4:48
GEFI 3D FS	4.0	20	64	30/4.8	10	512 × 384	78	Yes	1	1	—	42	24:34

PD, proton density; FOV, field of view; FS, fat suppression; GEFI, gradient-echo fast imaging; RARE, rapid acquisition with relaxation enhancement.

[a]Total scan time was about 45 min. Total exam time including animal installation, coil tuning, and matching, and scan time did not exceed 1 h.

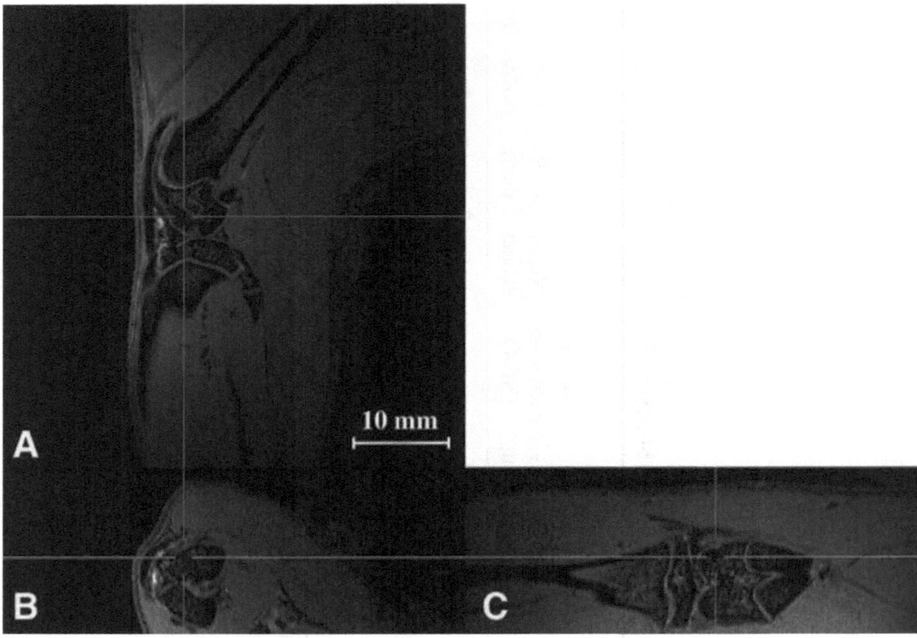

Fig. 4. Sagittal high-resolution image of knee cartilage (**A**) and reformatted axial (**B**) and coronal (**C**) images obtained from a 3D dataset. Thin slices from 3D acquisition allows multiplanar reconstruction and slice reorientation when acquisitions are not performed in strict anatomical directions.

time in all three directions, allowing precise slice location (**Fig. 4**). Moreover, thin slices from 3D acquisition allow slice reorientation in the required directions. Moving through slices and rotating around the region of interest are mandatory for image registration when comparing results in similar regions, as in longitudinal studies.

MRI provides an excellent, noninvasive method to investigate hard and soft tissue in the small animal joint. The image contrast achieved clearly depicts cartilage. Interest in evaluation of thickness and volume ***(10,11)*** in a human cross-sectional study was demonstrated for screening of osteoarthritis. The potential of such studies must still be demonstrated in small-animal models of diseases for accurate and reproducible staging of the pathology (*see* **Note 6**), as well as to monitor therapy response in joint disease.

4. Notes

1. Phased-array coils have become important in clinical MRI for improving the SNR in 1.5-T images. Increasing the magnetic field strength to improve SNR was the

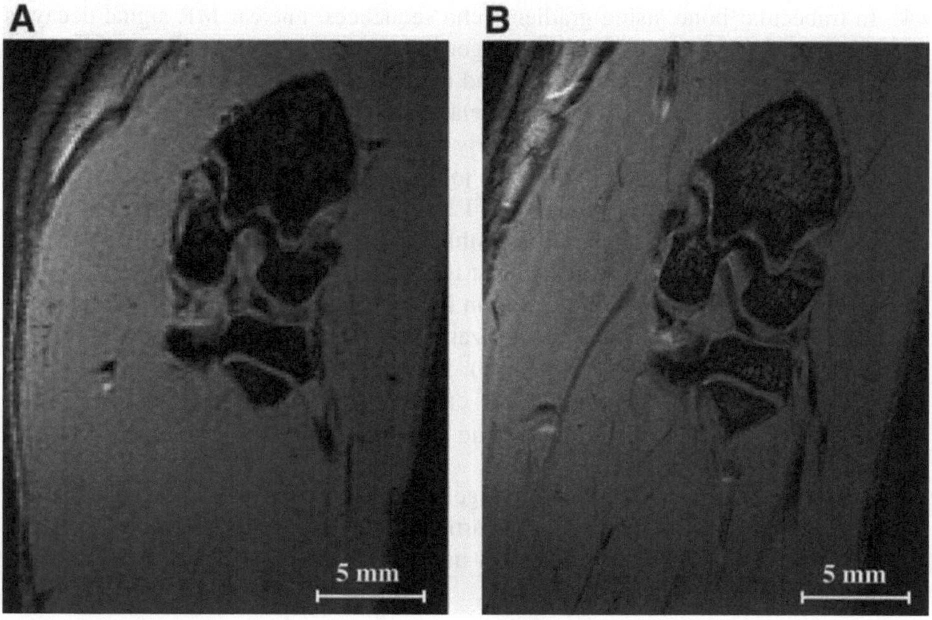

Fig. 5. MR images at two different in-plane resolutions. (**A**) 256-pixel matrix leading to 156 μm pixel size, 312 μm slice thickness. (**B**) 512-pixel matrix leading to 78 μm pixel size and identical slice thickness. Although the signal-to-noise ratio and contrast increase, the in-plane resolution in the image with lower resolution is clearly unsuitable for assessing focal cartilage alterations and cartilage boundaries. Also notice the impact on cruciate ligament visualization.

first step, and advantages obtained through phased-array technology are beginning to be implemented. The multiple-receiver channels needed are already available on spectrometers, and only dedicated phased-array coils are still required. Significant gains (15–30%) in SNR are expected with this technology *(12)* .

2. Owing to marked differences in the precession frequencies of water and fat (3.5 ppm is about 1000 Hz at 7 T), chemical shift artifacts at the cartilage (water)-bone (fat) interface are observed along the frequency-encoding direction. At 62 kHz rbw, with 256 frequency-encoding steps, the fat-water misregistration extends up to 4 pixels, causing blurring at the cartilage boundary. Increasing the rbw, minimizes this artifact and ensures better accuracy in registration but comes at the cost of SNR.
3. Effective fat suppression is undoubtedly an important issue for reliable quantification of cartilage. Because cartilage is adjacent to adipose-rich regions of the femur and tibia, inadequate fat suppression could potentially lead to chemical shift artifacts that would dilute the true boundary between the subchondral bone and articular cartilage.

4. In trabecular bone, using gradient echo sequences, nuclear MR signal decay is governed by magnetic field inhomogeneity arising from the difference in magnetic susceptibility between bone and marrow, leading to intravoxel phase dispersion *(13)*. Effective transverse relaxation time (T2*) dominates transverse relaxation time (T2) and scales linearly with field strength *(14)*. At 7 T, the effect on signal decay is strong in the knee joint and the following qualitative classification was made: T2* (epiphysis) < T2* (metaphysis) << T2* (diaphysis). This explains signal intensity variation within the tibia and femur but is to our advantage by improving the image contrast in the joint.
5. Developing and using high-resolution imaging schemes is clearly warranted for improved morphological characterization of cartilage changes postinjury and during longitudinal studies (**Fig. 5**). However, SNR decreases linearly with elementary volume or voxel. SNR can be expressed by following formula: $SNR \propto Voxel \cdot \sqrt{scan\ time}$. An adequate compromise has to be found among spatial resolution, SNR, and scan time.
6. Reproducibility and precision are largely affected by the dimension of the object to be measured. For example, the cartilage in osteoarthritis decreases in thickness and volume, and reproducibility under these circumstances would probably be different than in normal subjects.

References

1. Recht, M. P. and Resnick, D. (1998) Magnetic resonance imaging of articular cartilage: an overview. *Top. Magn. Reson. Imaging* **9,** 328–336.
2. Dawson, J., Gustard, S., and Beckmann, N. (1999) High-resolution three-dimensional magnetic resonance imaging for the investigation of knee joint damage during the time course of antigen- induced arthritis in rabbits. *Arthritis Rheum.* **42,** 119–128.
3. Recht, M., Bobic, V., Burstein, D., et al. (2001) Magnetic resonance imaging of articular cartilage. *Clin. Orthop.* **391(suppl.),** S379–S396.
4. Link, T. M., Majumdar, S., Peterfy, C., et al. (1998) High resolution MRI of small joints: impact of spatial resolution on diagnostic performance and SNR. *Magn. Reson. Imaging* **16,** 147–155.
5. Link, T. M., Lindner, N., Haeussler, M., et al. (1997) Artificially produced cartilage lesions in small joints: detection with optimized MRI-sequences. *Magn. Reson. Imaging* **15,** 949–956.
6. Watson, P. J., Hall, L. D., Carpenter, T. A., and Tyler, J. A. (1993) A magnetic resonance imaging study of joint degeneration in the guinea pig knee. *Agents Actions* **Suppl. 39,** 261–265.
7. Watson, P. J., Carpenter, T. A., Hall, L. D., and Tyler, J. A. (1997) MR protocols for imaging the guinea pig knee. *Magn. Reson. Imaging* **15,** 957–970.
8. Hennig, J. and Friedburg, H. (1988) Clinical applications and methodological developments of the RARE technique. *Magn. Reson. Imaging* **6,** 391–395.
9. Wald, L. L., Carvajal, L., Moyher, S. E., et al. (1995) Phased array detectors and an automated intensity-correction algorithm for high-resolution MR imaging of the human brain. *Magn. Reson. Med.* **34,** 433–439.

10. Eckstein, F., Adam, C., Sittek, H., et al. (1997) Non-invasive determination of cartilage thickness throughout joint surfaces using magnetic resonance imaging. *J. Biomech.* **30,** 285–289.
11. Stammberger, T., Eckstein, F., Englmeier, K. H., and Reiser, M. (1999) Determination of 3D cartilage thickness data from MR imaging: computational method and reproducibility in the living. *Magn. Reson. Med.* **41,** 529–536.
12. Beck, B., Plant, D. H., Grant, S. C., et al. (2002) Progress in high field MRI at the University of Florida. *MAGMA* **13,** 152–157.
13. Ford, J. C. and Wehrli, F. W. (1991) In vivo quantitative characterization of trabecular bone by NMR interferometry and localized proton spectroscopy. *Magn. Reson. Med.* **17,** 543–51.
14. Song, H. K., Wehrli, F. W., and Ma, J. (1997) Field strength and angle dependence of trabecular bone marrow transverse relaxation in the calcaneus. *J. Magn. Reson. Imaging* **7,** 382–388.

12

High-Resolution Imaging of Osteoarthritis Using Microcomputed Tomography

Lydia Wachsmuth and Klaus Engelke

Summary

Three-dimensional imaging of osteoarthritis is so far limited to late stages of the disease. In this chapter we introduce microcomputed tomography (μCT) as a new imaging tool that offers exciting features for diagnosis of earlier disease stages and for disease monitoring. μCT provides spatial resolution better than 100 μm, but the size of the objects that can be scanned is restricted to several centimeters. The strength of X-ray-based techniques like μCT is the excellent visualization of bone. Therefore, the main application of μCT in osteoarthritis (OA) will be the analysis of bone in small-animal models or of human bone biopsies.

As an example, we will exemplarily describe the application of μCT for the examination of knee joints of male STR1N mice. This inbred strain spontaneously develops OA that carries many characteristics of the human disease. With μCT it is possible to monitor the prominent bony alterations such as osteophyte formation, trabecular remodeling, subchondral bone plate thickening, and subchondral sclerosis. We discuss sample preparation, scanning procedures, data processing, and analysis as well as implications and restrictions for in vivo and in vitro applications.

Key Words: Microcomputed tomography (μCT); subchondral bone; osteoarthritis; genetic animal models; STR1N mice.

1. Introduction

Visualization and quantitative analysis of articular joint damage is of great importance for the clinical diagnosis of osteoarthritis (OA), for monitoring therapeutic interventions, and for pharmaceutical research. However, the ability of diagnostic imaging modalities to assess the initial stages of OA is still very limited. Currently radiography is the clinical standard for the diagnosis of advanced stages of human OA, depicting joint space narrowing, osteophyte formation, and subchondral sclerosis ***(1)***. Magnetic resonance imaging (MRI), which provides superior soft tissue contrast ***(2,3)***, or X-ray computed tomography (CT), which extends the capabilities of plain radiography into the third

From: *Methods in Molecular Medicine, Vol. 101: Cartilage and Osteoarthritis, Volume 2: Structure and In Vivo Analysis*
Edited by: F. De Ceuninck, M. Sabatini, and P. Pastoureau © Humana Press Inc., Totowa, NJ

dimension *(4,5)*, are largely restricted to research. A possibility for better understanding of osteoarthritis and potential prediction of its progression is the use of OA animal models. Obviously the spatial resolution of imaging techniques must be improved when investigating small laboratory animals such as mice or rats because the articular joints are much smaller than in humans. Here we enter the field of microcomputed tomography (μCT), which is the topic of the current chapter.

μCT is an X-ray technique based on the same principles as clinical CT. It offers spatial resolutions greater than 100 μm, but the size of the objects that can be scanned is restricted to several centimeters. The strength of X-ray methods is the excellent differentiation of bone from soft tissue, whereas cartilage can only be assessed indirectly, e.g., by measuring joint space narrowing. Therefore, the main application of μCT in OA will be the investigation of subchondral bone in mice and rats. Of course, bone biopsies of humans can also be imaged, but here applications are limited, as subchondral biopsies cannot be taken in vivo. A different application of μCT, not addressed here, is the phenotypic characterization of the skeletal system of transgenic mice to investigate the role of "cartilage-characteristic" molecules.

As an example, we describe the application of μCT to the investigation of knee joints of male STR1N mice. This inbred strain spontaneously develops OA that carries many characteristics of the human disease *(6)*. With μCT it is possible to monitor the prominent bony alterations such as osteophyte formation, trabecular remodeling, subchondral bone plate thickening, and subchondral sclerosis *(7)*. We discuss sample preparation, scanning procedures, data processing, and analysis as well as implications and restrictions for in vivo and in vitro applications.

The basic principles and parameters of μCT are outlined in detail in the Notes. This should provide the reader with the knowledge to estimate whether the addition of μCT to his/her research tools will be of benefit and to better understand and exploit the possibilities and options of a given μCT scanner.

2. Materials

1. OA strain: knee joints of STR1N mice at different ages (28, 46, 107, and 150 d) (*see* **Note 1**).
2. Strain with no OA prevalence: knee joints of 130-d-old CBA mice.
3. Sample holder: Perspex cylinders with inner diameters of 10 and 5 mm (*see* **Note 2**).
4. Fixative: 37% formaldehyde (Sigma) diluted 1:10 with tap water (*see* **Note 3**).
5. μCT scanner: we use a multipurpose cone beam scanner (for an overview of the principles of μCT, *see* **Notes 4–7**) that was developed at our institute. The geometry can be adapted to a large range of object sizes, and therefore it is well suited to demonstrate the capabilities of μCT in the diagnosis of OA. Although the μCT

scanner is not set up for in vivo investigations, the geometry (X-ray tube-object and object-detector distance) can be varied so that scans with realistic "in vivo" spatial resolutions can be acquired, which is adequate for the demonstration purposes of this chapter. The dedicated components of our scanner are listed below as an example, but the reader should consider that a considerable range of components may be used in other μCT scanners.

a. Transmission X-ray microfocus tube, focal spot size s = 5 μm (MediXtec, Wendelstein, Germany).
b. Cooled 2D 16-bit CCD area detector (Photometrics, Tucson, AR), with an integrated 3:1 fiberoptics taper resulting in an $n = 1024^2$ matrix and an isotropic pitch p = 57 μm. A spatial resolution k =5 μm (2% modulation transfer function [MTF] value) was measured using a magnification factor of 29 that resulted in a sampling distance of u = 1.97 μm *(8)*. Of course, spatial resolution deteriorates for the lower magnification factors that were used for the knee scans presented here (*see* **Note 6**).

3. Methods

1. For in vitro scanning, mice hind legs were disarticulated with intact soft tissue at the hip joint.
2. The knees were tightly fixed in a Perspex cylinder (diameter 10 mm) filled with 3.7% formaldehyde solution (*see* **Notes 2** and **3**).
3. The following scan parameters were used: 5° cone angle, 70 kV tube voltage, 40 μA tube current, 8 s scan time per projection.
4. Two different scan protocols were selected, one with a larger sampling distance (u = 22 μm) and one with a smaller sampling distance (u = 11 μm) (*see* **Note 8**).
5. For comparative purposes, the 46-d-old mouse was also scanned with the low spatial resolution protocol. The improved resolution required a reduction of the object diameter. A smaller Perspex cylinder (diameter 5 mm) was used, and all soft tissue was removed from the leg to fit the bone into the cylinder. The same scan parameters as above were used.
6. Reconstruction. A volumetric dataset of 512^3 voxels was reconstructed from 720 projections using a modified Feldkamp algorithm developed at the Institute of Medical Physics, Erlangen, Germany *(9)*. The voxel size in the reconstructed images (**Figs. 1–4**) is identical to the sampling distance, 22 and 11 μm, respectively (*see* **Notes 4–7** and **9**).
7. Data Analysis (*see* **Note 10**). Currently, there are no standard procedures for the quantitative analysis of subchondral bone. We refer the reader to the Notes for some discussion of quantitative analysis of μCT images. Here we compare μCT with histology, the standard tool for analyzing OA changes post mortem.
   a. **Fig. 1** shows coronal sections stained with safranin O (upper row) along with the site-matched images selected from the reconstructed volumetric μCT datasets (lower row). In the histological sections the cartilage of the articulating surfaces and the growth plates can easily be differentiated from bone,

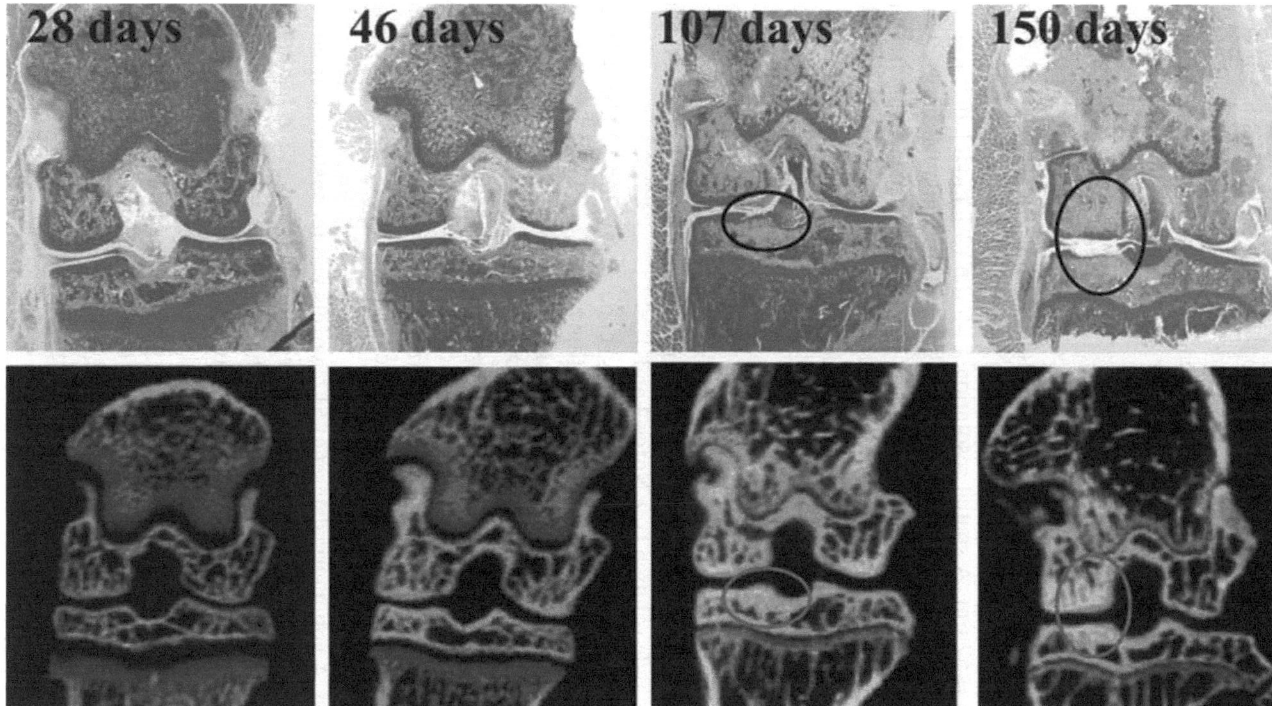

Fig. 1. Selected coronal histological sections (**upper row**) and corresponding site-matched μCT views reconstructed from the 3D dataset (lower row). Sampling distance in the μCT images was u = 22 μm. Immature mice at 28 and 46 d show a normal bone appearance of the femur and tibia. Cartilage surface deterioration is evident in the 107-d-old mouse. More severe structural degradation, together with cell loss and focal abrasion of the whole cartilage layer, occurs at 150 d. The μCT images show that local cartilage damage is accompanied by local trabecular remodeling and thickening of the subchondral bone plate (*see* marks).

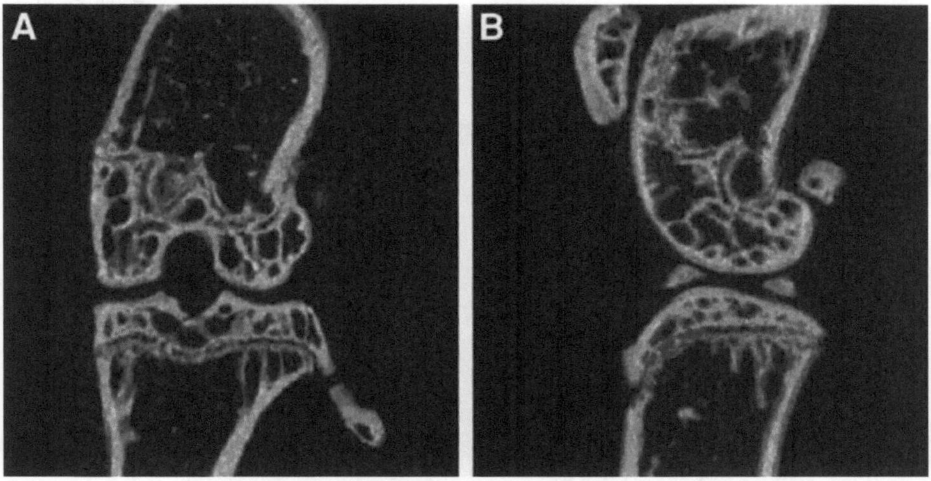

Fig. 2. μCT scan of the knee joint of a 130-d-old control mouse. (**A**) Coronal, and (**B**) sagittal multiplanar reconstructions. Skeletal maturity can be assessed by the growth plate, which is almost completely closed. Neither trabecular remodeling nor subchondral bone plate thickening nor sclerosis are visible. The inner part of the meniscus is typically calcified in mice. Same resolution as in **Fig. 1**.

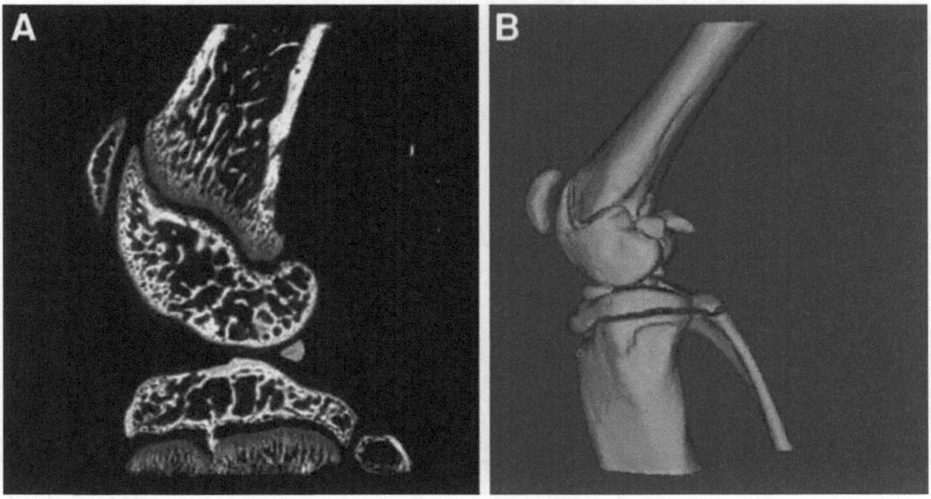

Fig. 3. μCT dataset of the knee of the 46-d-old mouse with improved resolution. (**A**) Sagittal multiplanar reconstruction. (**B**) Surface shaded display. Fine bone structures are more accurately depicted compared with **Figs. 1** and **2**. Even differences in the grade of calcification are evident in the growth plate cartilage.

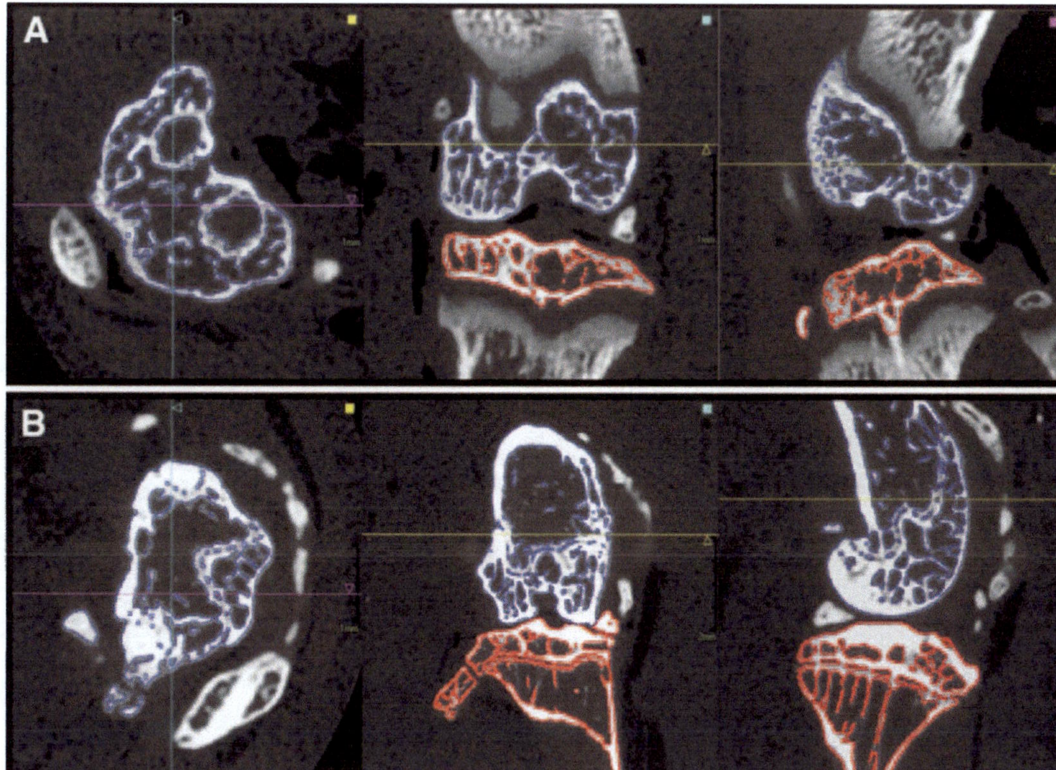

Fig. 4. Three dimensional segmentation of the subchondral bone is shown in (**left**) axial, (**middle**) coronal and (**right**) sagittal multiplanar reconstructions of knee joints of (**upper row**) 28-d and (**lower row**) 150-d-old mice. In the young mouse the segmentation worked fully-automatic. In the old mouse the epiphysis could no longer be automatically separated from the metaphysis because of the particulate calcification of the growth plate. Also sclerotic areas were separated manually from normal trabecular bone. Interestingly, a patella dislocation is evident in the old mouse (see axial reconstruction; lower row). Calcification of the patella tendon and ligaments is visible at 150 d.

joint capsule, and tendons. Surface destruction of the cartilage is evident in 107- and 150-d-old mice. As can be seen from the corresponding μCT images, the cartilage deterioration is accompanied by trabecular remodeling and subchondral bone plate thickening. Sclerotic areas within the epiphyses of the femur and the tibia expand with increasing age.

b. In comparison, the μCT scan of a CBA mouse at 130 d shows no abnormalities (**Fig. 2**).

c. Using histology, all joint tissues affected by the complex OA pathology can be assessed. However, the technique is tedious, and typically only a few grindings per joint are prepared. In contrast, μCT shows modifications of bone tissue only but covers the complete joint volumetrically. Although the resolution is not as good as in the histological sections, the μCT datasets depict osteophyte formation, trabecular remodeling, subchondral bone plate thickening, and subchondral sclerosis of the entire knee. From the examples presented here, the value of the volumetric approach of μCT is evident. In contrast to the stained sections, the spatial extension of the subchondral bone modifications can be quantified in 3D. As there is a local correspondence between cartilage deterioration and subchondral bone modification the total size of the deteriorated cartilage surface may also be derived indirectly using the μCT data. Of course methods for a differential analysis of the modifications that occur in subchondral bone must still be developed for the μCT data.

d. The impact of spatial resolution is demonstrated in **Fig. 3**. The lower resolution obtainable in vitro provides more details and reduces partial volume artifacts. Whether the improved resolution results in a substantially better diagnosis or whether the image quality of μCT images acquirable in vivo is satisfactory still needs to be determined. In general, in vivo imaging offers the option of continuously monitoring disease progression instead of an endpoint assessment by histological means.

4. Notes

1. Several inbred strains of small laboratory animals, i.e., mice and guinea pigs, spontaneously develop OA in the knee joints. There is evidence that in animals ***(4,6,10,11)*** and in humans ***(5,12–19)*** subchondral bone alterations have already occurred at the onset of OA, that is, well before joint space narrowing and macroscopic osseous changes can be observed. In mice or rats whole joints can easily be imaged. The subchondral bone plate, underlying trabecular bone, osteophyte formation, and calcification status of adjacent soft tissues can be assessed using a single dataset. Disease incidence and progression, and in particular the role of bony alterations, vary considerably among different animal models. However, it is not the aim of this chapter to present the broad range of pathological manifestations of OA but rather to exemplify the diagnostic power of μCT.
2. *Movement, coverage, and centering.*
   a. In tomography it is mandatory to prevent movements of the object during a scan. With improving spatial resolution, movements become more critical, and an appropriate object holder must be used.

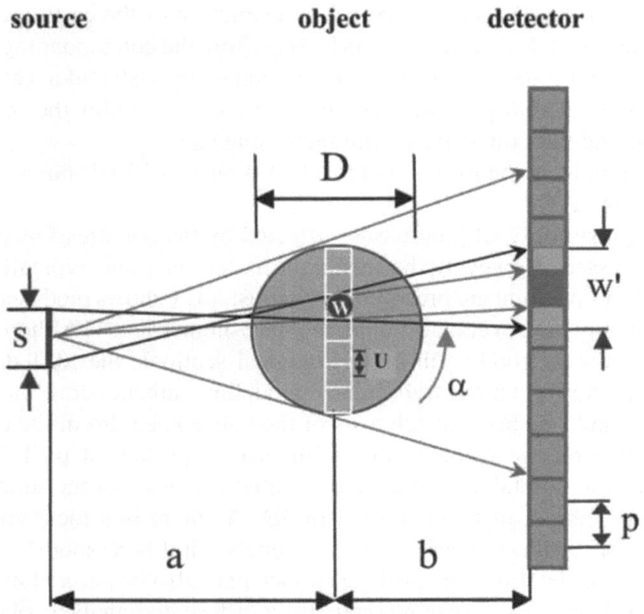

Fig. 5. Set-up for fan beam geometry. s, size of the focal spot of the X-ray tube; u, sampling distance; D, object diameter; w', image of a contrasting detail of size w on the detector; p, detector pitch; a, distance X-ray tube–object; b, distance object-detector.

b. Each tomographic projection must completely cover the rotating object. This may be a problem if the shape of the object to be scanned largely differs from a cylindrical shape. Then, for certain angles α (**Fig. 5**), the detector may not be large enough to cover the complete object, and so-called truncated projections are sampled, which cause artifacts in the reconstructed tomographic images.
c. The axis of rotation must be centered with respect to the projections; otherwise artifacts in the reconstructed images occur. In general, there are a variety of sources of mechanical scanner misalignment ***(9,20)***, but a detailed discussion is beyond the scope of this chapter. The user should be aware that the better the spatial resolution, the larger the image artifacts caused by a given misalignment.
d. Tissue can be stored frozen or in fixative. Scanning can be performed with frozen and thawed samples. However, it is important that during a μCT scan the tissue density does not change, which is the case in particular in soft tissues during the thawing process. Owing to density differences, quantitative results may differ in frozen and thawed objects. At the lower end of the resolution scale, even tissue dehydration that results in tissue shrinking may cause blurring artifacts in the reconstructed images. Thus it can be advantageous to

scan the object in fixative provided the fixative does not contain large amounts of elements with high atomic numbers ($Z > 8$).

4. *Components*. The main hardware components of a μCT scanner are the same as in clinical CT scanners: X-ray source, X-ray–sensitive detector, and sample stage. The software components consist of data acquisition, tomographic reconstruction (*see* **Note 9**), and 2D or 3D visualization and analysis modules. Most μCT systems are equipped with X-ray tubes, but for applications requiring ultra-high spatial resolution, synchrotron radiation (X-rays generated in large electron or positron storage rings) is more frequently is used. Here we focus on μCT scanners equipped with X-ray tubes, as this is most likely the equipment the reader will use. Synchrotrons are large stationary machines located in only a few centers worldwide, and user access is limited. In these centers a user will usually be supported by local experts. On the other hand, access to a laboratory μCT scanner is more convenient, but technical support is limited. Here the user depends more on his or her own knowledge.
5. *Setup*. In clinical CT scanners, the X-ray tube and detector rotate with high speed (≤1 s per rotation) around the patient, who is positioned horizontally in the center of the circular path. This setup is also beneficial for in vivo small animal tomography. However, more frequently a scanner design is encountered in which the object is rotated and the X-ray source and detector are stationary during a scan. The major advantage is flexibility, because magnification is variable and can be optimized for a large range of object sizes. Also, mechanically the rotating object design is less demanding and cheaper, and scanners can be more compact because it is easy to rotate a small object weighing typically less than a pound. The general setup of this scanner type is shown in **Fig. 5** for fan and in **Fig. 6** for cone beam geometry. Cone beam systems are equipped with area detectors and require more sophisticated tomographic reconstruction algorithms. On the other hand, they allow for shorter scan times, which is crucial for in vivo applications. The following discussion applies to both fan and cone beam systems but for simplicity will be mostly exemplified using fan beam geometry.
6. *Magnification*. From **Figs. 5** and **6** it is obvious that geometric magnification is an inherent feature in fan and cone beam systems. As can be seen, the shadow w' of a small structure of size w within an object of diameter D is given by displayed equation: $w' = (a + b)/a \cdot w + b/a \cdot s$.

   In case of a point source ($s = 0$) an arbitrarily high spatial resolution could be obtained by extending the distance b between object and detector. In reality ($s > 0$) spatial resolution is limited but can be optimized if $b \gg a$. In this so-called projection mode, the following approximation holds: $w' = b/a\ (w + s)$.

   The source size s should be smaller than w so that $w' \approx (b/a)\ w$. For $s \geq w$, in principle the so-called contact mode is more advantageous. Here b is minimized, and the spatial resolution is determined by the distance p of the detector elements that should then be in the order of w. A major limitation, of the contact mode is scatter, which can significantly reduce the image quality; thus for $s \geq w$, in practice a compromise between projection and contact geometries must be found.

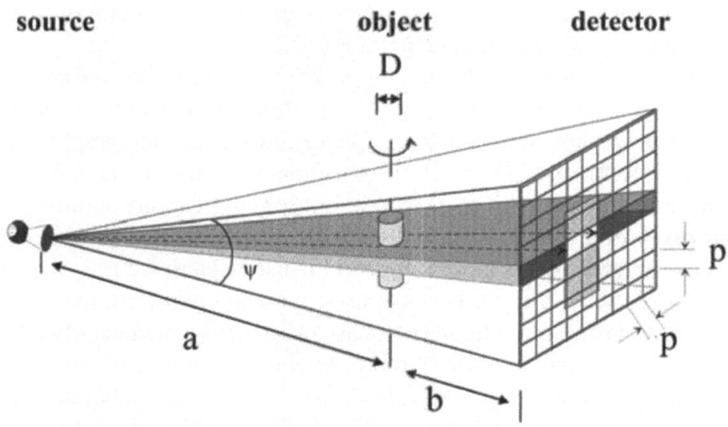

Fig. 6. Set-up for cone beam geometry. ψ, cone angle; p, detector pitch.

7. *Characteristic parameters of a μCT scanner.* From a user's perspective, probably the most important parameter of a μCT system is its spatial resolution. Other parameters of interest, especially for in vivo applications, are maximum object size, scan time, and radiation exposure. All these parameters are related to each other. For example, the contrast that adjacent structures can be imaged with depends on the spatial resolution and the signal-to-noise ratio (SNR). For a given scanner and magnification, low contrast detectability can be improved by increasing the SNR which typically requires a higher radiation exposure and longer scan times. A detailed explanation of the physics of an imaging system as well as of the mathematics of the tomographic reconstruction is beyond the scope of this chapter, and we must refer the reader to the literature ***(21–24)***.

   Let us just remind the reader that CT is a technique in which a slice of an object can be reconstructed from the measurement of projections taken from a large number of different angles α (**Fig. 5**) ***(24)***. The aim of this section is to discuss a few simple relationships and rules of thumb, which should enable the user to estimate whether a given scanner may serve as an adequate imaging tool for the desired application.

   a. *Discrete sampling and spatial resolution.* The term *spatial resolution* is used very ambiguously in medical imaging. One problem is the lack of a unique definition. Spatial resolution can be given as the full width at half the maximum value of the point spread function (PSF) of the imaging system ($FWHM_{PSF}$). Alternatively, spatial resolution is often defined by the 2, 5, or 10% value of the Fourier transform of the PSF, the modulation transfer function (MTF) ***(25,26)***. Using the first definition, spatial resolution is expressed in units of length, and a smaller value is better. Using the MTF-based definition, spatial resolution is expressed in line pairs per length; consequently a higher value is better. In this chapter we use the PSF-based definition.

Manufacturers as well as scientific publications often report *pixel or voxel sizes* of the reconstructed tomographic images for spatial resolution. Apart from the ambiguity in terminology discussed in the previous paragraph, this occurs for the following reasons: (1) pixel sizes are easier to comprehend than parameters specifying the spatial resolution; (2) pixel sizes are easier to determine; and (3) pixel sizes are almost always smaller than the spatial resolution. Thus, using pixel size can easily lead to a misstatement of the resolution of a given system. It is important to understand that pixel (or in the 3D case voxel) size, spatial resolution, and sampling distance are three different quantities that depend nonlinearly on each other.

A basic characteristic of an electronic imaging system is *discrete sampling* because the detector consists of a finite number of discrete X-ray-sensitive elements typically arranged uniformly along a line or across an area (**Figs. 5** or **6**). The distance between the detector elements denoted as p is sometimes called detector pitch. In fan and cone beam systems, the sampling distance u is smaller than p: $p = u\ (a + b)/a$ where $(a + b)/a$ is the magnification factor. According to the Nyquist theorem ***(27–29)***, the spatial resolution k is limited by the sampling distance u. It states that $k \geq 2\ u$, where k and u are given in units of length. For example, if the sampling distance is 50 μm, the spatial resolution is 100 μm at best. In practice, this value will never be achieved, as other components of the imaging system such as scatter additionally limit the spatial resolution.

To understand *the difference between sampling distance and pixel size* in the reconstructed image, we assume the following special situation: let each projection consist of n samples corresponding to n detector elements, and let the reconstructed image consist of n^2 pixels with a side length of u. In this case sampling distance and pixel size are the same. In general, the pixel or voxel size in the reconstructed image is arbitrary and can be chosen independently of the sampling distance and the spatial resolution. For example, only a part of the n detector elements may be used for the tomographic reconstruction, and subsampling may be applied in the projections or in the reconstructed images.

The *relation between sampling distance and spatial resolution largely* depends on the scanner components. The Nyquist condition only gives a lower limit. Typically the pixel size in the reconstructed images is slightly smaller than the sampling distance and a discrepancy by a factor of 3 to 4 exists between spatial resolution and pixel size.

b. *Object size, noise, and scan time*. What are the implications if we want to improve spatial resolution? To answer this question we have to distinguish three scenarios that can easily be understood by inspecting **Fig. 7**, where (A) repeats the setup shown in **Fig. 5**, with which we compare the three scenarios shown in (B), (C), and (D).

In scenario 1 (**Fig. 7B**), we want to improve (that is, decrease) spatial resolution in a given object (D = const) by a factor of m. In this case we have to

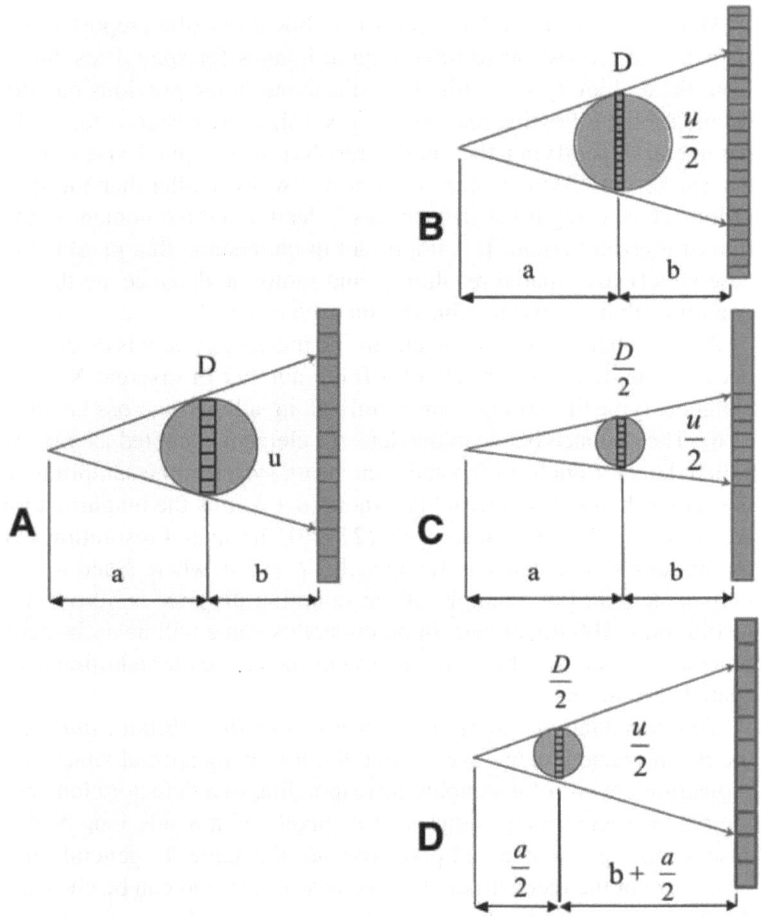

Fig. 7. Options to decrease spatial resolution. **(A)** Start point, same geometry as in **Fig. 1. (B–D)** Improvement, i.e., decrease of spatial resolution by a factor of two. **(B)** Decrease of resolution in a given object (D = const). The sampling distance and detector pitch must be reduced; twice the number of detector elements is required. **(C)** Smaller resolution in smaller objects (D/u = const); compared to (a) sampling distance and detector pitch must be reduced but the number of detector elements that cover the object are unchanged. **(D)** Increase of magnification; compared to (a) the sampling distance is reduced but detector pitch and the number of detector elements are unchanged.

decrease the sampling distance u by also increasing the number of detector elements by a factor of m. **Figure 7** illustrates $m = 2$. In scenarios 2 (**Fig. 7C**) and 3 (**Fig. 7D**), we improve spatial resolution by the same factor but keep the number of samples n per projection (that is, D/u) constant. Obviously, this is only possible in smaller objects.

In scenario 2 we scan the object in the same position as in scenario 1. This is the situation in scanners when the X-ray tube and detector are rotated and there is no possibility of translating the object between source and detector. Scenario 3 is representative for a scanner with variable magnification when the object is rotated. For simplicity, in the following we assume that the percentage improvement in spatial resolution is identical to the percentage decrease in sampling distance.

μCT systems are routinely operated with area detectors of 1024 × 1024 elements. Thus, as a rule of thumb the maximum object diameter *D* in mm is equal to the sampling distance *w* in μm. For example, a sampling distance of 10 μm would limit the object size to 10 mm. Of course, area detectors of 2048 × 2048 and even more elements exist and are, for example, used in mammography, but in radiographic applications only a small number of images are taken, whereas in μCT volumetric datasets are generated.

If we increase the number of samples isotropically by a factor of *m*, the tomographic reconstruction time increases by m^4, partly because there are more samples per projections and partly because the number of projections should also be increased by a factor of *m*. Additionally, the size and storage requirements of the reconstructed images increase dramatically. A volumetric dataset that consists of 1000^3 voxels containing 2 bytes of information each requires 2 GB of storage, which is approximately half the capacity of a DVD-R, whereas a 2048^3-element dataset requires 8 GB of storage.

The main limitations of spatial resolution are scan time and radiation exposure, which can best be discussed in terms of the number of required X-ray quanta. In scenario 1 ($D = \text{const}$), a decrease of sampling distance by a factor of *m* requires an increase in X-ray quanta by m^4 in order to keep the image quality constant. Thus, if for a given object diameter *D* the spatial resolution is to be improved isotropically by a factor of 2 without deteriorating image quality, the number of quanta and therefore the radiation exposure must be increased by a factor of 16 ***(23,30)***. In scenarios 2 and 3 (constant *n*), only an increase by a factor of m^2 is necessary.

In scenarios 1 and 2, the increase in scan time scales with the demand on additional X-ray quanta unless the tube current can be increased. However, most likely the opposite case is realistic, and scan times have to be increased, as a decrease in sampling distance should typically be accompanied by a decrease in focal spots size *s* (**Fig. 5**). This requires a reduction of tube current because the heat and cooling capacities of the anode material are limited.

In scenario 3, each sampling element covers the same solid angle as in scenario 1, and in principle the required increase in X-ray quanta is offset by the higher magnification. In practice, a smaller focal spot is also mandatory, which results in longer scan times in this scenario as well.

As can be concluded from the last paragraph, in μCT it is of extreme interest to optimize the utilization of the available photons. Therefore cone beam systems employing area detectors are attractive. If an area detector with a matrix of n^2 elements is used, the scan time is reduced by a factor of n compared with a fan beam system using a line scan detector of n elements.

For in vivo imaging, both scan time and radiation exposure are limiting parameters. Therefore ultra-high resolution scans are limited to in vitro imaging. Scan time is limited by maximum anesthesia times, which for small laboratory animals such as rats or mice is on the order of 30–60 min. The limit of acceptable radiation exposure in vivo in these animals has not been exactly specified so far and depends on the specific scientific question. Reported radiation exposure values vary from 100 mGy (total body exposure *[31]*) to 900 mGy (rat hind leg *[32]*). Although upper limits are missing, it is obvious that dose minimization is an important issue for in vivo applications. For clinical CT, a number of techniques that significantly reduce dose without reducing image quality such as noise filtering ***(33)*** or tube-current modulation ***(34)*** have been developed, but so far these methods have not been transferred to µCT.

8. In principle, the 22-µm sampling distance protocol is suitable for in vivo scans of the extremities once scan times are reduced (*see* **Notes 4–7**), for example, by employing a more powerful X-ray tube. Also, the rotating mouse should then be positioned horizontally in the scanner with a vertically extended leg. For an in vivo whole-body scan of a mouse, an even larger sampling distance (> 50 µm) is required.
9. The tomographic reconstruction is typically performed automatically, and only a small number of parameters have to be set by the user. One of them is the reconstruction kernel. From a user's perspective, the most important property of the kernel is the determination of the relation between noise and spatial resolution. At the extremes, a smoothing filter can be selected to reduce noise and blur sharp edges. This is advantageous if relatively large features with small contrast are to be detected in the images. On the other hand, a sharpening filter maximizes spatial resolution at the expense of noise. The sharpening filters are typically used for assessment of bone in order to improve the location of the bone edges. In practice, there are a large variety of filters in between the extremes. The algorithms implemented in a given scanner are manufacturer-specific, and therefore the number, names, and specification of available kernels vary.
10. A number of 3D structural parameters have been developed for the analysis of bone biopsies in the field of osteoporosis ***(35–38)***. Most of them are 3D extensions to the well-known parameters obtained in conventional 2D histomorphometry ***(39)***, such as trabecular spacing or thickness. Additionally, bone microarchitecture can be specified with new parameters, for example, the so-called structure model index ***(40–42)***. The relevance of these parameters in OA has not yet been shown. In knee joints of small animals, the analysis is complicated by the fact that the bone microstructure is not just a scaled-down human trabecular structure. Not only trabecular structures but also subchondral bone plate thickness, osteophyte formation, and soft tissue

calcification are of interest in OA. An appropriate segmentation of the femur and tibia (in the knee), and of the epiphysis and metaphysis is nessessary. In STR1N mouse subchondral bone sclerosis is so prominent during disease progression that individual trabeculae can no longer be distinguished in advanced stages of OA.

Thus, we propose the use of a combination of parameters that consists of (1) the 3D histomorphometry-like parameters mentioned above for the quantification of subchondral trabecular bone; (2) a parameter quantifying the volume of sclerotic bone; (3) a parameter to quantify cortical thickness; and (4) a parameter grading the number and size of osteophytes. All these parameters should be independently analyzed in the epiphyses of the distal femur and the proximal tibia.

The differentiation of several volumes of interest requires an initial segmentation step, which is also needed to distinguish subchondral trabeculae from soft tissue. Here, automated procedures are not yet widely available. As an example, in **Fig. 4** we have used advanced multistep gradient-based segmentation algorithms that are largely operator-independent ***(43)***.

Acknowledgments

Mouse scans presented here were obtained within the scope of a project supported by the Federal Ministry of Education and Research (BMBF) and the Intedisciplinary Center for Clinical Research (IZKF) at the University Hospital of the University of Erlangen-Nuremberg.

References

1. Resnick, D. and Niwayama, G. (1988) *Diagnosis of Bone and Joint Disorders*. WB Saunders, Philadelphia.
2. Eckstein, F., Reiser, M., Englmeier, K.-H., and Putz, R. (2001) In vivo morphometry and functional analysis of human articular cartilage with quantitative magnetic resonance imaging—from image to data, from data to theory. *Anat. Embryol.* **203,** 147–173.
3. Burstein, D., Bashir, A., and Gray, M. L. (2000) MRI techniques in early stages of cartilage disease. *Invest. Radiol.* **35,** 622–638.
4. Layton, M., Goldstein, S., Goulet, R., Feldkamp, L., Kubinsky, L., and Bole, G. (1988) Examination of subchondral bone architecture in experimental osteoarthritis by microscopic computed axial tomography. *Arthritis Rheum.* **31,** 1400–1405.
5. Shimizu, M., Tsuji, H., Matsui, H., and Sano, A. (1993) Morphometric analysis of subchondral bone of the tibial condyle in osteoarthrosis. *Clin. Orthop.* **293,** 229–239.
6. Benske, J., Schunke, M., and Tillmann, B. (1988) Subchondral bone formation in arthrosis. Polychrome labeling studies in mice. *Acta Orthop. Scand.* **59,** 536–541.
7. Engelke, K., Wachsmuth, L., Taubenreuther, U., et al. (2001) High resolution in vitro μCT of osteoarthritis in a mouse model. *High Resolution Imaging in Small Animals Meeting*, Maryland, USA.

8. Engelke, K., Karolczak, M., Lutz, A., Seibert, U., Schaller, S., and Kalender, W. A. (1999) High spatial resolution 3D x-ray cone-beam microtomography. *RSNA 85th Scientific Assembly and Annual Meeting*, Radiology, Chicago, Il, p. 194.
9. Karolczak, M., Schaller, S., Engelke, K., et al. (2001) Implementation of a cone-beam reconstruction algorithm for the single-circle source orbit with embedded misalignment correction using homogeneous coordinates. *Med. Phys.* **28,** 2050–2069.
10. Jiang, Y., Zhao, J., White, D., and Genant, H. (2000) Micro CT and micro MR imaging of 3D architecture of animal skeleton. *J. Musculoskel. Neuronal Interaction* **1,** 45–51.
11. Dedrik D, Goldstein S, Brandt K, O'Connor B, Goulet R, Albrecht M. (1993) A longitudinal study of subchondral bone plate and trabecular bone in cruciate-deficient dogs with osteoarthritis followed up for 54 month. *Arthritis Rheum.* **36,** 1460–1467.
12. Buckland-Wright J. (1994) Quantitative radiography of osteoarthritis. *Ann. Rheum. Dis.* **53,** 268–275.
13. Buckland-Wright, J., Lynch, J., and Macfarlane, D. (1996) Fractal signature analysis measures cancellous bone organisation in macroradiographs of patients with knee osteoarthritis. *Ann. Rheum. Dis.* **55,** 749–755.
14. Imhoff, H., Sulzbacher, I., Grampp, S., Czerny, C., Youssefzadeh, S., and Kainberger, F. (2000) Subchondral bone and cartilage disease. A rediscovered functional unit. *Invest. Radiol.* **35,** 581–588.
15. Li, B. and Aspden, R. (1997) Mechanical and material properties of the subchondral bone plate from the femoral head of patients with osteoarthritis or osteoporosis. *Ann. Rheum. Dis.* **56,** 247–254.
16. Li, B., Marshall, D., Roe, M., and Aspden, R. (1999) The electron microscope appearance of the subchondral bone plate in the human femoral head in osteoarthritis and osteoporosis. *J. Anat.* **195,** 101–110.
17. Radin, E. and Rose, R. (1986) Role of subchondral bone in the initiation and progression of cartilage damage. *Clin. Orthop.* **213,** 34–40.
18. Yamada, K., Healey, R., Amiel, D., Lotz, M., and Couttts, R. (2002) Subchondral bone of the human knee joint in aging and osteoarthritis. *Osteoarthritis Cartilage* **10,** 360–369.
19. Yamashita, T., Nabeshima, Y., and Noda, M. (2000) High-resolution micro-computed tomography analyses of the abnormal trabecular bone structures in klotho gene mutant mice. *J. Endocrinol.* **164,** 239–245.
20. Taubenreuther, U., Engelke, K., Karolczak, M., Lutz, A., Noo, F., and Kalender, W. A. (2001) Practical misalignment correction in circular and spiral cone beam tomography. *RSNA 87th Scientific Assembly and Annual Meeting*, Radiology, Chicago, IL, p. 543.
21. Barrett, H. B. and Swindell, W. (1981) *Radiological Imaging*. Academic, New York.
22. Beutel, J., Kundel, H. L., and Van Metter, R L. (2000) Volume 1. *Physics and Psychophysics*, vol. 1. *Handbook of Medical Imaging*. SPIE, Bellingham, WA.
23. Graeff, W. and Engelke, K. (1991) Microradiography and microtomography, in: *Handbook on Synchrotron Radiation*. (Ebashi, E., Koch, M., and Rubenstein, E., eds.) North-Holland, Amsterdam, pp. 361–405.

24. Kalender, W. A. (2000) *Computed Tomography*. Wiley, New York.
25. Metz, C. E. and Doi, K. (1979) Transfer function analysis of radiographic imaging systems. *Phys. Med. Biol.* **24,** 1079–1106.
26. Rossmann, K., Haus, A. G., and Doi, K. (1972) Validity of the MTF of magnification radiography. *Phys. Med. Biol.* **17,** 648–655.
27. Nyquist, H. (1928) Certain topics in telegraph transmission theory. *Trans. Am. Inst. Elec. Eng.* **47,** 617–644.
28. Shannon, C. (1948) A mathematical theory of communication. Part 2. *Bell Sys. Tech. J.* **27,** 623–656.
29. Shannon, C. (1948) A mathematical theory of communication. Part 1. *Bell Sys. Tech. J.* **27,** 379–423.
30. Bonse, U. and Busch, F. (1996) X-ray computed microtomography (μCT) using synchrotron radiation (SR). *Prog. Biophys. Mol. Biol.* **65,** 133–169.
31. Engelke, K., Karolczak, M., Fuchs, H., de Angelis, M. H., Ulzheimer, S., and Kalender, W. A. (2003) An in-vivo Cone Beam Micro-CT Scanner for Whole Body Investigation of Mice. *25th Annual Meeting of the American Society for Bone and Mineral Research*, Minneapolis, MI. *JBMR* **18(suppl. 1),** 320.
32. Kinney, J. H., Lane, N. E., and Haupt, D. L. (1995) In vivo, three-dimensional microscopy of trabecular bone. *J. Bone Miner. Res.* **10,** 264–270.
33. Kachelrieß M, Kalender WA. (1999) Dose reduction by generalized 3D adaptive filtering for conventional and spiral single-, multirow and cone-beam CT. *RSNA 85th Scientific Assembly and Annual Meeting*, Radiology, Chicago, IL, pp. 283–284.
34. Kalender, W. A., Wolf, H., Suess, C., Gies, M., Greess, H., and Bautz, W. A. (1999) Dose reduction in CT by on-line tube current control: principles and validation on phantoms and cadavers. *Eur. Radiol.* **9,** 323–328.
35. Hahn, M., Vogel, M., Pompesius-Kempa, M., and Delling, G. (1992) Trabecular bone pattern factor—a new parameter for simple quantification of bone microarchitecture. *Bone* **13,** 327–330.
36. Laib, A., Beuf, O., Issever, A., Newitt, D. C., and Majumdar, S. (2001) Direct measures of trabecular bone architecture from MR images. *Adv. Exp. Med. Biol.* **496,** 37–46.
37. Laib, A., Newitt, D. C., Lu, Y., and Majumdar, S. (2002) New model-independent measures of trabecular bone structure applied to in vivo high-resolution MR images. *Osteoporosis Int.* **13,** 130–136.
38. Majumdar, S., Link, T. M., Augat, P., et al. (1999) Trabecular bone architecture in the distal radius using magnetic resonance imaging in subjects with fractures of the proximal femur. *Osteoporosis Int.* **10,** 231–239.
39. Parfitt, A. M., Drezner, M. K., Glorieux, F. H., et al. (1987) Bone histomorphometry: standardization of nomenclature, symbols, and units. *J. Bone Miner. Res.* **2,** 595–610.
40. Laib, A., Hildebrand, T., Hauselmann, H. J., and Rügsegger, P. (1997) Ridge number density: a new parameter for in vivo bone structure analysis. *Bone* **21,** 541–546.

41. Hildebrand, T. and Rügsegger, P. (1997) A new method for the model independent assessment of thickness in three-dimensional images. *J. Microsc.* **185,** 67–75.
42. Hildebrand, T. and Rügsegger, P. (1997) Quantification of bone microarchitecture with the structure model index. *CMBBE* **1,** 15–23.
43. Kang, Y., Engelke, K., and Kalender, W. A new accurate and precise 3D segmentation method for skeletal structures in volumetric CT data. *IEEE Med Ima.* **22,** 586–598.

13

High-Resolution Ultrasonography for Analysis of Age- and Disease-Related Cartilage Changes

Amena Saïed and Pascal Laugier

Summary

Because of their limited spatial resolution, current clinical noninvasive imaging modalities (radiography, computed tomography, conventional echography, and magnetic resonance imaging) are able to detect only the late stages of the cartilage degradation. To detect early lesions and follow their evolution in time with imaging, higher resolution is necessary. Recent work suggest that high-frequency ultrasound may serve as a useful means for the investigation of cartilage matrix structural changes occurring under various experimental and clinical circumstances, like the growing process and osteoarthritis. In this chapter, an experimental 50–100-MHz ultrasound scanner is described for high-resolution echographic imaging of articular cartilage. The procedures of data acquisition and signal processing are detailed for the quantitative evaluation of ultrasonic reflection and backscatter coefficients, which have been reported to be sensitive to subtle surface and internal disease-related alterations. Further technological developments and miniaturization of the echographic probes may lead to extension of this technique to the study of living small animals or to the clinical field in combination with conventional arthoscopy.

Key Words: Attenuation; backscatter; cartilage; echography; osteoarthritis; reflection; sound velocity; ultrasound.

1. Introduction

Current imaging modalities such as radiography, computed tomography, conventional ultrasonography in the 5–20-MHz frequency range, and recently magnetic resonance imaging (MRI) are routinely used for the assessment of late-stage lesions of osteoarticular stuctures. Because of their limited resolution and sensitivity, they do not allow imagery of subtle morphological and structural changes of the joint tissues, nor do they permit accurate measurement of cartilage thickness. Improvement in quantitative imaging of osteoarthritis (OA) requires the introduction of very high resolution and reliable imaging modalities that allow assessment of surface microdamages, internal

From: *Methods in Molecular Medicine, Vol. 101: Cartilage and Osteoarthritis, Volume 2: Structure and In Vivo Analysis*
Edited by: F. De Ceuninck, M. Sabatini, and P. Pastoureau © Humana Press Inc., Totowa, NJ

structure alteration, thickness variation, and bone remodeling. High-frequency ultrasound has raised a great deal of interest since it provides much higher resolution than conventional echography. Micro-ultrasonography, coupled with quantitative evaluation of the tissue structure, has proved to be successful for the investigation of cartilage diseases.

Ultrasonic waves are elastic waves that can penetrate the body without difficulty. They are used to probe mechanical or elastic properties of the propagating medium, which in the case of cartilage are associated with various tissue features, including extracellular matrix composition (collagen and proteoglycans contents) and microarchitecture (collagen fiber orientation and thickness). When an ultrasound wave impinges on the articular cartilage surface, it is partly reflected back and partly transmitted to the internal structures. Reflection on a smooth cartilage surface (normal cartilage) is highly directional, in contrast to diffuse reflection from rough surfaces such as altered osteoarthritic cartilage (fibrillations). The transmitted wave propagates through the cartilage depth to the subchondral bone. During propagation, wave interactions with the cartilage matrix gives rise to ultrasonic scattering, which results from interaction with small obstacles such as collagen fibers or cells. Finally, the transmitted wave is reflected from the subchondral bone boundary. Reflection events play an important role in the formation of ultrasound images by contributing organ morphology. Scattering events are also of primary importance for echographic image formation or for assessing microstructural properties of the medium (scatterer size, scatterer number density, orientation) ***(1)***. In addition, acoustic properties such as wave velocity, attenuation coefficient (*see* **Subheading 5., Glossary**), backscatter, and reflection coefficients may be used to assess tissue composition and microarchitecture quantitatively.

In ultrasound imaging, high resolution is reached by using high ultrasonic frequencies. However, because ultrasound attenuation experienced in articular cartilage is dependent on a frequency with an approximately linear variation, the maximum operating frequency is determined by the depth of wave penetration in the tissue, i.e., cartilage thickness. Several investigators have reported that frequencies ranging between 20 and 80 MhZ are suitable for studies in human or animal cartilage ***(2–6)***. In this frequency range, the cartilage structures are analyzed with a spatial resolution down to approx 30 μm along the propagation direction and 80 μm in the transverse direction.

In this chapter, we describe sample preparation, data acquisition procedures steps, and signal processing used for cartilage ultrasonic pulse echo imaging and quantitative measurements of backscatter and reflection coefficients in approx the 20–80-MHz frequency bandwidth (*see* **Subheading 5., Glossary**).

2. Materials

1. Water tank in transparent plastic (e.g., Plexiglas). The dimensions of the water tank must be adapted to contain the reflector plane, the specimen holder, and the sample. Dimensions used in the experiment setup described below are 9 cm in height, 20 cm in length, and 12 cm in width.
2. Saline solution. The water tank is filled with saline. The measured sample must be immersed in the solution such that the height of liquid covering the sample must be greater than the focal length of the ultrasonic transducer (*see* **Subheading 5., Glossary**). Here, for a focal length of 7.5 mm, the sample surface was 1 cm below the saline surface.
3. Sample holder such as modeling clay or dental paste.
4. Thermostat with stirring system.
5. Vacuum pump (Brandt RD4), 4.3 m^3/h.
6. Perfect reflector plane such as steel or glass plate, placed in the bottom of the water tank. Dimensions must fit within the water tank described above. Dimensions used in the experiment setup described in **Subheading 3.2.1.** below are 2 cm in height, 10 cm in length, and 5 cm in width.
7. Piezoelectric transducer, 80-MHz nominal central frequency, 3-mm diameter, 7.5-mm focal length (Toray Techno, Sonoyama, Japan).
8. Ultrasonics pulser receiver electronics (Panametrics, Waltham, MA, model PR 5900).
9. Analog-to-digital (A/D) signal convertor. The A/D convertor can be a plug-in PC board or a digital oscilloscope (e.g., LeCroy, NY; oscilloscope model 9450A).
10. Electronic cables of electrical impedance 50 Ω. The cable connection to the electronic equipment is made via BNC connectors. The cable connection to the transducers will depend on the transducer and will be specified by the manufacturer.
11. Personal computer, IBM compatible.
12. Tilt stage and water tank holder, stepping motors XYZ, motor controller (Micro Controle Newport, Evry, France).
13. Drivers for pulser receiver, motor displacement, and A/D convertor. Drivers are supplied by the manufacturers. Custom software with labview "basic package" for control of data acquisition and motor displacement.
14. Signal processing and image analysis software with custom software for signal and image reconstruction, visualization, and processing. Otherwise, commercially available signal and image processing tools such as Matlab can be used.

3. Methods

3.1. Sample Preparation

In contrast to conventional ultrasonography, which can be achieved transcutaneously on articular cartilage, the high-frequency ultrasonography discussed here requires removal of all intervening tissues between the probe and cartilage surface. The technique described here is appropriate to the exploration of in vitro or ex vivo cartilage specimens (*see* **Note 1**). However, the procedure could be extended to an open articulation of living animals, so that the probe is in direct contact or close to the cartilage surface. In this case, a coupling medium is required to transmit the emitted sound wave to the tissue. The coupling medium may be saline- or water-based ultrasonic coupling gel such as those used for clinical echographic examinations.

For in vitro or ex vivo experiments, the specimens can be taken from sacrificed animals and immediately explored or frozen and stored at –20°C until further investigations. In this latter case, the specimens must be thawed at room temperature in degassed saline before ultrasound data acquisition. It has been shown that freeze-thawing does not alter the acoustic properties of the tissues *(6)*. For sample preparation, proceed as follows:

1. Remove gas bubbles that may have been trapped during excision. It is recommended to place the saline tank in partial vacuum for approx 1 h.
2. Mount the specimens on a holder (e.g., modeling clay or dental cement) that permits one to maintain and position the cartilage surface facing the transducer.
3. Position the specimen such that the cartilage surface is roughly oriented perpendicularly to the ultrasound beam axis.
4. Control the temperature. This is recommended for experimental measurements because tissue acoustic properties vary with temperature *(7)*. In this case, the saline-filled container must be nestled within a larger water bath equipped with a thermostated heating and stirring system. For comparison purposes, it is important to note that the experiments must be carried out at the same temperature.

3.2. Ultrasound Exploration

3.2.1. Experimental Setup

The experimental setup is illustrated in **Fig. 1.** A single-element piezoelectric transducer operates in the transmit receive mode. A focused transducer is preferred to achieve an optimal spatial resolution.

1. Place the transducer on a mechanical support connected to micrometric stepping motors allowing lateral (*xy*) and vertical (*z*-axis, corresponding to the ultrasound beam axis) translation.
2. Place the saline tank beneath the transducer on a mechanical tilt stage mounted on a support enabling sample orientation relative to the ultrasound beam axis.
3. Connect the transducer to a broadband ultrasonic pulser–receiver. The excitation voltage pulse delivered by the pulser is transformed by the piezoelectric transducer into an ultrasound pulse that propagates through the coupling medium. Echoes reflected or backscattered by the cartilage structures are converted by the transducer into an electrical radiofrequency (RF) signal. This echographic signal is amplified by the receiver electronics.
4. Connect the RF output of the pulser-receiver to the input of the A/D convertor. The received signal is then digitized at a sampling frequency that is at least 5–10 times the central frequency of the transducer.

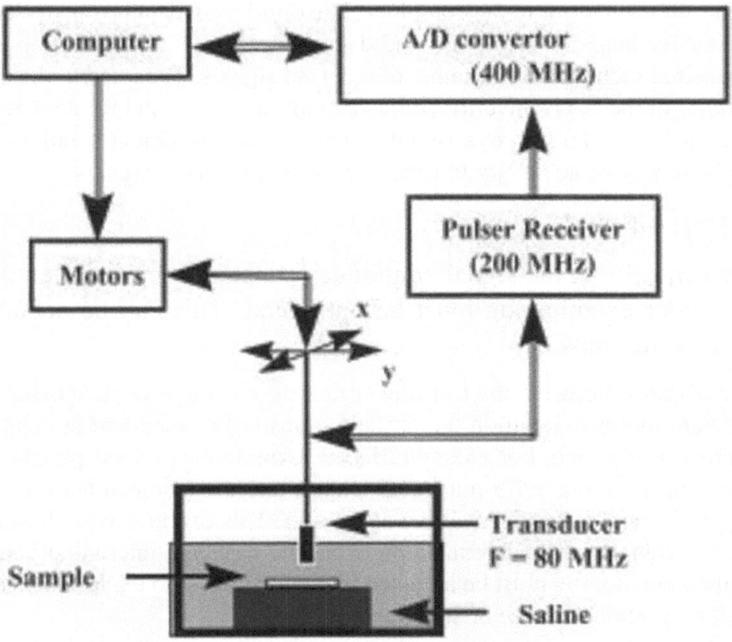

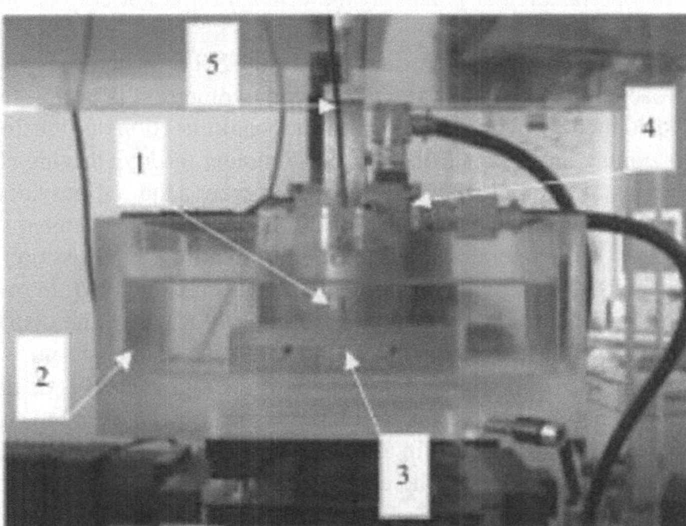

Fig. 1. Experimental setup. 1, transducer; 2, water tank filled with saline; 3, plane reflector; 4, stepping motors; 5, cables.

5. Connect the A/D convertor to the computer. The digitized signal is transferred to the computer for image construction and data processing. The acquisition gain must be adjusted such that the dynamic of received signals is adapted to the voltage sensitivity of the A/D convertor while keeping samples in the RF data below the saturation limits. To improve signal-to-noise ratio and detect small-amplitude signals, it may be necessary to time-average the received signals.

3.2.2. Data Acquisition

Before data acquisition, the signal amplitude reflected or backscattered by the structures under examination must be optimized. This can be achieved through the following steps:

1. Adjust the distance between the transducer and the cartilage surface using the *z*-displacement motor to position the tissue regions to be examined at approximately the focal distance. For example, in our experiments on rat patella, we used a transducer having a 7.5-mm focal length, and the distance between the probe and the specimen surface was set at 7.4 mm. This distance was chosen to maximize the signal amplitude emanating from the cartilage internal structure. The specimen positioning must be adjusted in the focal zone to explore different layers such as articular surface or subchondral bone.
2. Position the cartilage surface of the specimen perpendicularly to the insonification axis. This can be achieved by tilting the tank support in the focal zone. The orientation of the specimen relative to the ultrasound beam axis is then evaluated across the region to be scanned by performing two preliminary scans in two perpendicular planes. If the orientation is not correct, the sample must be remounted.
3. Once the sample is correctly positioned, i.e., when the signal amplitude has reached its maximum, the ultrasound exploration is performed by scanning the specimen in two translational orthogonal directions (*xy*) using the micrometric stepping motors controlled by the computer through driving electronics so that a series of parallel adjacent scan planes were acquired providing 3D information about the cartilage and subchondral bone. The displacement step must be of the order of the lateral resolution (*see* **Subheading 5., Glossary**) of the transducer, which is given by the beam width at half maximum ***(8)***. In our investigations of rat patella at 80MHz (lateral resolution of 80 μm), the displacement step was 50 μm ***(5)***. The RF signal is acquired at each scan position.
4. Select the beginning and the length of the digitized RF signals to include all the tissue depth of interest. Considering a mean speed of sound (*see* **Subheading 5., Glossary**) of 1650 *m/s* in articular cartilage and a typical rat patellar cartilage of 300 μm in thickness, the echographic signal duration from the whole cartilage thickness is approx 365 ns. Hence, the length of the digitized RF signals must be larger than this value. For example, at least 400 samples are required at a 1-GHz sampling rate.

3.3. Signal Processing

3.3.1. Echographic Image Formation

3.3.1.1. Echographic A-Mode

Reflected and backscattered signals propagate back to the transducer and generate an electrical signal (called an RF signal) when striking the transducer front face. The video signal is obtained by envelope detection (i.e., only the amplitude modulation is kept) of the RF signal and may be displayed in several modes *(9)*. Envelope detection can be achieved by calculating the Hilbert transform of the RF signal *(10)*.

The A-mode (A for amplitude) is a time-base display of received echo amplitude. The measured amplitude indicates tissue "reflectivity," i.e., the variation in acoustic properties encountered at the boundaries of the echo-generating objects. The A-mode can be used to determine the depth z of a reflector by measuring the time of flight t (*see* **Subheading 5.**, **Glossary**) of the corresponding echo. Depth z is given by:

$$z = \frac{ct}{2} \tag{1}$$

where c is the speed of sound, assumed to be a constant in the cartilage. The factor 2 in the equation comes from the fact that the pulse has traveled to and returned from the target. Usually, a value of approx c = 1650 m/s is used for articular cartilage. The A-mode provides a useful tool for accurate measurements of cartilage thickness along the axis of the ultrasound beam at the position of the A-line.

3.3.1.2. Echographic B-Mode

By steering the beam into a plane (scan plane), a cross-sectional image of echo-generating structures cut by the plane can be obtained. B-mode (B for brightness) is the display of the detected amplitude (video signal) of echo signals in a gray scale on a computer video screen. Typical B-mode images of normal and osteoarthritic rat patellar cartilages are shown in **Fig. 2**.

Vertical and horizontal dimensions are related to the transducer scanning and the ultrasound propagation (cartilage depth) directions, respectively. Ultrasound images show an excellent discrimination between the cartilage interfaces. For normal cartilage (**Fig. 2**, left), the articular surface (saline/cartilage interface; denoted by cs) is regular, smooth, and marked by a thin band of intense echo arising from a specular reflection of the ultrasound wave at this surface. The second broad band delineates the cartilage-calcified cartilage/bone

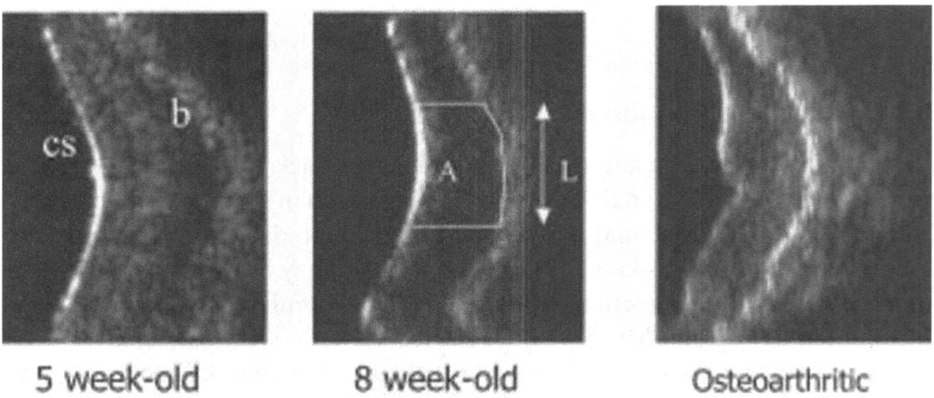

Fig. 2. Typical 50-MHz B-mode images of rat patellar cartilage. (**Left**) Immature rat patellar cartilage displaying the echoic cartilage matrix. b, cartilage-calcified cartilage and bone interface; cs, cartilage surface at the cartilage-saline interface. (**Middle**) Mature rat patellar cartilage showing cartilage thinning and hypoechoic matrix. On this image, we illustrate the delimited area used for cartilage thickness estimation. A, delimited area of measurement; L, length of region. (**Right**) Osteoarthritic patella showing an irregular cartilage surface and increased signal level reflected from subchondral bone.

(*b*) interface. This boundary is irregular, dense, less smooth, and less echoic than the articular surface. It consists of calcified cartilage, trabecular bone, and marrow. Deep layers of subchondral bone could not be visualized because of high reflection of ultrasound at the interface and/or high attenuation (*see* **Note 2**) of ultrasound in this tissue. The cartilage surface and cartilage/bone interface are separated by the cartilage internal structure, which is echoic. For most of the specimens, the first two-thirds of the internal cartilage tissue are the most echogenic, displaying an echostructure on the ultrasound image.

Alterations of the cartilage surface are well detected on the ultrasound image of the osteoarthritic specimen (**Fig. 2**, right). The cartilage subchondral bone interface is hyperechoic and discontinous. It consists of new fibrovascular repair tissue with an increased collagen and osseous cell content. The proliferation of this tissue extended to the deep layer of the cartilage and resulted in an echoic band on the ultrasound image whose texture appeared different from that of normal cartilage and denoted the fibrous nature of the tissue.

3.3.2. Cartilage Thickness Measurement

Local measurement of the cartilage thickness (*see* **Note 3**) can be performed on A-mode line by calculating the difference in time of flight of detected echoes corresponding to the cartilage and subchondral bone surfaces. An average estimate of cartilage thickness (*see* **Note 3**) can be obtained from B-mode images ***(11)***.

1. Select a region, which is adjusted manually to the cartilage boundaries, for example, in the central part of the cartilage (**Fig. 2**, middle).
2. Calculate the area of this region in pixels
3. Divide the area by the length L of the region measured along the transducer scanning axis to estimate the average thickness of the cartilage (also in pixels).
4. Convert the average thickness in pixels into micrometers using a scaling factor, which is determined by the sampling frequency and the speed of sound (*see* **Note 2**), as in the following equation:

$$Scaling\ factor = \frac{c}{2F_e} \qquad (2)$$

where c is the sound velocity in cartilage and F_e the sampling frequency of the digitized radiofrequency signal.

3.3.3. Acoustic Parameter Measurements

The echogenicity or reflectivity level of ultrasound signal reflects the interaction between ultrasound and tissue structures. Therefore, quantitative analysis of the echogenicity variation is a means of evaluating the modification of the tissue characteristics. An example of analysis is given in the following paragraphs for rat patellar cartilage. However, this analysis can be easily applied to cartilage specimens taken from other articular sites or species (*see* **Note 1**).

The RF signals can be processed in the frequency domain in order to estimate the reflection coefficient from the cartilage surface (called the integrated reflection coefficient [IRC]) and the backscatter coefficient from the cartilage internal structure and from the cartilage/bone interface (called the apparent integrated backscatter [AIB]) ***(11)***. These parameters, which are device- and operator-independent, are measured using a standard substitution method that compensates for the apparatus transfer function ***(11)***.

The reflection coefficient is a quantitative index of the acoustic energy level reflected from cartilage surface that is mainly related to the composition and microarchitecture of the superficial layer of cartilage and to surface roughness (*see* **Note 4**).

1. Select the first 32 samples of the signal reflected by the cartilage surface using an appropriate Hamming time window (**Fig. 3**).
2. Calculate the power spectrum $|S_c(f,z_0)|^2$ of the windowed signal using the Fourier transform.
3. Divide the calculated spectrum by the power spectrum $|S_r(f,z_0)|^2$ of the signal reflected by a perfect acoustic mirror (steel or glass plate) in order to compensate for the signal for system transfer function. The acoustic mirror is positioned at the same distance z_0 from the transducer as the cartilage surface.

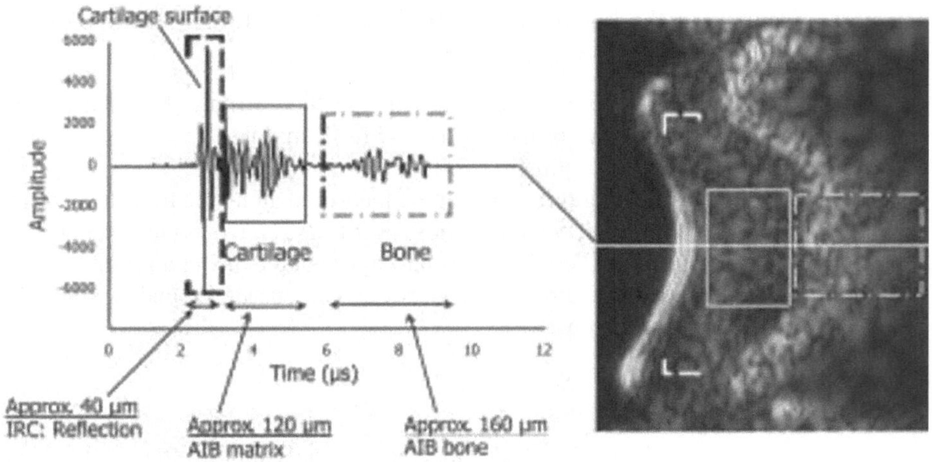

Fig. 3. A 50-MHz rat patellar echographic cartilage image (**right**) and radiofrequency signal (**left**) at one scan position displaying the echoes reflected from the cartilage surface, matrix, and subchondral bone. The analysis of reflected signals is restricted to a segment of the radiofrequency signal defined by a time gate, as shown on the left. The time gate is used to select the data from a reflecting or scattering volume, i.e., cartilage surface, matrix, and subchondral bone respectively, as shown on the right. IRC, integrated reflection coefficient; AIB, apparent integrated backscatter.

4. The ratio of both spectra is averaged spatially over a region of interest (ROI) that is selected in the central part of the specimen, where the cartilage surface is perpendicular to the direction of sound propagation.
5. Then the mean ratio is converted into dB and integrated over the –6-dB frequency bandwidth f of $|S_c(f,z_0)|^2$ to estimate the integrated reflection coefficient (**Fig. 4**). All calculations are summarized by the following equation:

$$R_c^{dB}(f) = 10 \log_{10} \left\langle \frac{|S_c(f,z_0)|^2}{|S_r(f,z_0)|^2} \right\rangle \tag{3}$$

where $R_c{}^{dB}(f)$ is the intensity reflection coefficient at the cartilage surface in dB, and <...> indicates the spatial average calculated over 45 A-lines corresponding to a ROI of 120 µm in the transverse direction by 600 µm in the sagittal direction. The integrated reflection coefficient is defined by the following integral equation:

$$IRC = \frac{1}{\Delta f} \int R_c^{dB}(f)\,df \tag{4}$$

where Δf corresponds to the frequency range of 30–75 MHz.

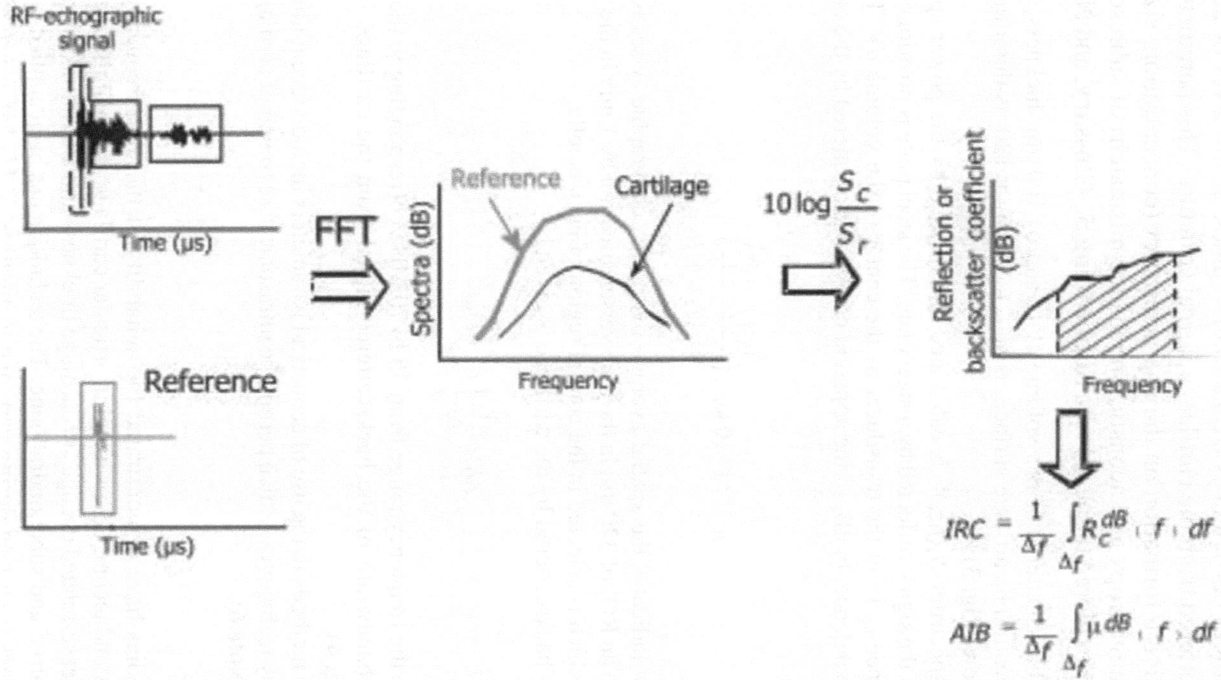

Fig. 4. Illustration of signal processing steps for the estimation of the integrated reflection coefficient (IRC) and apparent integrated backscatter (AIB). FFT, fast Fourier transform; RF, radiofrequency.

The backscatter coefficient is a quantitative index of the level of acoustic energy backscattered from the cartilage internal structure. This parameter provides quantitative information on the characteristics (concentration, size, orientation, e.g., anisotropy and acoustic impedance mismatch) of subresolution scatterers of the explored tissue *(1)* (*see* **Subheading 5.**, **Glossary**, and **Note 5**).

1. The signal backscattered from a volume dV of approx 100 µm-thickness, located 32 µm beneath the cartilage surface, is selected using a 120-ns-duration Hamming window (**Fig. 3**).
2. Its power spectrum $|S_v(f,z_v)|^2$ is calculated and divided by the power spectrum $|S_r(f,z_v)|^2$ of the signal reflected by a steel plate. The steel plate is positioned at the same distance z_v from the transducer as the center of the volume dV. The frequency dependence, in dB, of the apparent energy backscattered by the cartilage is equal to:

$$\mu^{dB}(f) = 10\log_{10}\left\langle \frac{|S_v(f,z_v)|^2}{|S_r(f,z_v)|^2} \right\rangle \tag{5}$$

where <...> indicates the spatial average over 200 echographic A-scans corresponding to an ROI of 320 µm in the transversal direction by 1 mm in the sagittal direction, which is selected in the central region of each patella.
3. The energy backscattered by the cartilage is given by:

$$AIB = \frac{1}{\Delta f}\int_{\Delta f} \mu^{dB}(f)\,df \tag{6}$$

where f is the frequency range from 35 to 70 MHz corresponding to the –6-dB frequency bandwidth of the backscattered signal from the cartilage internal matrix (**Fig. 4**).

Alternative methods to the use of acoustical parameters include recent ultrasonic elastography techniques, which permit the ultrasonic assessment of cartilage elasticity (*see* **Note 6**).

4. Notes

1. Several studies have demonstrated the suitability of the high-frequency pulse echo ultrasound technique for imaging articular cartilage and quantitative evaluation of disease-related changes in cartilage thickness and alterations of cartilage surface, matrix, and subchondral bone. The technique has been applied to investigate changes occurring during cartilage maturation *(4,11–13)*, OA *(2,3,5,11)*, and arthritis and during treatment *(14)*. The methodology described above has been specifically applied to the investigation of rat patellar cartilage; however, slight modifications (e.g., ultrasonic frequency, transducer, and electronics specifications) may be introduced to make the methodology suitable for studies of human or large animal (canine, porcine, or bovine) cartilage *(2,4,6,15)*. For

example, subsurface characteristics of normal and OA human femoral condyle of human osteoarthritic cartilage have been visualized *(3)*.

2. Several modifications to the described methods can be made to extract additional acoustical parameters such as attenuation coefficient or sound velocity. The focusing settings described above were specific for echographic imaging and quantitative assessment of reflection and backscatter coefficients. A different adjustment of the specimen in the focal zone is required for the measurement of attenuation coefficient and sound velocity. To this end, the ultrasonic beam must be focused on the reference plate, and the echo signals reflected by the cartilage surface and the plate are acquired first without and then with the cartilage sample interposed between the transducer and the plate. The attenuation coefficient and sound velocity values can be calculated following the standard substitution method described in detail in **ref. *19***. The attenuation coefficient and sound velocity in articular cartilage are sensitive to modification of the matrix collagen ***(20)*** and proteoglycans. The enzymatic degradation of the matrix proteoglycans in human or bovine articular cartilage significantly increased the attenuation coefficient ***(17,21)*** and decreased the speed of sound ***(6,17,21)*** in the 20–40-MHz range.
3. Regarding cartilage thickness estimation, it is worth noting the dependence of the estimated thickness on the value of ultrasound velocity (**Eq. 2**). Therefore, accurate estimation of cartilage thickness relies on the knowledge of accurate velocity values. Velocity values may vary with cartilage state (normal or pathologic), skeletal sites, or species. These variations are generally considered to be negligible, and therefore an average constant value (e.g., 1650 *m/s*) obtained from literature may be used for thickness determination. A 1.3% reproducibility has been reported for thickness measurement in B-scan images ***(11)***. Measurements of ultrasonic cartilage thickness have been found to be sensitive to variations occurring during animal maturation or disease-related cartilage state ***(6,11,12)***.
4. The reflection coefficient (IRC) is sensitive to surface fibrillation and changes occurring in the superficial layer ***(6,11,14,16–18)***. The thickness of the superficial layer assessed using IRC is determined by the axial resolution (*see* **Subheading 5., Glossary**) of the transducer. The reproducibility (defined as the coefficient of variation of repeated measurements with interim repositioning) of IRC measurements has been found to be of the order 3.5% ***(11)***. It should be noted that IRC values may be subject to measurement errors, including the acquisition system function, the position of the articular cartilage surface with respect to the focal zone, and the incidence angle. Careful adjustment of the distance between the probe and the cartilage surface and correct acquisition of the reference signal on a plate are mandatory to ensure accurate and precise estimates. The major source of error remains the beam incidence angle with respect to the cartilage surface. The orientation must be carefully optimized following the procedure described in **Subheading 3.2.**, otherwise the IRC would be underestimated.
5. The echogenecity level and the quantitative evaluation of ultrasonic backscatter (AIB) are useful for the investigation of cartilage matrix or subchondral bone

structural changes occurring under various experimental or clinical circumstances, like the growing process *(12)*, osteoarthritis *(5,11)*, arthritis, and drug effects *(14)*. In particular, this parameter has been shown to be related to collagen network organization *(12,14)* but was not sensitive to changes in proteoglycan content *(13)*. In rats, ultrasonic backscatter increases during the progression of OA but decreases with aging *(11,12)*. This parameter has also been used to detect changes in subchondral bone related to chemically induced arthritis and to monitor anti-inflammatory treatment effects in rats *(14)*. The reproducibility of AIB measurements has been found to be of the order 1% *(11)*. This integrated backscatter coefficient is referred to as *apparent* because it is not compensated for by the attenuation effects caused by tissue between the cartilage surface and the window studied. Hence, to minimize these effects, measurements must be obtained in the region located just beneath the cartilage surface.

6. Alternative methods to the use of acoustical parameters include recent ultrasonic elastography techniques, which permit the ultrasonic assessment of cartilage elasticity. Ultrasound compression systems for high-resolution assessment of articular cartilage elasticity have been developed *(22,23)*. Laasanen et al. *(24)* developed an arthroscopic-type ultrasound indentation probe to determine the stiffness of articular cartilage tissues. Ultrasonic measurement of elastic modulus can detect changes occurring in enzymatically degraded bovine cartilage *(22,24)*. With the rapid advances in this field, the combination of elastic and acoustic properties may be utilized effectively toward a more complete quantitative evaluation of cartilage quality *(18)*.

5. Glossary

Acoustic impedance The acoustic impedance is a characteristic of the medium defined as:

$$Z = \rho c$$

where ρ is the mass density and c the speed of sound.

Attenuation coefficient The relative change in the acoustic wave amplitude per unit path length in a medium. Unit: cm^{-1} or $dB \cdot cm^{-1}$. The attenuation experienced in biological tissues is dependent on a frequency with an approximately linear variation. In biomedical ultrasonics, ultrasonic attenuation is commonly characterized by its frequency slope in $dB \cdot cm^{-1} \cdot MHz^{-1}$ (*see also Slope of attenuation coefficient*).

Axial resolution The axial resolution can be estimated by measuring the –6-dB width of the envelope of a pulse reflected by a steel plate positioned at the focus and perpendicular to the probe axis.

Frequency bandwidth Portion of the frequency response of a transducer or of the complete measuring chain (including transmitting and receiving electronics) that falls within given limits. The conventional limits used to characterize the frequency bandwidth of a measuring device are at a –3 dB (also –6 dB) level of the maximum value of the response. However, different limits (–20 dB) may be used to define total usable bandwidth of the measuring device depending on the signal-to-noise ratio.

Lateral resolution The lateral resolution can be estimated by measuring the −6-dB full width of the transverse (off-axis) profile of the signal reflected by a thread (e.g., nylon or metal) at the focal distance of the transducer. The diameter of the thread must not exceed half a wavelength (q.v.).

Slope of attenuation coefficient Assuming a linear variation with frequency of the attenuation, the slope of a linear regression fit to the frequency-dependent attenuation coefficient. Unit: $cm^{-1} \cdot MHz^{-1}$ or $dB \cdot cm^{-1} \cdot MHz^{-1}$.

Spectral analysis A method of analyzing a waveform signal such as an ultrasonic pulse, by providing the amplitude and phase as a function of frequency of its component waves. Fourier analysis is frequently used and is based on determining the harmonic content of a waveform.

Time of flight The time elapsed between the transmission of the incident pulse (time origin) and the reception of the signal. The time of flight is assumed to be proportional to the distance between the echo source and the receiving transducer.

Ultrasonic transducer The device used to convert electrical energy to mechanical energy and, reciprocally, to convert mechanical energy to electrical energy.

Speed of sound Speed at which the vibrational energy is propagating. Sound waves propagate with a definite velocity, called the speed of sound, which is a characteristic of the medium. In general, sound velocity can be determined by both the geometrical and material properties of the medium.

Wavelength The wavelength represents the spatial extent of a cycle of vibration and is the distance between two consecutive points of the wave, which are mutually in phase. The wavelength can be obtained from the ultrasonic frequency f following:

$$\lambda = \frac{c}{f}$$

where c is the sound velocity. Given the typical value of sound velocity in cartilage of approx 1650 $m \cdot s^{-1}$, the wavelength is about 30 μm at 50 MHz.

References

1. Shung, K. K. and Thieme, G. A., eds. (1993) *Ultrasonic Scattering in Biological Tissues.* CRC Press, Boca Raton, FL.
2. Sanghvi, N. T., Snoddy, A. M., Myers, S. L., Brandt, K. D., Reilly, C. R., and Franklin, T. D., Jr. (1990) Characterization of normal and osteoarthritic cartilage using 25 MHz ultrasound, in *IEEE Ultrasonics Symposium Proceedings* (Schneider, S. C., Levy, M., and McAvoy, B. R., eds.), IEEE, Piscataway, NJ, pp. 1413–1416.
3. Myers, S. L., Dines, K., Brandt, D. A., Brandt, K. D., and Albrecht, M. L. (1995) Experimental assessment by high frequency ultrasound of articular cartilage thickness and osteoarthritic changes. *J. Rheumatol.* **22,** 109–116.
4. Kim, H. K. W., Babyn, P. S., Harasiewicz, K. A., Gahunia, H. K., Pritzker, K. P. H., and Foster, F. S. (1995) Imaging of immature articular cartilage using ultrasound backscatter microscopy at 50 MHz. *J. Orthop. Res.* **13,** 963–970.

5. Saïed, A., Chérin, E., Gaucher, H., et al. (1997) Assessment of articular cartilage and subchondral bone: subtle and progressive changes in experimental osteoarthritis using 50 MHz echography in vitro. *J. Bone Miner. Res.* **12,** 1378–1386.
6. Töyräs, J., Rieppo, J., Nieminen, M. T., Helminen, H. J., and Jurvelin, J. S. (1999) Characterization of enzymatically induced degradation of articular cartilage using high frequency ultrasound. *Phys. Med. Biol.* **44,** 2723–2733.
7. Goss, S., Johnston R., and Dunn, F. (1980) Compilation of empirical ultrasonic properties of mam-malian tissues. II. *J. Acoust. Soc. Am.* **108,** 68–93.
8. Hunt, J. W., Arditi, M., and Foster, F. S. (1983) Ultrasound transducers for pulse-echo medical imaging. *IEEE Trans. Biomed. Eng.* **30,** 453–481.
9. Fish, P., ed. (1990) Physics and instrumentation of diagnostic medical ultrasound. John Wiley & Sons, New York.
10. Gammell, P. M. (1981) Improved ultrasonic detection using the analytic signal magnitude. *Ultrasonics* **19,** 73–76.
11. Chérin, E., Saïed, A., Laugier, P., Netter, P., and Berger, G. (1998) Evaluation of acoustical parameter sensitivity to age-related and osteoarthritic changes in articular cartilage using 50-MHz ultrasound. *Ultrasound Med. Biol.* **24,** 341–354.
12. Chérin, E., Saïed, A., Pellaumail, B., et al. (2001) Assessment of rat articular cartilage maturation using 50-MHz quantitative ultrasonography. *Osteoarthritis Cartilage* **9,** 178–186.
13. Pellaumail, B., Watrin, A., Loeuille, D., et al. (2002) Effect of articular cartilage proteoglycan depletion on high frequency ultrasound backscatter. *Osteoarthritis Cartilage* **10,** 535–541.
14. Jaffre, B., Watrin, A., Loeuille, D., et al. (2003) Effects of anti-inflammatory drugs on arthritic cartilage: a high frequency quantitative ultrasound study in rats. *Arthritis Rheum.* **48,** 1594–1601.
15. Agemura, D. H., O'Brien, W. D., Olerud, J. E., Chun, L. E., and Eyre, D. E. (1990) Ultrasonic propagation properties of articular cartilage at 100 MHz. *J. Acoust. Soc. Am.* **87,** 1786–1791.
16. Adler, R. S., Dedrick, D. K., Laing, T. J., et al. (1992) Quantitative assessment of cartilage surface roughness on osteoarthritis using high frequency ultrasound. *Ultrasound Med. Biol.* **18,** 51–58.
17. Nieminen, H.J., Toyras, J., Rieppo J., et al. (2002) Real-time ultrasound analysis of articular cartilage degradation in vitro. *Ultrasound Med. Biol.* **28,** 519–525.
18. Toyras, J., Nieminen, H. J., Laasanen, M. S., et al. (2002) Ultrasonic characterization of articular cartilage. *Biorheology* **39,** 161–169.
19. D'Astous, F. and Foster, F. S. (1986) Frequency dependence of ultrasound attenuation and backscatter in breast tissue. *Ultrasound Med. Biol.* **12,** 795–808.
20. Pellaumail, B., Dewailly, V., Loeuille, D., Netter, P., Berger G., and Saïed, A. (1999) Attenuation coefficient and speed of sound in immature and mature rat cartilage: a study in the 30–70 MHz frequency range, in *IEEE Ultrasonics Symposium Proceedings* (Schneider, S.C., Levy, M., and McAvoy, B. R., eds.), IEEE, Piscataway, NJ, pp. 1361–1364.

21. Joiner, G. A., Bogoch, E. R., Pritzker, K. P., Buschmann, M. D., Chevrier, A., and Foster, F. S. (2001) High frequency acoustic parameters of human and bovine articular cartilage following experimentally-induced matrix degradation. Ultrason. *Imaging* **23,** 106–116.
22. Zheng, Y. P., Ding, C. X., Bai, J., and Mak, A. F. T. (2001) Measurement of nonhomogeneous compressive properties of trypsin treated articular cartilage: an ultrasound investigation. *Med. Biol. Eng. Comput.* **39,** 534–541.
23. Zheng, Y. P, Mak, A. F. T, Lau, K. P., and Qin, L. (2002) An ultrasonic measurement for in vitro depth-dependent equilibrium strains of articular cartilage in compression. *Phys. Med. Biol.* **47,** 3165–3180.
24. Laasanen, M. S., Toyras, J., Hirvonen, J., et al. (2002) Novel mechano-acoustic technique and instrument for diagnosis of cartilage degeneration. *Physiol. Meas.* **23,** 491–503.

14

Evaluation of Cartilage Composition and Degradation by High-Resolution Magic-Angle Spinning Nuclear Magnetic Resonance

Jürgen Schiller, Daniel Huster, Beate Fuchs, Lama Naji, Jörn Kaufmann, and Klaus Arnold

Summary

Rheumatic diseases are accompanied by a progressive destruction of the cartilage layers of the joints. Although the number of patients suffering from rheumatic diseases is steadily increasing, degradation mechanisms of cartilage are not yet understood, and methods for early diagnosis are not available. Although some information on pathogenesis could be obtained from the nuclear magnetic resonance (NMR) spectra of degradation products in the supernatants of cartilage specimens incubated with degradation-causing agents, the most direct information on degradation processes would come from the native cartilage as such. To obtain highly resolved NMR spectra of cartilage, application of the recently developed high-resolution magic-angle spinning (HR-MAS) NMR technique is advisable to obtain small line-widths of individual cartilage resonances. This technique is nowadays commercially available for most NMR spectrometers and has the considerable advantage that the same pulse sequences as in high-resolution NMR can be applied. Except for a MAS spinning equipment, no solid-state NMR hardware is required. Therefore, this method can be easily implemented. Here, we describe the most important requirements that are necessary to record HR-MAS NMR spectra. The capabilities of the HR-MAS technique are discussed for the ^{1}H and ^{13}C NMR spectra of cartilage.

Key Words: Cartilage; HR-MAS; collagen; proteoglycans; enzymatic digestion; magic angle.

1. Introduction

The progressive diminution of the thickness of the cartilage layers of the joints is a feature of rheumatic diseases, although the mechanisms of cartilage degradation processes remain widely unknown *(1)*. The nuclear magnetic resonance (NMR) spectroscopic analyses of pathologically modified synovial fluids (SF) from patients suffering from rheumatic diseases were helpful to gain further insights into these mechanisms since fragmentation products of carti-

From: *Methods in Molecular Medicine, Vol. 101: Cartilage and Osteoarthritis, Volume 2: Structure and In Vivo Analysis*
Edited by: F. De Ceuninck, M. Sabatini, and P. Pastoureau © Humana Press Inc., Totowa, NJ

lage accumulate in the SF *(2,3)*. These investigations indicated, for instance, that reactive oxygen species generated by neutrophilic granulocytes play a prominent role in cartilage degradation *(4)*.

A number of studies have investigated the relative importance of various molecular compounds involved in cartilage degradation. In these studies, cartilage specimens were incubated with degradation-causing agents *(5–7)* or activated neutrophils *(8)* and the supernatants were subsequently analyzed by NMR and other techniques *(9)*. Healthy cartilage is normally insoluble. However, as soon as degradation occurs, the branched polymer network of cartilage is destroyed, and polymers are transformed into a soluble form that can be identified in the supernatants *(9)*.

The sensitivity of NMR spectroscopy is enhanced by the presence of the relatively mobile and therefore intense *N*-acetyl groups of cartilage polysaccharides. When depolymerization of cartilage polysaccharides occurs, the comparable sharp resonances of degradation products are easily detectable compared with the broad lines of intact polysaccharides of healthy cartilage *(2)*.

However, these experiments were limited in the sense that they were nearly exclusively performed on the supernatants of cartilage samples treated with different agents. Therefore, the results obtained are strongly influenced by further parameters, especially the "extraction" behavior of cartilage: Fragmentation products may stick to the solid cartilage and thus be undetectable in the supernatant. Because of the negative charge density of cartilage and the resulting repulsive forces, this is only a minor problem for fragments of acidic polysaccharides *(1)*, but it represents a major problem for the fragmentation products of cartilage proteins. On the other hand, the characterization of the cartilage samples as such would provide a more direct approach to the in vivo situations relevant for cartilage degradation.

Unfortunately, standard high-resolution ^{1}H NMR spectroscopic analysis of cartilage is nearly impossible since only broad, less informative resonances can be obtained owing to significant chemical shift anisotropy and residual dipolar coupling contributions for motionally constrained species, leading to severe line broadening *(10)*. Therefore, ^{13}C NMR instead of ^{1}H NMR has mainly been used in the past for the characterization of cartilage specimens *(11–13)*. ^{13}C NMR spectra are far less influenced by sample heterogeneities than ^{1}H NMR spectra, and even a relaxation time study of the polysaccharides of cartilage proteoglycans could be performed *(14)*.

One modern approach to overcome problems with linewidths of ^{1}H NMR resonances is the application of the high resolution magic-angle spinning (HR-MAS) technique. Here, in contrast to standard solid-state NMR, strong decoupling is not used *(10)*. However, the solid-like sample is spun at high speeds under the magic angle of 54.7° with respect to the applied magnetic field B_0. This minimizes the line-broadening effects owing to isotropic magnetic susceptibility differences, and, therefore, sharper NMR resonances can be obtained. One further advantage of this method is the small size of MAS rotors and thus, the small amounts of sample required *(15)*. For scientists who would like to use HR-MAS for the first time, it is also an advantage that all the pulse sequences of high-resolution NMR can be used and there is no need to apply special, sophisticated solid-state NMR pulse sequences *(10)*.

To these authors' knowledge, cartilage has been characterized only three times so far by HR-MAS NMR *(14,16,17)*. Therefore, a more detailed description of the related methodology seems necessary.

2. Materials

2.1. Chemicals

1. Purchase all chemicals with the highest available purity. In contrast to biochemical methods, the content of low-molecular-weight compounds in particular (e.g., detergents, solvents, and others) should be as low as possible since such compounds are most sensitively detected by NMR.
2. Collagenase, papain, and chondroitin sulfate (from bovine trachea) were from Fluka. These compounds contained only low amounts of impurities.

2.2. Solutions

1. Prepare all solutions (buffers, enzymes, and others) in deuterated water (D_2O) with a high isotopic purity to minimize the water content of the sample.
2. When an internal (frequency as well as concentration) standard is necessary, 3-trimethylsilyl-propionate (TSP) is most often used. Although this compound is known to bind to proteins *(18)*, it has often been used in cartilage research *(14)*. This is done either by adding a small catheter that contains the standard or—when only a frequency standard is required—by rinsing the cartilage sample with an aqueous TSP solution.

2.3. Cartilage Preparation

The cartilage used depends on particular research interests. Pig articular (PAC) and bovine nasal cartilage (BNC) are frequently used *(12)*. The former closely resembles human articular cartilage and presents higher pathological interest *(9)* than the latter, which has the advantages of availability in larger quantities and more homogeneity. Therefore, BNC is often used as "model cartilage" *(12)*. Another advantage is that it is a completely isotropic material *(14)*. Preparation of cartilage is crucial for performing reliable NMR studies, and it is very important that pure cartilage is used.

1. Carefully remove all traces of bone in the case of PAC and the cartilage membrane (the so-called perichondrium) in the case of BNC *(16)*. Since both are lipid-rich tissues, their presence might lead to intense interfering resonances.

2. Cut the cartilage into sufficiently small pieces so as to pack the rotors as homogeneously as possible. In this study, cubic cartilage slices of about 1.5 mm diameter were used.
3. Rinse cartilage samples with D_2O to decrease the water content and to provide a field-frequency lock *(16)*.

2.4. Enzymatic Digestion of Cartilage

To obtain a tissue that resembles pathologically modified cartilage, healthy cartilage was digested with the enzymes collagenase and papain. These enzymes are known to affect collagens or proteoglycans of cartilage, respectively *(7,16)*.

1. Mix 100-mg (wet weight) cartilage specimens with 0.8 mL of 50 m*M* phosphate, 154 m*M* NaCl, pH 7.4, containing 1 mg/mL of the enzyme (corresponding to about 1 U enzymatic activity).
2. Incubate for 4 h at 37°C
3. Perform a control incubation in the absence of enzymes.

2.5. NMR Spectroscopy

All NMR measurements were conducted on a Bruker DRX-600 spectrometer operating at 600.13 MHz for ^1H and 150.86 MHz for ^{13}C. All spectra were recorded at 37°C (310 K) using a 4-mm dual (^{13}C-^1H) MAS probe and a spin rate of 5000 Hz. The residual water signal (HDO) was suppressed by presaturation on the water resonance frequency. In all cases, 128 transients were acquired for each spectrum using a repetition time of 5 s. All spectra were recorded with a spectral width of 6000 Hz (10 ppm) and 32,000 k data points. No window functions were used prior to Fourier transformation. The lactate resonance at 1.31 ppm was used for frequency calibration *(16)*.

Partially relaxed ^{13}C NMR spectra were recorded with a spectral width of 200 ppm, 32,000 k time-domain data points with a pulse angle of 45° (3.3-μs pulse), and a repetition time of 2 s. Usually 8000 k transients were accumulated with low-power broadband ^1H decoupling (Waltz-16). All free induction decays were processed with a 5-Hz line-broadening.

Since it is known that the *N*-acetyl methyl group of chondroitin sulfate is only slightly influenced by changes in the chemical environment, this resonance was used for calibration of the ^{13}C NMR spectra *(16)*.

3. Methods

The most important advantage of HR-MAS is that the same pulse sequences as in standard high-resolution NMR may be used *(19)*: the user will not notice differences in comparison with high-resolution NMR as soon as the sample is spinning within the magnet. Modern probes are normally computer-controlled, and there is no need to remove the probe from the magnet when the sample has

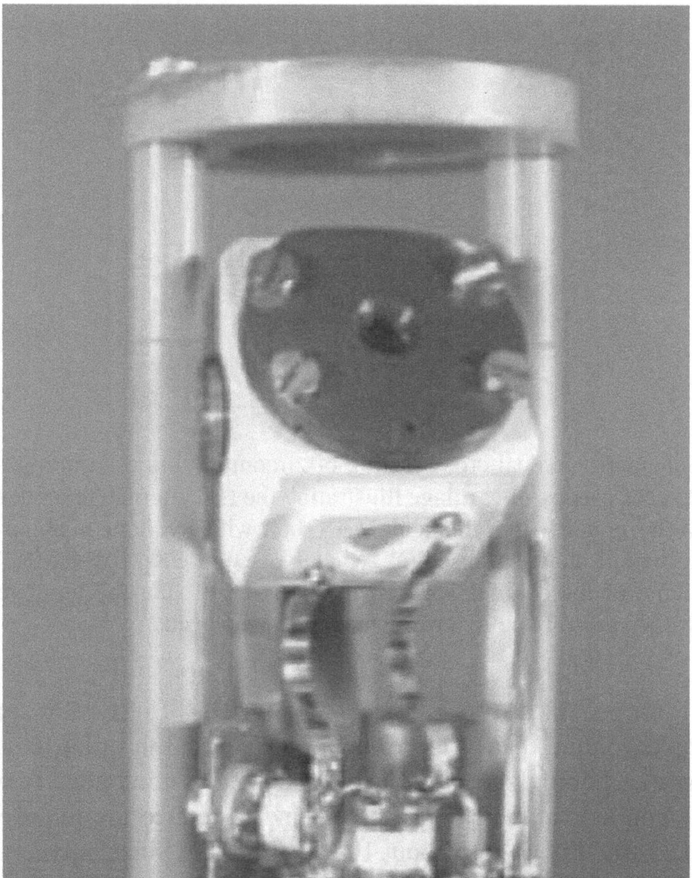

Fig. 1. Image of an open HR-MAS probe (Bruker). The upper probe chamber with the MAS stator in magic angle position is shown. For inserting and ejecting the sample, the stator is moved into a vertical position.

to be exchanged. In **Fig. 1** the upper part of a typical HR-MAS probe is shown. The stator is shown in the magic angle position. For inserting and ejecting the sample, the stator is automatically set in a vertical position, and the rotor can be loaded conveniently via a special transfer tube.

3.1. Filling the Rotor

Normally, for HR-MAS, small rotors (often with a diameter of 4 mm) are used (**Fig. 2**). The rotors used for MAS are often made of zirconium oxide (zirconia). The maximum spinning rate of about 6 kHz (quite low in comparison with normal MAS) is limited by the sealing of the sample compartment

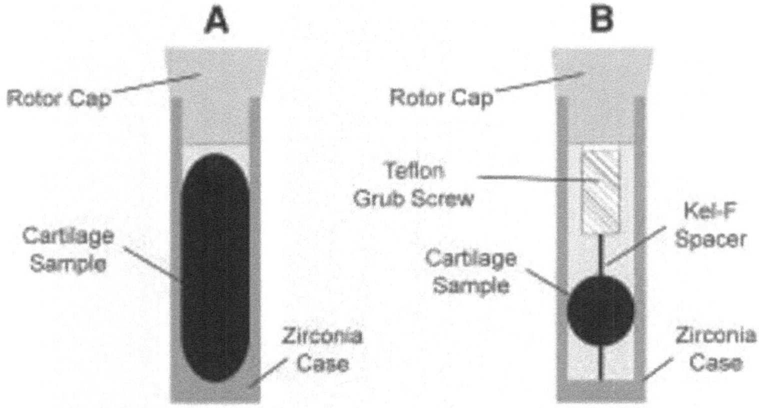

Fig. 2. Schematic vertical cross-section of zirconia rotors used in high-resolution MAS NMR spectroscopy of cartilage illustrating the two alternative modes of sample handling. **(A)** A regular 4-mm-diameter MAS rotor with a volume of about 65 μL. **(B)** A MAS rotor with a spherical insert, as typically used in HR-MAS NMR. With spacers, the volume of the rotor is reduced to about 16 μL but the homogeneity and, accordingly, the spectral quality are considerably improved.

inside the rotor provided by the "spacers" (**Fig. 2B**). These rotor spacers provide a sample volume that is approximately spherical in order to support the "shimming" (i.e., optimization of the magnetic field homogeneity with reference to the applied sample) of the probe and to reduce the required volume from about 65 μL (**Fig. 2A**) to about 16 μL (**Fig. 2B**). Since only small quantities of sample are applied, ^{1}H NMR is most often used since the proton represents the most sensitive nucleus. A large number of scans are required for ^{13}C NMR spectra, leading to considerable measurement times.

The rotor cap has two different functions, first, to close the rotor and second, to provide the spinning of the rotor. Several types of caps are available (*see* **Note 1**). The standard caps are made of Kel-F, which can be used in a temperature range from about 10 to 50°C and should not be spun faster than 6500 Hz at any temperature. Kel-F will shrink at lower temperatures and soften at more elevated temperatures. However, for a more extended temperature range (–30 to 100°C), caps made from "macor" or boron nitride can be used. The most critical factor in spinning reliability is the dynamic balance of the filled rotor. In contrast to, e.g., powders, cartilage specimens cannot be packed very homogeneously. Therefore, cartilage should be cut into small pieces or—even better—punced into many disks, each having the inside diameter of the rotor, with stacking of the disks into the rotor until full. One might also think about filling the voids between cartilage pieces with a fine powder that does not give any NMR resonances, e.g., sulfur flowers (*see* **Note 2**).

Hand pressure is always sufficient to adjust rotor packing. Hard packing of the sample using a press or a hammer is not necessary and may even damage the rotor. The cap works best if it is in slight contact with the top of the sample material. **Caution:** spinning a rotor for more than a few minutes in a vibrating state can cause permanent damage to the bearing surface of both the stator and the rotor.

3.2. Spinning the Rotor

Standard samples will easily spin in a 4-mm HR-MAS system, and problems are normally only encountered for solid heavy samples and when the rotor is not carefully balanced. In case of problems with spinning the cartilage sample, the spectrometer manual should be consulted and the bearing and drive pressure carefully adjusted according to the manufacturer's information. Sometimes, the best solution is to repack the fractious rotor. In all circumstances, however, gas pressures higher than recommended by the manufacturer must be avoided *(19)*.

3.3. Adjusting the Magic Angle

The precise setting of the magic angle is mandatory to obtain a maximum of spectral resolution. To adjust the magic angle, a sample with an NMR resonance that is highly sensitive to angle misadjustment is needed. A suitable and readily available sample is KBr: the ^{79}Br resonance frequency (150.32 MHz at a ^{1}H frequency of 600.13 MHz) is very close to the ^{13}C resonance frequency (150.86 MHz), and thus no or only slight retuning of the radiofrequency circuit is necessary. Furthermore, KBr provides a sensitive signal with a very short T_1 relaxation time, allowing a fast repetition rate. At moderate spin rates the intense side bands can already be observed; these must be as narrow as possible for the optimum angle setting *(19)*.

In **Fig. 3** two ^{79}Br spectra of the aforementioned KBr sample are shown: the upper spectrum (**Fig. 3B**) was obtained with an angle deviating from the magic angle and the lower one at correct angle setting (**Fig. 3A**). As can easily be seen, the deviation from the magic angle leads to a splitting of the center band as well as to a splitting of each side band. The angle adjusted with the micrometer screw at the probe is correctly set when the splitting disappears and the center band and side bands have minimum widths *(19)*.

3.4. Shimming an HR-MAS Probe

In contrast to standard high-resolution NMR spectroscopy, shimming is not as important for HR-MAS since line widths of resonances of solid-like material are in any case broader than resonances of liquids. For the first shimming of a probe, a cartilage sample should be prepared using a rotor with a spherical insert (**Fig. 2B**). This sample is inserted into the probe and rotated under the

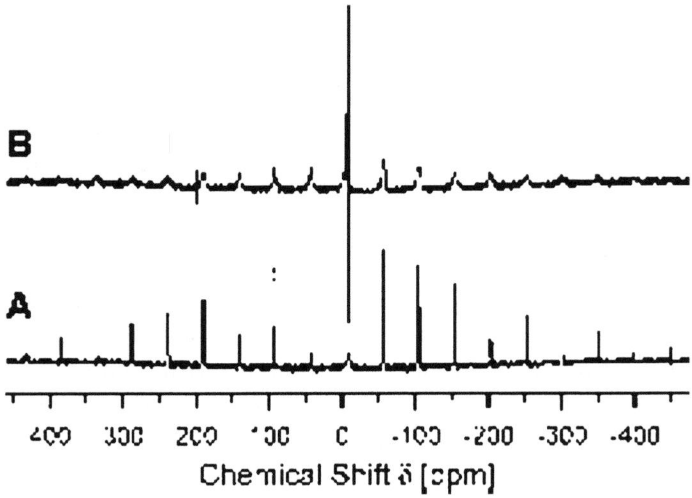

Fig. 3. ^{79}Br spectrum of KBr that is advantageously used to determine the magic angle. **(A)** The sample is exactly in the magic angle. **(B)** The sample is out of the magic angle.

magic angle using a spinning speed that depends on the field strength of the magnet. To prevent spinning side bands from appearing in the spectral regions of interest, the higher the field strength, the higher the spinning speed must be set. Therefore, at 300 MHz, at least 2400 Hz should be used, whereas at 600 MHz the spinning rate should not be lower than 4800 Hz. Special care must also be taken in controlling the temperature (*see* **Note 3**).

The success of the shimming procedure can best be controlled by using the lock line and the spectral quality simultaneously as criteria. For shimming an HR-MAS probe, it is often sufficient to use the z, z^2, z^3, z^4, x, and y directions exclusively. One should keep in mind that cartilage will not yield a half-line width better than typically 2 Hz. Therefore, it might be a waste of time to shim the probe to the absolute optimum. However, there is a considerable difference if rotors (**Fig. 2**) are used with or without spacers. Both require different shim sets that should be stored separately. Having established a suitable basic shim, all other samples should be usable with these shims, and it might only be necessary to readjust z and x.

3.5. Determination of Pulse Lengths

Using the correct pulse lengths is crucial for performing reliable NMR experiments. This especially holds for more complex pulse sequences. For calibration of the pulse length of the transmitter pulse (the "90° pulse"), normally the free induction decay (FID) or the corresponding spectrum is observed and the excitation pulse varied until the integral intensity is zero ***(19)***. This pulse length corresponds to the 180° pulse and the division by a factor of two yields the corresponding excitation (90°) pulse ***(19)***. It is important to use always the same parameter set for Fourier transformation and to wait a sufficiently long time between two pulses to allow complete relaxation. For a first rough knowledge of suitable pulse lengths, one should always have a manual describing the probe currently used and the corresponding pulse lengths. The determination of the 90° decoupler pulse that is important for ^{13}C NMR spectroscopy can be performed in the same way ***(19)***.

Cartilage spectra are always characterized by a strong contribution of water even after cartilage has been rinsed with D_2O. Different water suppression techniques are routinely available ***(20,21)***. As a starting point, the less experienced user is advised to use the "traditional" presaturation technique: the water resonance is attenuated by the application of a short, broad pulse in the time interval between two excitation pulses. This method can be implemented easily and gives reasonable results. However, saturation transfer may occur, and it is recommended to check the intensities of resonances under normal as well as presaturation conditions and to seek out any differences ***(19)***.

3.6. Performing the HR-MAS NMR Experiment

3.6.1. ^{1}H NMR Spectra of Cartilage

If all parameters described above are properly set, cartilage spectra can be easily recorded. Because of the small amounts of cartilage used in rotors with spacers, one should start with the acquisition of the corresponding ^{1}H NMR spectra ***(16)***. Initially, simple pulse-acquire spectra in combination with a water suppression technique, e.g., presaturation, should be recorded. If desired, broad lines may be eliminated or attenuated by applying a T_2 filter sequence, for instance, a spin echo sequence that suppresses rapidly relaxating compounds ***(2)***.

Two selected ^{1}H NMR spectra of BNC are shown in **Fig. 4**. The spectrum in **Fig. 4A** was recorded without MAS, that in **Fig. 4B** and was recorded with a MAS spinning frequency of 5 kHz. It is obvious that both spectra differ considerably. The intense resonance at about 2.0 ppm that is clearly detectable in both spectra is caused by the *N*-acetyl side groups of the polysaccharides of cartilage. These possess a tremendous mobility and are therefore most easily detectable owing to their comparably long T_2 relaxation times ***(2)***. This is the reason why this resonance is more easily detectable than the residual –C–H groups of the polysaccharides of cartilage, which show much broader resonances between about 3.5 and 4.0 ppm ***(9)***. Since chondroitin sulfate is the most abundant polysaccharide of cartilage ***(12)***, it primarily contributes to

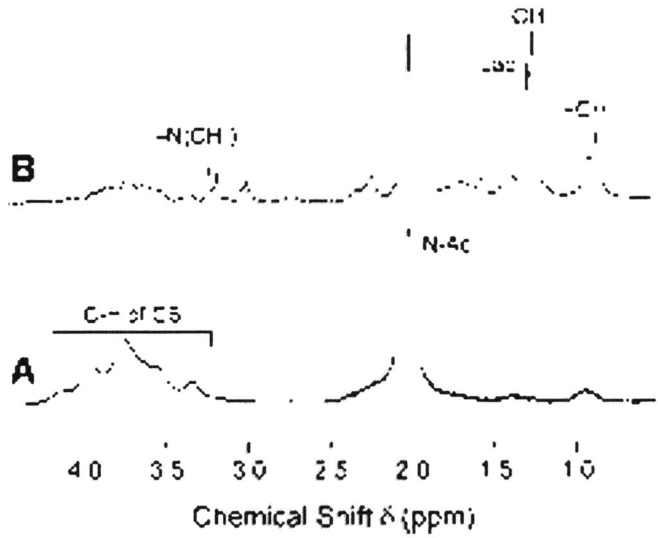

Fig. 4. Comparison of two ^1H NMR spectra of bovine nasal cartilage. In both cases the same sample was used. **(A)** Recorded without MAS. **(B)** The sample was spun with a frequency of 5 kHz in the magic angle. CS, chondroitin sulfate; Lac, lactate; $–CH_2–$ and $–CH_3$, the fatty acid residues of lipids; $–N(CH_3)_3^+$, quaternary ammonia groups.

the spectra, whereas keratan sulfate and hyaluronan are not detected ***(16)***. To be able to assign all resonances, it is a good idea to investigate the isolated polymers of cartilage. All these compounds (collagen, hyaluronan, and chondroitin and keratan sulfate) are commercially available and can be readily used as reference compounds (*see* **Note 4**). One should also note that healthy cartilage does not provide any collagen resonances under HR-MAS conditions ***(17)***. Collagen resonances are detectable only following enzymatic digestion (see below).

Spectra recorded under MAS conditions are dominated by three peaks at about 2.0, 1.3, and 0.9 ppm whereby the methyl resonance of the lactate at 1.31 ppm is also clearly detectable as a doublet ***(22)***. This confirms the considerable improvement of spectral quality under HR-MAS conditions since coupling constants of at least 7 Hz can be resolved. Of course, a more precise assignment of even minor metabolites of cartilage can be performed by 2D NMR (data not shown) ***(16)***. A survey of all detectable metabolites is provided in **Table 1**. 2D NMR correlated spectroscopy has also shown that the peaks at 1.3 and 0.9 ppm are caused by the methylene and methyl groups, respectively, of the fatty acids of lipids. Although cartilage represents a tissue whose lipid content is rather low ***(23)***, intensities of lipid resonances are markedly enhanced

Table 1
Chemical Structures and ^{1}H Chemical Shifts of Compounds Detectable in the Nuclear Magnetic Resonance (NMR) Spectra of Cartilage

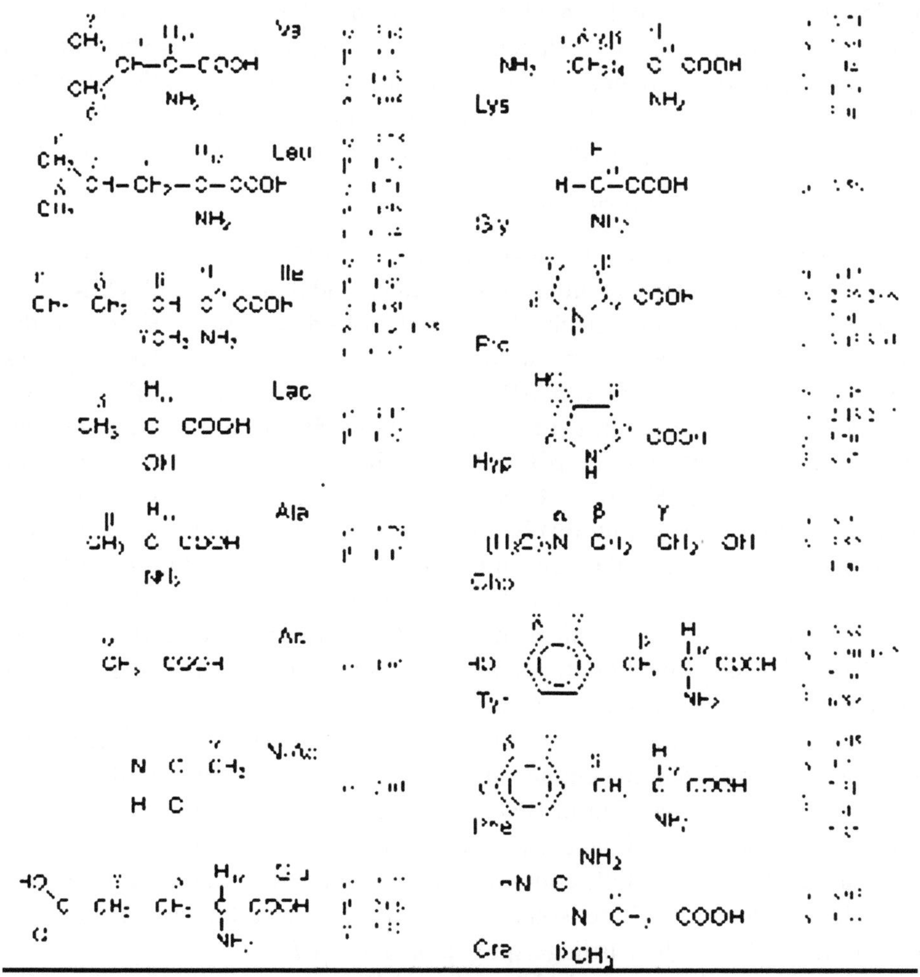

by HR-MAS. Lipids form micelles and vesicles in an aqueous environment and are, therefore, only detectable with rather low intensities under standard NMR conditions *(24)*. Accordingly, the sharp singlets at 3.25 and 3.19 ppm shown in **Fig. 4** represent the polar choline head groups of phospholipids like phosphatidylcholine or sphingomyelin *(16,24)*.

However, the resonances at 1.3 and 0.9 ppm are not exclusively caused by lipids but are superimposed by the methyl groups of amino acids like leucine, valine, isoleucine, and alanine *(16)*. Although these amino acids are not very abundant in cartilage collagen *(1)*, they give comparably intense peaks since their side groups possess a higher mobility than the more abundant but motionally constrained amino acids (mainly lysine, glutamic acid, glycine, proline, and hydroxyproline) of collagen *(25)*. Similar spectra can also be obtained with other types of cartilage and not only with BNC. However, BNC yields the most convincing spectra, whereas spectra of articular cartilage are less well resolved because of higher collagen and lower glycosaminoglycan contents *(14)*.

3.6.2. ^{13}C NMR Spectra of Cartilage

In contrast to ^{1}H NMR, the resolution of ^{13}C NMR spectra of cartilage is less influenced by heterogeneities of the sample, and therefore, ^{13}C NMR spectra do not have to be recorded absolutely under MAS conditions. However, the quality of the ^{13}C NMR spectra can be improved using MAS. **Figure 5** shows a comparison between the ^{13}C NMR spectra of BNC (**Fig. 5A** and **B**) and PAC (**Fig. 5C** and **D**). The spectra (**Fig. 5A**) and (**Fig. 5C**) were recorded without MAS and the spectra in (**Fig. 5B**) and (**Fig. 5D**) under MAS conditions. For comparison, in (**Fig. 5E**) the ^{13}C NMR spectrum of an aqueous chondroitin sulfate sample (8 wt% solution) is also shown. This concentration was used since it is comparable to the concentration of chondroitin sulfate in cartilage *(26)*. The chemical structures of both chondroitin sulfate isomers (the 4- and 6-sulphates) as well as the chemical shifts of all ^{13}C resonances are shown at the top of **Fig. 5**. Assignment of all resonances was performed according to previously published data (*27–29*; *see* **Note 4**).

Although spectra resemble each other closely, comparison of cartilage spectra (**Fig. 5A** and **B**) and the chondroitin sulfate spectrum (**Fig. 5E**) shows that some resonances are lacking in BNC. This especially concerns the resonance of the C-6 of the *N*-acetylgalactosamine residue in chondroitin-6-sulfate (68.7 ppm) and confirms that BNC contains only low amounts of chondroitin-6-sulfate. This chondroitin sulfate isomer as well as keratan sulfate and hyaluronan are not detectable in the cartilage spectra of BNC *(14)*.

By comparing the spectra in **Fig. 5A** and **B**, and especially the spectra in **Fig. 5C** and **D**, it is obvious that HR-MAS conditions (**Fig. 5B** and **D**) lead to

Fig. 5. (*opposite*) ^{13}C NMR spectra of bovine nasal cartilage (**A**, **B**), pig articular cartilage (**C**, **D**), and chondroitin sulfate (8 wt% in D_2O; **E**). Both types of cartilage were allowed to swell free in D_2O. Spectra **(B)** and **(D)** were recorded under conditions of HR-MAS, and all other spectra were recorded with a conventional 5-mm high-resolution NMR probe. Since primarily chondroitin sulfate resonances are detectable, at the top of the figure both chondroitin sulfate isomers and the corresponding ^{13}C chemical shifts of all carbon atoms are shown.

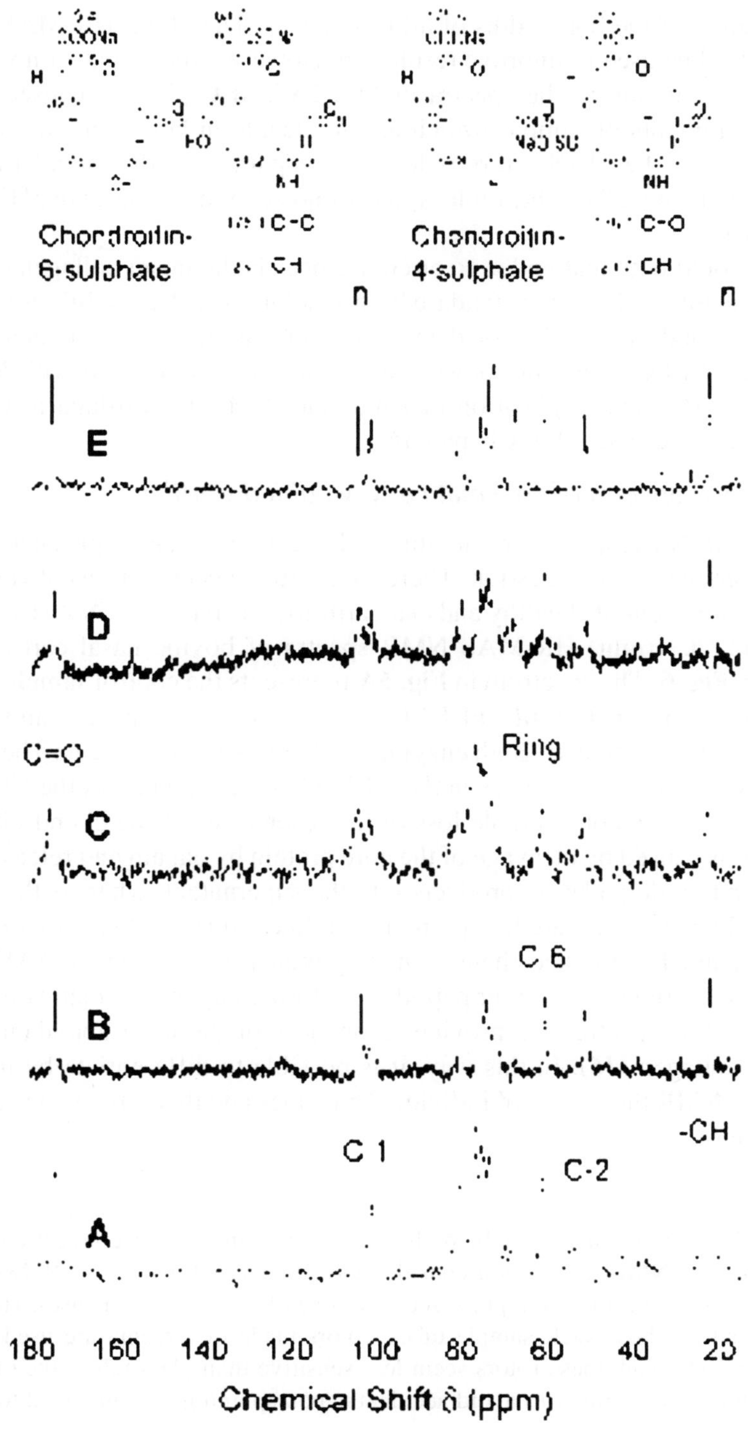
Chondroitin-
6-sulphate
Chondroitin-
4-sulphate
NH
C-O
CH
E
D
C=O
Ring
C
C 6
B
C 1
C-2
-CH
A
180 160 140 120 100 80 60 40 20
Chemical Shift δ (ppm)

a diminution of the line widths of all resonances. Therefore, HR-MAS conditions should be used to improve resolution. However, the signal-to-noise ratio is more convincing in the spectra in **Fig. 5A** and **C**. This is caused by the different amounts of sample, which are applicable in both techniques. Since the volume of the MAS rotors is low in comparison with a standard 5-mm NMR sample tube, the achievable signal-to-noise ratio is poor under HR-MAS conditions.

One should note that under no circumstances is the intact collagen of cartilage detectable under either standard high-resolution NMR conditions or under HR-MAS conditions ***(17)***. For detection of the rigid, native collagen, "real" solid-state NMR using high-power decoupling in combination with MAS is necessary ***(30)***. The application of solid-state NMR to cartilage research is described in more detail in Chapter 16.

3.6.3. NMR Spectra of Enzymatically Modified Cartilage

HR-MAS NMR spectra are suitable to detect fragmentation products of cartilage after enzymatic digestion. Therefore, further specifications of HR-MAS will be to differentiate healthy and osteoarthritic cartilage (*see* **Note 5**). The ^{1}H (left) and ^{13}C (right) HR-MAS NMR spectra of bovine nasal cartilage are shown in **Fig. 6**. The spectrum in **Fig. 6A** represents the control sample treated with buffer; that in **Fig. 6B**, of BNC, was digested with papain and that in **Fig. 6C** with collagenase. Both enzymes yield marked differences: The papain leads to only small differences in the ^{1}H NMR spectra, whereas the ^{13}C NMR spectrum shows a considerable loss of the resonances of the chondroitin sulfate. This is caused by cleavage of the core protein by papain and release of the corresponding degradation products into the supernatant, whereas the effects on the collagen moiety are less pronounced. In contrast, collagenase digestion is accompanied by marked changes in the proton as well as the ^{13}C NMR spectrum since a number of smaller peptides are formed upon enzymatic digestion. The ^{13}C NMR spectra also provide resonances of the most abundant amino acids of collagen ***(16)***. In this way, it is possible to differentiate by mean of HR-MAS NMR the effects of individual enzymes and their effects on cartilage (*see* **Note 6**).

4. Notes

1. HR-MAS experiments can be performed in the same way as conventional high-resolution NMR, and it is a considerable advantage for the less NMR-experienced user that the same pulse sequences can be used in both cases. However, instead of glass NMR sample tubes, rotors made of zirconia are used in HR-MAS. Although these rotors seem less sensitive than glass tubes, they must be treated very carefully to avoid accidents upon spinning that may lead to expen-

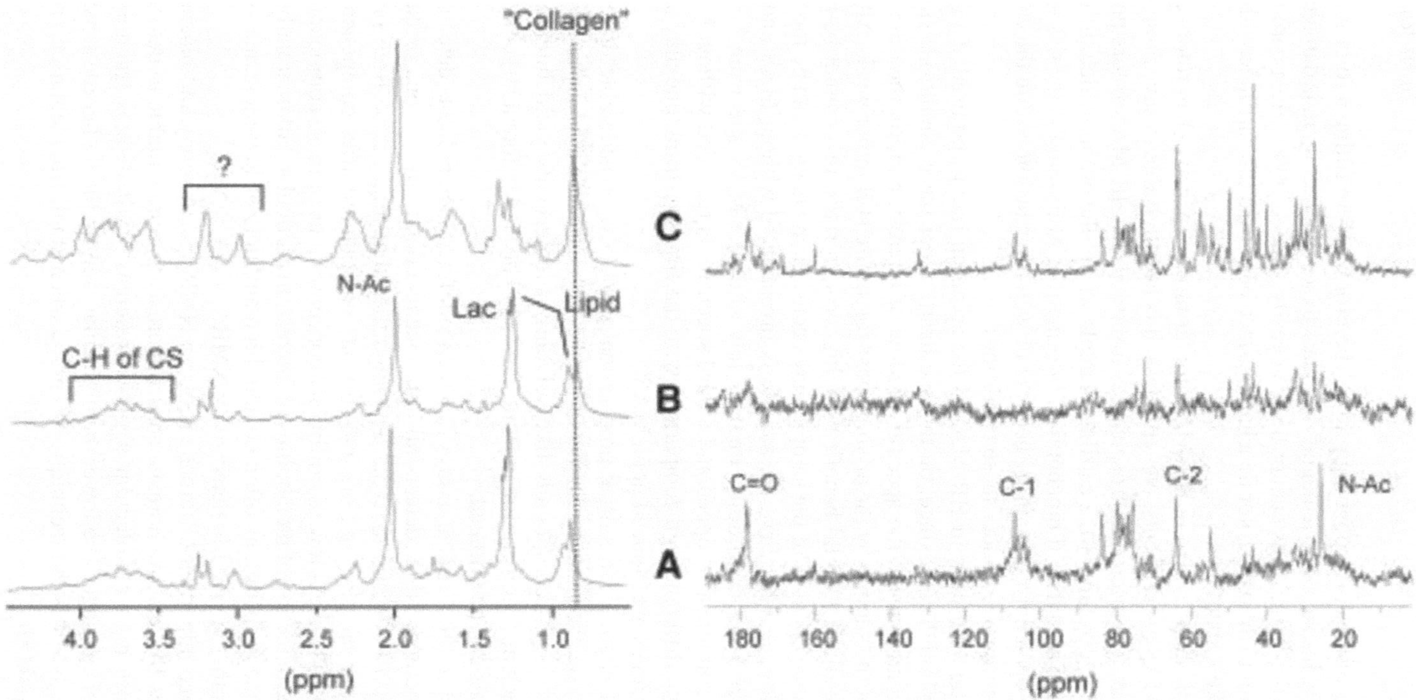

Fig. 6. ^{1}H (**left**) and ^{13}C (**right**) NMR spectra of bovine nasal cartilage in dependence on pretreatment conditions. **(A)** Cartilage sample that was exclusively treated with buffer. **(B)** Digested with papain. (C) Digested with collagenase.

sive repair of the corresponding probe. Therefore, before filling a rotor it should be carefully inspected by a magnifying glass to see whether there is damage to its surface. Micro-crackings cannot be seen easily. Accordingly, great care should be taken not to drop the rotor on a hard surface or to treat the cartilage with metal devices like a spatula.

2. Rotors with spacers used in HR-MAS are far more expensive than rotors used in standard MAS experiments. Nevertheless, it is not advisable to save money with these rotors. The use of microspherical inserts in the HR-MAS rotors provides optimum localization of the cartilage sample within the probe, which ultimately enhances the recovery of biochemical information. Additionally, the risk that the rotor may open during spinning because of water expansion within the cartilage sample is minimized under these conditions.
3. An important question in HR-MAS is the spinning rate to be used: 5 kHz is a suitable spinning rate, since, on the one hand, under these conditions spinning side bands are outside the spectral window of interest, and, on the other hand, changes of the sample by the arising shear forces are still rather weak. Although spectral resolution would benefit from higher spin rates, this cannot be recommended since changes of the sample may occur. Such changes can be monitored in the following way: first, the sample is investigated without MAS and afterward under MAS conditions. Immediately after the MAS spectrum has been recorded, spinning is stopped and a third spectrum is recorded without MAS. If there are no differences in comparison with the first spectrum, one may assume that no changes are induced upon MAS.
4. Individual chondroitin sulfate preparation may show considerable differences depending on the manufacturer and on the lot number. Since especially low-molecular-weight compounds like solvents or detergents yield intense resonances, each new preparation must be carefully checked before a larger series of experiments can be initiated.
5. In contrast to biochemical assays in which a defined metabolite is detected by a specific method, NMR detects all components containing protons or carbons. Therefore, it is crucial to avoid any impurities that might arise from pretreatments of the sample, e.g., organic solvents or organic buffer components like HEPES or EDTA. As low as millimolar concentrations of these compounds may prevent the detection of metabolites of interest. In particular, commercially available enzyme preparations often contain high amounts of low-molecular-weight impurities that are readily detected by NMR.
6. There is one important difference between NMR spectroscopy and biochemical approaches like electrophoresis: electrophoresis is more suitable to detect compounds with higher molecular weights, whereas NMR detects fragmentation products of cartilage. The lower the molecular weight, the higher the sensitivity. Therefore, NMR is the technique of choice when small fragmentation products are expected ***(9)***.

Acknowledgments

This work was supported by the Deutsche Forschungsgemeinschaft (SFB 294/G5) and the Bundesministerium für Bildung und Forschung (BMB+F), Interdisciplinary Center for Clinical Research (IZKF) at the University of Leipzig (01KS9504/1, Project A17). We thank Prof. Dr. Häntzschel and Dr. Ulf Wagner (Clinics of Rheumatology, University of Leipzig) for their kind help and many fruitful discussions. The helpful advice of Prof. Berger and Dr. Findeisen (Faculty of Chemistry and Mineralogy, Institute of Analytical Chemistry, University of Leipzig) is also gratefully acknowledged.

References

1. Flugge, L. A., Miller-Deist L., and Petillo P. A. (1999) Towards a molecular understanding of arthritis. *Chem. Biol.* **6,** R157–R166.
2. Grootveld, M., Henderson, E. B., Farrell, A., Blake, D. R., Parkes, H. G., and Haycock, P. (1991) Oxidative damage to hyaluronate and glucose in synovial fluid during exercise of the inflamed rheumatoid joint. *Biochem. J.* **273,** 459–467.
3. Damyanovich, A. Z., Staples, J. R., and Marshall, K. W. (1999) ^{1}H NMR investigation of changes in the metabolic profile of synovial fluid in bilateral canine osteoarthritis with unilateral joint denervation. *Osteoarthritis Cartilage* **17,** 165–172.
4. Schiller, J., Arnhold, J., Sonntag, K., and Arnold, K. (1996) NMR studies on human, pathologically changed synovial fluid: role of hypochlorous acid. *Magn. Reson. Med.* **35,** 848–853.
5. Schiller, J., Arnhold, J., and Arnold, K. (1995) NMR studies of the action of hypochlorous acid on native pig articular cartilage. *Eur. J. Biochem.* **233,** 672–676.
6. Schiller, J., Arnhold, J., Schwinn, J., Sprinz, H., Brede, O., and Arnold, K. (1998) Reactivity of cartilage and selected carbohydrates with hydroxyl radicals—an NMR study to detect degradation products. *Free Radic. Res.* **28,** 215–228.
7. Schiller, J., Arnhold, J., and Arnold, K. (1998) Nuclear magnetic resonance and mass spectrometric studies on the action of proteases on pig articular cartilage. *Z. Naturforsch.* **53c,** 1072–1080.
8. Hilbert, N., Schiller, J., Arnhold, J., and Arnold, K. (2002) Cartilage degradation by stimulated human neutrophils: elastase is the enzyme most responsible for cartilage breakdown. *Bioorg. Chem.* **30,** 119–132.
9. Schiller, J., Benard, S., Reichl, S., Arnhold, J., and Arnold, K. (2000) Cartilage degradation by stimulated human neutrophils: reactive oxygen species decrease markedly the activity of proteolytic enzymes. *Chem. Biol.* **7,** 557–568.
10. Tomlins, A. M., Foxall, P. J. D., Lindon, J. C., et al. (1998) High resolution magic angle spinning ^{1}H nuclear magnetic resonance analysis of intact prostatic hyperplastic and tumour tissues. *Anal. Commun.* **35,** 113–115.
11. Brewer, C. F. and Keiser, H. (1975) Carbon-13 nuclear magnetic resonance study of chondroitin 4-sulfate in the proteoglycan of bovine nasal cartilage. *Proc. Natl. Acad. Sci. USA* **72,** 3421–3423.

12. Torchia, D. A., Hasson, M. A., and Hascall, V. C. (1977) Investigation of molecular motion of proteoglycans in cartilage by ^{13}C magnetic resonance. *J. Biol. Chem.* **252,** 3617–3625.
13. Jelicks, L. A., Paul, P. K., O'Byrne, E., and Gupta, R. K. (1993) Hydrogen-1, sodium-23, and carbon-13 MR spectroscopy of cartilage degradation in vitro. *J. Magn. Reson. Imaging* **3,** 565–568.
14. Naji, L., Kaufmann, J., Huster, D., Schiller, J., and Arnold, K. (2000) ^{13}C NMR relaxation studies on cartilage and cartilage components. *Carbohydr. Res.* **327,** 439–446.
15. Waters, N. J., Garrod, S., Farrant, R. D., et al. (2000) High-resolution magic angle spinning ^{1}H NMR spectroscopy of intact liver and kidney: optimization of sample preparation procedures and biochemical stability of tissue during spectral acquisition. *Anal. Biochem.* **282,** 16–23.
16. Schiller, J., Naji, L., Huster, D., Kaufmann, J., and Arnold, K. (2001) ^{1}H and ^{13}C HR-MAS NMR investigations on native and enzymatically digested bovine nasal cartilage. *MAGMA* **13,** 19–27.
17. Huster, D., Schiller, J., and Arnold, K. (2002) Comparison of collagen dynamics in articular cartilage and isolated fibrils by solid-state NMR spectroscopy. *Magn. Reson. Med.* **48,** 624–632.
18. Kriat, M., Confort-Gouny, S., Vion-Dury, J., Sciaky, M., Viout, P., and Cozzone, P. J. (1992) Quantitation of metabolites in human blood serum by proton magnetic resonance spectroscopy. A comparative study of the use of formate and TSP as concentration standards. *NMR Biomed.* **5,** 179–184.
19. Braun, S., Kalinowski, H.-O., and Berger, S. (eds.) (1998) *150 and More NMR Experiments.* Wiley-VCH, Weinheim.
20. Hore, P. J. (1989) Solvent suppression. *Methods Enzymol.* **176,** 64–77.
21. De Certaines, J. D., ed. (1989) *Magnetic Resonance Spectroscopy of Biofluids: A New Tool in Clinical Biology.* World Scientific, Singapore.
22. Agar, N. S., Rae, C. D., Chapman, B. E., and Kuchel, P. W. (1991) ^{1}H NMR spectroscopic survey of plasma and erythrocytes from selected marsupials and domestic animals of australia. *Comp. Biochem. Physiol.* **99B,** 575–597.
23. Bonner, W. M., Jonsson, H., Malanos, C., and Bryant, M. (1975) Changes in the lipids of human articular cartilage with age. *Arthritis Rheum.* **18,** 461–473.
24. Schiller, J. and Arnold, K. (2002) Application of high resolution ^{31}P NMR spectroscopy to the characterization of the phospholipid composition of tissues and body fluids—a methodological review. *Med. Sci. Monit.* **8,** MT205–MT222.
25. Ebert, G., ed. (1993) *Biopolymere.* Teubner, Stuttgart.
26. Maroudas, A. and Kuettner, K. (eds.) (1990) *Methods in Cartilage Research.* Academic, London.
27. Hamer, G. K. and Perlin, A. S. (1976) A ^{13}C NMR spectral study of chondroitin sulfates A, B, and C: evidence of heterogeneity. *Carbohydr. Res.* **49,** 37–48.
28. Mucci, A., Schenetti, L., and Volpi, N. (2000) ^{1}H and ^{13}C nuclear magnetic resonance identification and characterization of components of chondroitin sulfates of various origin. *Carbohydr. Polymers* **41,** 37–45.

29. Bociek, S. M., Darke, A. H., Welti, D., and Rees, D. A. (1980) The ^{13}C-NMR spectra of hyaluronate and chondroitin sulphates. *Eur. J. Biochem.* **109,** 447–456.
30. Saito, H. and Yokoi, M. (1992) A ^{13}C NMR study on collagens in the solid state: hydration/dehydration-induced conformational change of collagen and detection of internal motions. *J. Biochem.* **111,** 376–382.

15

Pulsed-Field Gradient Nuclear Magnetic Resonance (PFG NMR) to Measure the Diffusion of Ions and Polymers in Cartilage

Applications in Joint Diseases

Jürgen Schiller, Lama Naji, Robert Trampel, Wilfred Ngwa, Robert Knauss, and Klaus Arnold

Summary

Since cartilage contains neither blood nor lymph vessels, diffusion is the most important transport process for the supply of cartilage with nutrients and for the removal of metabolic waste products. Therefore, diffusion measurements are of high interest in cartilage research. Different techniques of diffusion measurements exist. Here we describe methods based on pulsed-field gradient nuclear magnetic resonance (PFG NMR). This technique offers the considerable advantage that neither concentration gradients nor labeling of the diffusing species are required. In addition to the description of the fundamentals and the applicability of PFG NMR studies in cartilage research, emphasis is on the influence of the observation time, Δ, on the diffusion coefficient, D: at short times, diffusion is primarily determined by the water content of the sample, and great care is needed to keep this parameter constant. However, by varying the diffusion time, data on the internal structure of cartilage, e.g., the distance of the collagen fibrils, can also be obtained. In addition to classical water diffusion, the diffusion behavior of selected ions and polymers in cartilage is described. The capabilities, the limitations, and the clinical relevance of diffusion measurements for the assessment of joint diseases are discussed.

Key Words: Cartilage; PFG NMR; diffusion; restricted diffusion; collagen; swelling; osmotic pressure; water content; polymer diffusion; cation diffusion.

1. Introduction

The biomechanical properties of cartilage are of high relevance for joint movement, and especially for retention of tissue shape *(1)*. The inner structure of cartilage is determined by the arrangement of the collagen molecules into collagen fibrils and fibers and by the filling of the gaps between collagen fibers

From: *Methods in Molecular Medicine, Vol. 101: Cartilage and Osteoarthritis, Volume 2: Structure and In Vivo Analysis*
Edited by: F. De Ceuninck, M. Sabatini, and P. Pastoureau © Humana Press Inc., Totowa, NJ

by water and proteoglycan aggregates *(2)*. The biophysical properties of these main components of cartilage differ considerably: the polysaccharides of cartilage (e.g., chondroitin and keratan sulfate) behave like a sponge and are able to absorb large quantities of water, and the stiff collagen molecules limit the swelling ability of cartilage and therefore its water content *(3)*.

Cartilage contains neither blood nor lymph vessels *(4)* and therefore represents a bradytrophic tissue. Nutrients and compounds required for the synthesis of cartilage components, on the one hand, and metabolic waste products, on the other hand, are exchanged exclusively by diffusion processes caused by brownian motion. Because of the importance of diffusion processes in cartilage physiology, it is assumed that degenerative joint diseases are also caused by—among other factors—changes in the metabolic transport systems of cartilage *(5)*. However, details of these mechanisms are so far not completely understood *(6)*.

1.1. How Can the Diffusion Processes Be Monitored?

There are two different approaches toward measuring diffusion in cartilage. The first technique, and the one that is still most frequently applied *(1)*, uses frozen cartilage as a membrane; the transport of radioactive tracers across this cartilage membrane is determined. Under these conditions, Fick's first law holds, and the corresponding diffusion coefficient can easily be derived if the concentration gradient of the metabolite of interest is known *(7)*. Unfortunately, this technique has the disadvantages that self-diffusion coefficients (SDCs) cannot be determined and the use of radioactive isotopes is required.

The application of pulsed-field gradient nuclear magnetic resonance (PFG NMR) overcomes both problems: in the case of unrestricted diffusion, the mean square displacement $\langle z^2 \rangle$ of the diffusing species obeys Einstein's equation:

$$\langle z^2 \rangle = 2\,D\Delta \qquad (1)$$

where Δ is the diffusion (observation) time and D the diffusion coefficient of the diffusing species. If diffusion is restricted, however, $\langle z^2 \rangle$ increases with less than the first power of the diffusion time *(6)*. With a polymer matrix such as cartilage, it would be expected that the measured D depends on the time over which the displacement was observed (**Fig. 1**). For instance, for short observation times (when the nuclei encounter only solvent and solute molecules), the measured SDC will be higher than for longer times (when the molecules also encounter cells and extracellular matrix molecules). This is examined experimentally by the measurement of D for different diffusion times *(6)*.

Typical displacements monitored by PFG NMR are of the order of micrometers. In PFG NMR, the molecular displacements can be monitored only in the

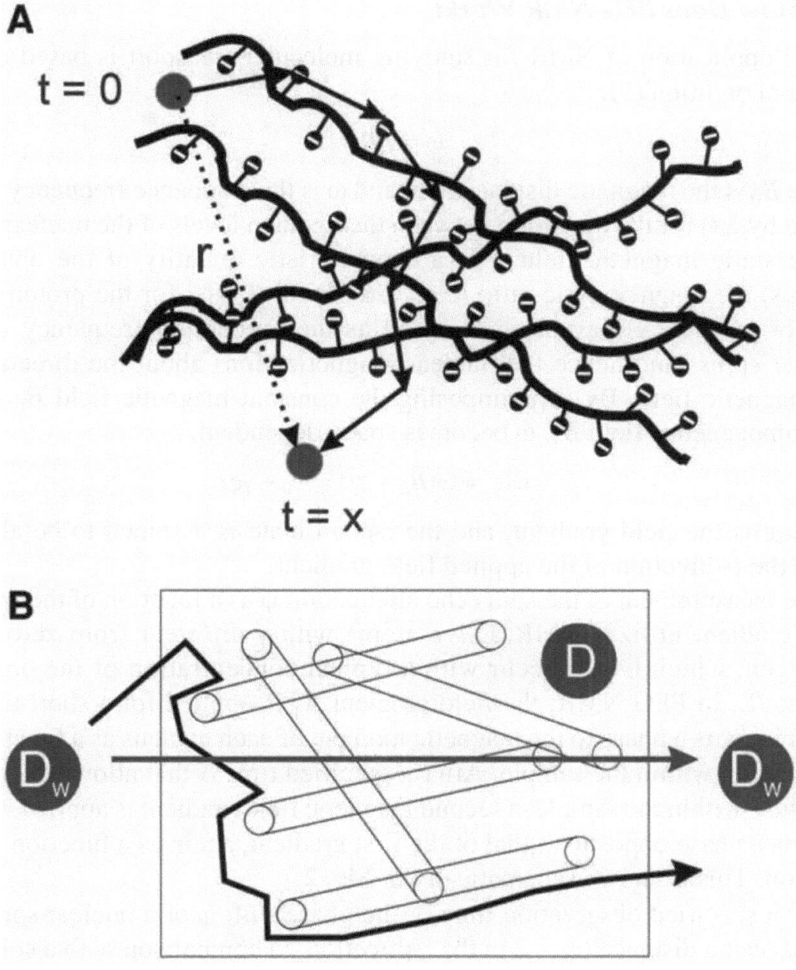

Fig. 1. **(A)** Self-diffusion of water independent of diffusion time. **(B)** Restricted diffusion of water in an environment with barriers. D_W represents the self-diffusion coefficient of free water (about 2.3×10^{-9} m^2s^{-1}) and D the self-diffusion coefficient of water in the presence of barriers. It is obvious that the diffusion coefficient is slowed down, especially at longer observation times and in the presence of solid barriers.

direction of the magnetic field gradient, commonly assumed to coincide with the *z*-direction. PFG NMR also has the advantage that it allows one to determine the mean square displacement of molecules in a noninvasive manner ***(8)***. This technique can be adapted to magnetic resonance imaging (MRI), and diffusion effects may be exploited as a means of contrast enrichment in clinical MRI ***(8)***.

1.2. How Does PFG NMR Work?

The application of NMR for studying molecular transport is based on the Larmor condition ***(9)***:

$$\omega = \gamma \boldsymbol{B}_0 \quad (2)$$

where $\boldsymbol{B}_0$ is the magnetic displacement and ω is the resonance frequency (multiplied by 2π) for the transition between the Zeeman levels of the nuclear spins in the static magnetic field. γ is a characteristic quantity of the observed nucleus, the magnetogyric ratio (e.g., 2.67×10^8 T^{-1} s^{-1} for the proton). The Larmor frequency may be understood as the precession frequency of the nuclear spins (and hence the nuclear magnetization) about the direction of the magnetic field. By superimposing the constant magnetic field $\boldsymbol{B}_0$ on an nonhomogeneous field $\boldsymbol{B}_1$, ω becomes space-dependent:

$$\omega = \omega(z) = \omega(\boldsymbol{B}_0 + \boldsymbol{g}z) = \omega_0 + \gamma \boldsymbol{g}z \quad (3)$$

where g is the field gradient, and the z-coordinate is assumed to be aligned along the z-direction of the applied field gradient.

The measurement of the spin echo attenuation ψ as a function of the applied field gradient utilizes NMR active atoms with γ different from zero, e.g., hydrogen, which has to occur with a typical concentration of the order of 0.1 mol/L. In PFG NMR, the field gradient $\boldsymbol{B}_1$ is applied for a short time δ, which imparts a phase to the magnetic moment of each nucleus as a function of the position within the sample. After a specified time Δ that allows the nuclei to diffuse within the sample, a second magnetic field gradient is applied, which imparts a phase opposite to that of the first gradient, again as a function of the position. This is shown schematically in **Fig. 2**.

For a specified observation time Δ, the phase shift φ of a nuclear spin displaced over a distance $(z_1–z_2)$ in the z-direction, in comparison with a spin that has remained in the same position, is given by the following equation ***(9)***:

$$\varphi = \gamma \boldsymbol{g}\, \delta\, (z_1 - zs_2) \quad (4)$$

Since the intensity of the NMR signal (the spin echo as generated, e.g., in the spin echo or the stimulated echo pulse sequence) is proportional to the total magnetization, the application of the field gradient pulses leads to signal attenuation, i.e., the vector sum of the contributions of the individual spins is diminished.

Following the assumption that the nuclei are moving with free brownian motion described by a single $\boldsymbol{D}$, it has been shown that attenuation of the spin echo amplitude ψ with the diffusion-sensitizing magnetic field gradients can be written as ***(10)***:

$$\mathbf{ln}\,(\psi) = -(\gamma\, \delta\, \boldsymbol{g})^2 \times (\Delta - \delta/3)\boldsymbol{D} \quad (5)$$

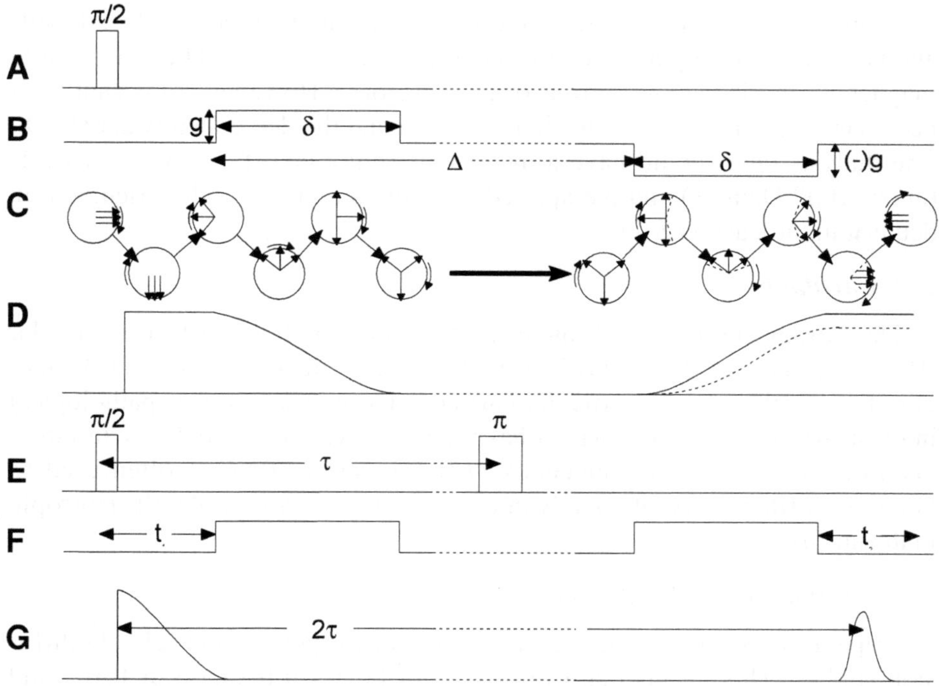

Fig. 2. Sketch of the basics of PFG NMR measurements. (**A**) and (**E**) indicate the HF (observation) pulses, and (**B**) and (**F**) the applied field gradients. In (**C**), the dephasing and refocusing of the spins and in (**D**) the course of the total magnetization are shown. In (**G**), the course of the magnetization during the spin echo (one 90° and one 180° pulse) technique is shown.

The experiment is typically performed so that ψ is measured for different values of $\boldsymbol{g}$ while the other variables are held constant. $\boldsymbol{D}$ is thus calculated from a fit of the data to **Eq. 5**. It is important to realize that in this technique, motion is measured along the direction of the magnetic field gradient, which can be set arbitrarily. For a more complete introduction to the general theory and experimental techniques of NMR spectroscopy, *see* refs. ***11*** and ***12***.

2. Materials

2.1. Chemicals

1. Deuterated water with 99.8% ^{2}H (Sigma-Aldrich, Taufkirchen, Germany).
2. Polyethylene glycol (PEG) 20,000 (Sigma-Aldrich).
3. Na-ethyl-mercuri-thiosalicylate (Merthiolate; Sigma-Aldrich).
4. Spectra/Por cellulose ester dialysis membrane with a molecular weight cutoff of at least 1000 g/mol (Spectrum, Houston, TX).
5. Spectra/Por dialysis membrane closure (Spectrum).

There is no need to take particular care of the applied chemicals. All salts and polymers can be purchased from any company but should be free of paramagnetic impurities (e.g., ferrous or cuprous ions). However, some caution is necessary when purchasing the dialysis tubes and the deuterated water (D_2O). The dialysis tube should have a molecular weight cutoff as low as possible (about 1000 Daltons) and the applied D_2O should have a high enrichment in deuterium (at least 99.8%).

2.2. Cartilage

The cartilage used depends on the particular research interests. Pig articular (PAC) and bovine nasal cartilage (BNC) are frequently used. The former closely resembles human articular cartilage and presents higher pathological interest ***(6)*** than the latter, which has the advantages of availability in larger quantities and greater homogeneity ***(13)***. Therefore, BNC is often used as "model cartilage." Another advantage is that it is a completely isotropic material ***(6)***.

2.2.1. Preparation of Cartilage

Preparation of the cartilage tissue is crucial for performing reliable diffusion studies. This means that even traces of bone (in the case of PAC) and cartilage membrane, the so-called perichondrium (in the case of the BNC), must be removed. Since the bone as well as the membrane are lipid-rich tissues ***(14)*** and lipids can easily be detected by NMR, their presence may lead to wrong results. The purity of each cartilage preparation can be monitored by recording the high-resolution NMR spectra of cartilage, in which lipids can be identified by the intense resonance at 1.3 ppm that corresponds to the methylene groups of the fatty acid residues ***(14)***. It is also important to note that articular cartilage has a considerable anisotropy ***(15)***, i.e., diffusion as well as relaxation properties of PAC strongly depend on the orientation of the sample with respect to the magnetic field. Therefore, it is important to consider the orientation of the cartilage or—if only the overall diffusion properties are studied—to cut the cartilage into sufficiently small pieces. Rectangular cartilage pieces of about 1.5 mm are suitable. Smaller pieces are more susceptible to degradation processes because of higher surface area ***(6)***.

2.3. Adjusting the Water Content of Cartilage

The water content of cartilage has the highest impact on the diffusion properties of molecules within cartilage. This is true for water diffusion but also for the diffusion of polymers and cations (following subheadings).

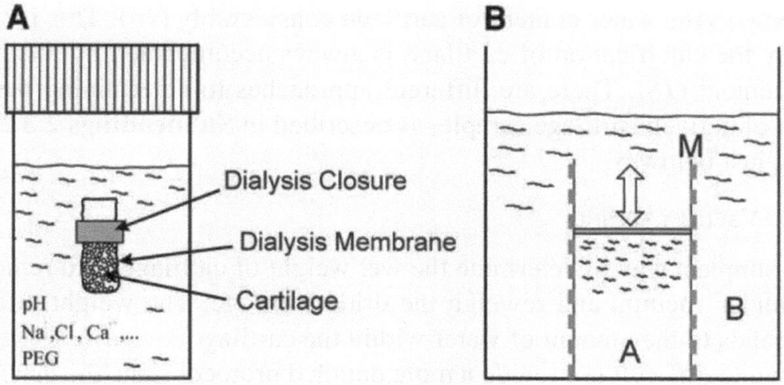

Fig. 3. (**A**) Typical experimental setup for obtaining a defined water content of cartilage (**B**) physical basics of the osmotic stress technique: a given cartilage sample will absorb or lose water until its osmotic pressure is in equilibrium with the environment. Aqueous solutions of polyethylene glycol (PEG) are well suited since they exert a well-defined osmotic pressure ***(17)***.

2.3.1. Osmotic Stress Technique

A defined water content of cartilage can be set by using the osmotic stress technique ***(16)***. A sketch of this technique is shown in **Fig. 3**. The cartilage is incubated in an aqueous polymer solution (**Fig. 3A**). For this, PEG is often used since its osmotic pressure is known in detail ***(17)***. The cartilage absorbs (or loses) water until its osmotic pressure π is in equilibrium with the surrounding solution (**Fig. 3B**). About 1 d of incubation of cartilage in the PEG solution is sufficient to establish equilibrium ***(16)***. However, we normally wait 2 d to ensure equilibrium, and the incubation is performed in the presence of Merthiolate. This compound possesses bactericidal properties and prevents the growth of microorganisms ***(6)***.

To prevent the PEG from penetrating the cartilage, the cartilage must be entrapped in a dialysis tube with a sufficiently low molecular weight cutoff (at least 1000 g/mol or lower). If the aim is to measure the diffusion of PEG, the dialysis tube can be omitted. In comparison with mechanical compression, an additional advantage of the osmotic stress technique is that the ion content can be controlled easily ***(6)***.

2.3.2. Determination of the Water Content of Cartilage

The water content of cartilage depends on its ion content: Since water is primarily bound to the negatively charged polysaccharides of cartilage, the neutralization of these charges by ions and especially by bivalent ions like

Ca^{2+} reduces the water content of cartilage considerably *(16)*. This is the reason why the calcification of cartilage is always accompanied by a decreased water content *(18)*. There are different approaches to determining the water content of a given cartilage sample, as described in **Subheadings 2.3.2.1.** and **2.3.2.2.** just below.

2.3.2.1. Vacuum Drying

The simplest way to determine the wet weight of cartilage is to remove the water under vacuum and reweigh the dried cartilage. The weight difference corresponds to the amount of water within the cartilage

It is quite difficult to provide a more detailed protocol since the drying time will depend the vacuum quality and on the size of the cartilage surface. We use a rapid evaporation system (Jouan RC, 10-22, Germany) that provides a pressure of about 5 torr. Under slight heating (60°C), about 4 h are necessary to obtain a constant cartilage weight *(6)*.

Typical water contents of different cartilage types as a function of the osmotic pressure are given in **Fig. 4**. It is obvious that, at similar osmotic pressure, the water content of BNC is higher compared with that of PAC. Also, the water content of young PAC is higher than that of adult cartilage. This result reflects the higher concentration of ions in the adult cartilage *(1)*.

2.3.2.2. Application of Organic Solvents

It remains possible that, upon vacuum drying, part of the water may be retained within cartilage, since some tight binding to cartilage polymers may prevent its removal.

Another way to determine the water content is to treat the cartilage with about a 10-fold excess of organic solvents (e.g., methanol or dimethylsulfoxide [DMSO]). The organic solvent removes the water from the cartilage, and the water content within the organic solvent can be determined by Karl-Fischer titration *(19)* or other specific assays.

3. Methods

It is quite difficult to provide a detailed description of diffusion measurements by PFG NMR without knowing what equipment is available in the NMR laboratory of the reader: it makes a considerable difference whether a clinical MR tomograph, a commercial high-resolution NMR spectrometer, or a home-built device for diffusion measurements is used *(20)*. This concerns not only the available gradient strengths and the achievable spectral resolution but also the software and pulse programming. Therefore, only a crude description of the most relevant steps necessary to perform diffusion measurements can be given, and the reader is strongly advised to consult the manual of his/her NMR device.

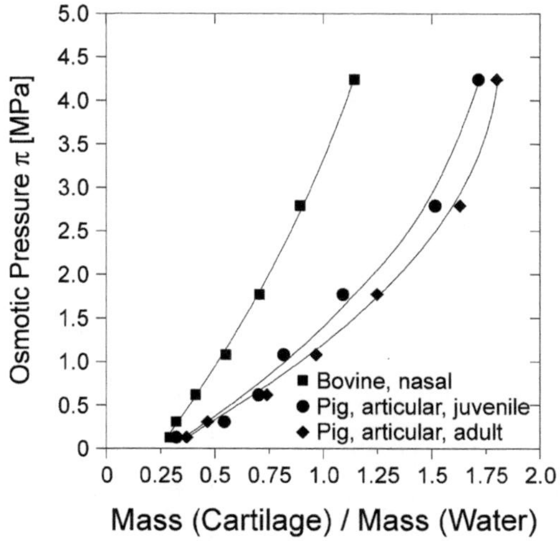

Fig. 4. Ratios between the cartilage and the water mass of different kinds of cartilage plotted against the osmotic pressure π that is necessary to establish the corresponding water contents. It is evident that the osmotic pressure is different for the individual cartilage types and, therefore, individual cartilage types can be easily differentiated. Data were obtained by drying and weighing the cartilage samples.

Our diffusion data were obtained on the home-built diffusion NMR spectrometer FEGRIS 400 at the Institute of Experimental Physics at the University of Leipzig. This device is remarkable, owing to the extreme field gradients applicable (up to 25 T/m), allowing the observation of even very small diffusion coefficients *(9)*.

3.1. Positioning of the Cartilage Sample

In contrast to standard high-resolution NMR spectroscopy, in which solutions are investigated, diffusion measurements must be performed with cartilage slices. Because of the considerable field gradient strengths that must be applied when small diffusion coefficients are studied, the related energy transfer may lead to vibrations of the sample that would alter the measurements. Therefore, such vibrations should be avoided. Typical PFG NMR equipment that helps to overcome problems of fixation of the cartilage sample is shown in **Fig. 5**.

3.1.1. Avoiding Diffusion Artifacts

There is an additional important consideration in NMR: all material brought into the space within the coils must be completely free of protons since such materials contribute to the NMR resonance. Therefore, all fittings must be made of special plastics. Vespel® (a polyimide from pyromellitic acid dianhydride

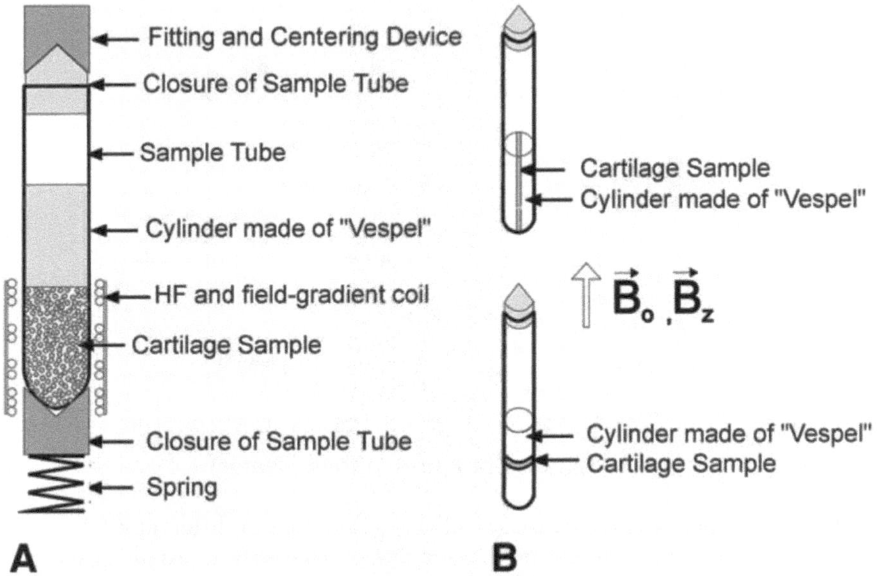

Fig. 5. (**A**) Positioning of cartilage samples during the PFG NMR experiment. (**B**) Experimental setup to determine effects of sample orientation with respect to the external magnetic field.

and 4,4'-diamino-diphenyl-ether; available from Dupont) can be advantageously used since this material does not provide any resonance detectable by NMR. Although this material is quite expensive, its use is more advisable than that of Teflon (*see* **Note 1**).

3.2. Determination of Pulse Lengths and Gradient Strengths

3.2.1. Calibration of the Observation Pulses

The use of correct pulse lengths and gradient pulses is crucial for performing reliable diffusion experiments. For calibration of the pulse length of the transmitter pulse (the "90° pulse") normally the free induction decay (FID) or the corresponding spectrum is observed, and the excitation pulse is varied until the integral intensity is zero.

This pulse length corresponds to the 180° pulse and the division by a factor of 2 yields the corresponding excitation (90°) pulse ***(21)***. It is very important to always use the same parameter set for the Fourier transformation and to wait a sufficiently long time between two pulses to allow complete relaxation. About five times the T_1 value of the slowest relaxating compound is a suitable parameter. The T_1 relaxation of water varies between about 10 and 200 ms and strongly depends on the water content and thus on the kind of cartilage used ***(16)***.

3.2.2. Calibration of the Gradient Pulses

The most challenging task in PFG NMR is the correct setting of both required gradient pulses, i.e., the determination of the correct width δ and field strength g. If these values are not properly set, an additional attenuation of the echo-attenuation curve (that may be misinterpreted as a change of the corresponding diffusion coefficient) occurs. The second gradient pulse is particularly critical since the temperature of the coil may rise, because the first pulse results in a change of the ohmic resistance of the coil. Therefore, gradient pulses must be recalibrated each time the field strength of the gradients is changed. This is also true when the sample is exchanged. For calibration purposes, a known sample (e.g., distilled water) should be used. If polymers or ions are studied, a concentrated aqueous solution of these compounds should be used.

3.3. Performing the PFG NMR Experiment

First the operator must check what kind of data acquisition and processing are available on his/her NMR device. Two different approaches are available, as described in **Subheadings 3.3.1.** and **3.3.2.**

3.3.1. Observing the FID

The first method uses the attenuation of the FID for determination of the corresponding diffusion coefficients: the intensity of the total FID is determined as a function of the applied field gradients at a certain diffusion time, i.e., a fixed pulse interval. This technique is most often used in medical applications since the major molecular compound in biological tissues is water. Owing to its high concentration (about 55 mol/L), there are normally no problems of sensitivity.

This technique is still most widely used on devices that allow the application of very high field gradients *(12)*: upon the application of such strong field gradients (up to 25 T/m), the homogeneity of the static magnetic field B_0 is considerably reduced, and spectroscopically resolved (i.e., high-resolution) NMR experiments can no longer be performed.

3.3.2. Recording Spectroscopically Resolved Data

Using lower field gradients, "normal" high-resolution NMR spectra can be recorded, i.e., the initially recorded FID can be Fourier-transformed. This is an advantage if mixtures must be analyzed by PFG NMR. However, on commercially available high-field NMR spectrometers, only rather weak gradients are available, and the molecular mass of the diffusing species is limited to about 1000 Daltons *(22)*. Slowly diffusing compounds with a higher molecular weight cannot be observed under these conditions. It should be at least briefly mentioned that diffusion-ordered spectroscopy (DOSY) is used more in mod-

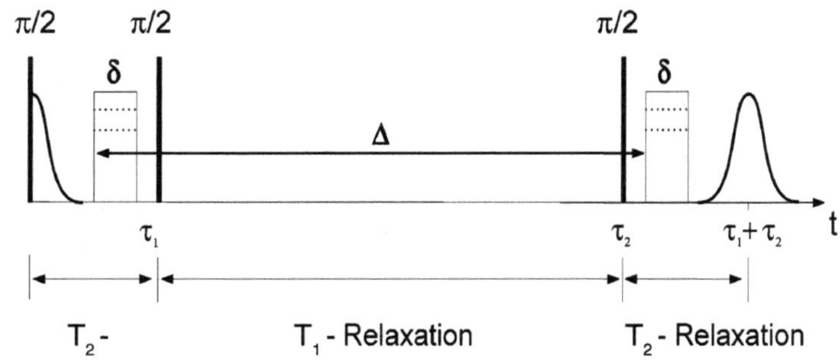

Fig. 6. Pulse sequence of the stimulated-echo experiment that is most often used in diffusion NMR studies of cartilage *(6)*. Intervals where T_1 and T_2 relaxation takes place are indicated in the figure.

ern chemistry and there is also an increasing number of applications in which heteronuclei (nuclei other than protons) are observed. Of course, these techniques are characterized by lower sensitivities *(22)*.

3.3.3. Observing Restricted Diffusion

One interesting (and unique) feature of PFG NMR is that internal barrier distances within the cartilage can be determined by varying the observation time (*see* **Note 2**). However, some caution is needed since, by increasing the observation time, the effect of the relaxation time T_1 is more pronounced, and it may lead to a considerable diminution of the observed NMR signal even without any diffusion effects *(6)*. **Figure 6** gives a schematic representation of one commonly used pulse sequence, the so-called stimulated echo (in comparison with the spin echo experiment, the second 180° pulse is replaced by two 90° pulses), as well as the intervals where relaxation occurs.

Therefore, to obtain reliable diffusion data, PFG NMR measurements should always be combined with the corresponding relaxation time measurements to exclude any relaxation effects. It is obvious from **Fig. 6** that the risk of intensity loss by relaxation is more pronounced when the diffusion time is longer (*see* **Note 3**).

3.4. Data Analysis

3.4.1. Monoexponential Decay

The easiest way to obtain PFG NMR data is to record the corresponding spin echo attenuation curve and to fit this echo decay with the corresponding function. Therefore, it is necessary to record the spin echo attenuation until a decay of about $1/e$ of the initial intensity is observed *(6)*. Fitting the data can be

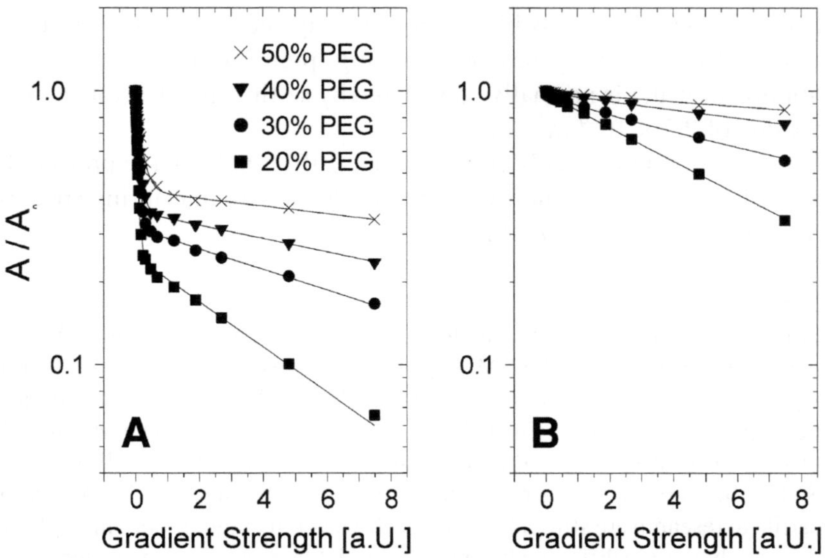

Fig. 7. Echo attenuation curves of differently concentrated solutions of polyethylene glycol (PEG) 6000 in (**A**) water and (**B**) deuterated water. *A* is the intensity of the spin echo amplitude when a certain gradient is applied, and A_0 is the intensity without an additional gradient. The fast-decaying component is caused by water and can be minimized in deuterated water.

done by most data analysis programs. However, to ensure accuracy of the method applied, a sufficient number of data points should be recorded, about 8–10 in the case of a monoexponential decay and about 16–20 if a biexponential decay is expected.

3.4.2. Polyexponential Decay

Extracting the diffusion coefficients from the obtained PFG NMR data is more difficult if several diffusing species exist. For instance, this is important when the diffusion of polymers in cartilage is investigated. Under these conditions it is important to prepare all solutions in D_2O since an attenuation of the intense water resonance can be achieved (**Fig. 7**).

It is obvious that upon the use of D_2O the signal of residual water can be completely suppressed. However, this method does not always provide reasonable results since a number of compounds such as carbohydrates show exchange with D_2O and lead to the formation of HDO. However, this may also be overcome: normally, diffusion coefficients or relaxation times of individual components within a mixture differ strongly, and therefore a separation of individual components is possible by considering the differences in diffusion properties or by performing the corresponding "prerelaxation" experiment. The contribution of water is normally considered by setting its diffusion coefficient to the value of 2.3×10^{-9} m^2 s^{-1}.

It is often a good idea to observe a nucleus different from the proton. Sensitivity is reduced in these conditions, but problems with interfering species can be overcome easily (*see* **Note 4**).

4. Notes

1. Since NMR is a less selective method, all materials must be carefully checked for potential contribution to the NMR signal. This is also highly relevant when studying the diffusion of sodium ions. At 9.935 T (400 MHz ^1H resonance frequency) the copper of the coils (^{63}Cu: 106.020 MHz) contributes to the NMR signal, and this might be misinterpreted as a sodium signal (^{23}Na: 105.805 MHz).
2. So far, diffusion NMR has been classically used in brain research; applications in cartilage research are still rather scarce. However, it could be convincingly shown that the short-time diffusion behavior is a reliable measure of the water content of cartilage ***(6)***. PFG NMR diffusion data are reliable measures of transport properties within cartilage. However, two different time scales should be differentiated: the short-time diffusion behavior is primarily influenced by the water content of the sample and can be used for the determination of the water content of a given sample ***(23)***. These data can be more reliably obtained since under these conditions interfering influences of relaxation effects are negligible. On the other hand, PFG NMR is also a quite useful technique to obtain information on the distance between two collagen fibrils within the cartilage by measuring the corresponding long-time SDC ***(24)*** until the phenomenon of restricted diffusion occurs.
3. Because diffusion data depend on the water content of the sample, data obtained with enzymatically digested cartilage should be regarded with caution ***(25)***. For instance, upon digestion of the collagen network ***(26)***, the cartilage sample will absorb much more water than under native conditions. Therefore, if the diffusion measurement is carried out without control of the water content, a higher diffusion coefficient will be measured. If the water content is carefully adjusted to the previous content, then one will not notice any differences, nor will it matter whether or not cartilage was digested with an enzyme ***(27)***.
4. Dependence of the diffusion coefficient on water content is observed in the case of the water diffusion but also when the diffusion of cations ***(28)*** or artificial polymers ***(29)*** within the cartilage is investigated. Therefore, it must concluded that the composition of cartilage has only a minor impact on the diffusion behavior within the cartilage since neutral and charged molecules behave similarly: independent of whether diffusion of water, polymers, or cations is measured, the water content primarily affects diffusion processes in cartilage.

Acknowledgments

This work was supported by the Bundesministerium für Bildung und Forschung (BMB+F), Interdisciplinary Center for Clinical Research (IZKF) at the University of Leipzig (grant number 01KS9504/1, project A 17). The very helpful cooperation of Prof. Kärger and Dr. Stallmach (Faculty of Physics and Earth Sciences, Institute of Experimental Physics, University of Leipzig) in the field of PFG NMR measurements is gratefully acknowledged.

References

1. Maroudas, A. and Kuettner, K., eds. (1990) *Methods in Cartilage Research.* Academic, London.
2. Stryer, L., ed. (1987) *Biochemie.* Vieweg-Verlag, Braunschweig.
3. Maroudas, A. and Bannon, C. (1981) Measurement of swelling pressure in cartilage and comparison with the osmotic pressure of constituent proteoglycans. *Biorheology* **18,** 619–632.
4. Freeman, M. A. R., ed. (1979) *Adult Articular Cartilage.* Pitman Medical, Turnbridge.
5. Flugge, L. A., Miller-Deist, L. A., and Petillo, P. A. (1999) Towards a molecular understanding of arthritis. *Chem. Biol.* **6,** R157–R166.
6. Knauss, R., Schiller, J., Fleischer, G., Kärger, J., and Arnold, K. (1999) Self-diffusion of water in cartilage and cartilage components as studied by pulsed field gradient NMR. *Magn. Reson. Med.* **41,** 285–292.
7. Maroudas, A., Weinberg, P. D., Parker, K. H., and Winlove, C. P. (1988) The distributions and diffusivities of small ions in chondroitin sulphate, hyaluronate and some proteoglycan solutions. *Biophys. Chem.* **32,** 257–270.
8. Callaghan, P. T., ed. (1991) *Principles of Nuclear Magnetic Resonance Microscopy.* Oxford Clarendon, Oxford.
9. Kärger, J., Heitjans, P., and Haberlandt, R. (1988) *Diffusion in Condensed Matter.* Vieweg Verlag, Braunschweig/Wiesbaden.
10. Stejskal, E. O. and Tanner, J. E. (1970) Spin diffusion measurements: spin echos in the presence of a time-dependent field gradient. *J. Chem. Phys.* **52,** 2523–2526.
11. Farrar, T. C. and Becker, E. D., eds. (1971) *Pulse and Fourier Transform NMR. Introduction to Theory and Methods.* Academic, New York.
12. Kärger, J., Pfeifer, H., and Heink, W. (1988) Principles and applications of self-diffusion measurements by nuclear magnetic resonance, in *Advances in Magnetic Resonance* (Waugh, J. S., ed.), Academic, London, pp. 1–89.
13. Torchia, D. A., Hasson, M. A., and Hascall, V. C. (1977) Investigation of molecular motion of proteoglycans in cartilage by ^{13}C magnetic resonance. *J. Biol. Chem.* **252,** 3617–3625.
14. Schiller, J., Naji, L., Huster, D., Kaufmann, J., and Arnold, K. (2001) ^{1}H and ^{13}C HR-MAS NMR investigations on native and enzymatically digested bovine nasal cartilage. *MAGMA* **13,** 19–27.

15. Henkelman, R. M., Stanisz, G. J., Kim, J. K., and Bronskill, M. J. (1994) Anisotropy of NMR properties of tissues. *Magn. Reson. Med.* **32,** 592–601.
16. Lüsse, S., Knauss, R., Werner, A., Gründer, W., and Arnold, K. (1995) Action of compression and cations on the proton and deuterium relaxation in cartilage. *Magn. Reson. Med.* **33,** 483‹489.
17. Gawrisch, K., Arnold, K., Dietze, K., and Schulze, U. (1988) Hydration forces between phospholipid membranes and the PEG-induced fudion, in *Electromagnetic Fields and Biomembranes* (Markov, M. and Blank, M., eds.), Plenum, New York, pp. 9–18.
18. Lesperance, L. M., Gray, M. L., and Burstein, D. (1992) Determination of fixed charged density in cartilage using nuclear magnetic resonance. *J. Orthop. Res.* **10,** 1–13.
19. Citterio, D., Minamihashi, K., Kuniyoshi, Y., Hisamoto, H., Sasaki, H., and Suzuki, K (2001) Optical determination of low-level water concentrations in organic solvents using fluorescent acridinyl dyes and dye-immobilized polymer membranes. *Anal. Chem.* **73,** 5339–5345.
20. Fukushima, E. and Roeder, S. W. (1981) *Experimental Pulse NMR—A Nuts and Bolts Approach.* Addison-Wesley, Reading, PA.
21. Braun, S., Kalinowski, H.-O., and Berger, S. (1998) *150 and More NMR Experiments.* Wiley-VCH, Weinheim.
22. Burstein, D., Gray, M. L., Hartman, A. L., Ripe, G., and Foy, B. D. (1993) Diffusion of small solutes in cartilage as measured by nuclear magnetic resonance (NMR) spectroscopy and imaging. *J. Orthop. Res.* **11,** 465–478.
23. Mackie, J. S. and Meares, P. (1955) The sorption of electrolytes by a cation exchange resin membrane. *Proc. R. Soc. A* **232,** 485–498.
24. Knauss, R., Fleischer, G., Gründer, W., Kärger, J., and Werner, A. (1996) Pulsed field gradient NMR and nuclear magnetic relaxation studies of water mobility in hydrated collagen II. *Magn. Reson. Med.* **36,** 241–248.
25. Xia, Y., Farquhar, T., Burton-Wurster, N., Ray, E., and Jelinski, L. W. (1994) Diffusion and relaxation mapping of cartilage-bone plugs excised discs using microscopic magnetic resonance imaging. *Magn. Reson. Med.* **31,** 273–282.
26. Xia, Y., Farquhar, T., Burton-Wurster, N., Vernier-Singer, M., Lust, G., and Jelinski, L. W. (1995) Self-diffusion monitors degraded cartilage. *Arch. Biochem. Biophys.* **23,** 323–328.
27. Naji, L., Trampel, R., Ngwa, W., Knauss, R., Schiller, J., and Arnold, K. (2001) Studium der Diffusion im Knorpel mit der PFG (pulsed-field gradient)-NMR-Technik. *Z. Med. Phys.* **11,** 179–186.
28. Ngwa, W., Geier, F., Stallmach, F., Naji, L., Schiller, J., and Arnold, K. (2002) Cation diffusion in cartilage measured by pulsed field gradient NMR. *Eur. Biophys. J.* **31,** 73–80.
29. Trampel, R., Schiller, J., Naji, L., Stallmach, F., Kärger, J., and Arnold, K. (2002) Self-diffusion of polymers in cartilage as studied by pulsed field gradient NMR. *Biophys. Chem.* **97,** 251–260.

16

Dynamics of Collagen in Articular Cartilage Studied by Solid-State NMR Methods

Daniel Huster, Jürgen Schiller, and Klaus Arnold

Summary

Methods for studying the fast molecular dynamics of the rigid macromolecules in cartilage are described. The strong dipolar couplings and chemical shift anisotropies of these molecules necessitate application of solid-state nuclear magnetic resonance (NMR) techniques such as magic-angle spinning, cross-polarization, and high-power dipolar decoupling to obtain resolved NMR spectra. The molecules in cartilage that are amenable to these techniques are collagen and the rigid portion of the glycosaminoglycans (mostly hyaluronan). Site-specific mobility information is obtained from scaled dipolar couplings measured in 2D NMR experiments. Motionally averaged dipolar couplings can be interpreted in terms of order parameters that provide information about the amplitudes of molecular motions. Qualitative dynamics information is obtained from the simple wideline separation experiment measuring ^{1}H-^{1}H widelines representing the strength of the ^{1}H-^{1}H dipolar coupling. Quantitative values for molecular order parameters are obtained from precise measurements of ^{1}H-^{13}C dipolar couplings along the C–H bond vector. Two experimental techniques, the Lee-Goldburg cross-polarization and the dipolar coupling/chemical shift experiment, are illustrated to measure these ^{1}H–^{13}C dipolar couplings. Unlike glycosaminoglycans in cartilage, the collagen moiety remains substantially ordered, undergoing fast small amplitude motions. As enzymes cleave the macromolecules in articular cartilage in the course of arthritis, solid-state NMR techniques are capable of characterizing the increased motions of their degradation products in diseased cartilage.

Key Words: CP MAS, WISE; DIPSHIFT; LG-CP; ^{13}C NMR; cartilage; collagen; glycosaminoglycan; hyaluronan; molecular dynamics; order parameter; macromolecules; magic-angle spinning.

1. Introduction

With the recent introduction of high-field magnets into solid-state nuclear magnetic resonance (NMR) applications, investigation of the structure and dynamics of largely immobile fibrous or membrane proteins has advanced significantly *(1–16)*. Because of these improvements in NMR technology, it is

From: *Methods in Molecular Medicine, Vol. 101: Cartilage and Osteoarthritis, Volume 2: Structure and In Vivo Analysis*
Edited by: F. De Ceuninck, M. Sabatini, and P. Pastoureau © Humana Press Inc., Totowa, NJ

now also possible to study native biological tissues such as cartilage without isotopic labeling at natural abundance *(17–19)*. As illustrated in Chapters 14 and 15 of this book, the dynamics of the highly mobile glycosaminoglycans of cartilage can be studied by solution NMR methods or high-resolution (HR) magic-angle spinning (MAS) NMR. Detection and dynamic characterization of the rigid cartilage collagen and hyaluronan requires knowledge of the solid-state NMR techniques discussed in this chapter. Owing to the rigidity of these molecules, anisotropic interactions such as dipolar coupling and chemical shift anisotropy that are averaged in solution result in NMR spectra several tens of kHz wide. To obtain high resolution, MAS in combination with high-power decoupling has to be applied to average out these interactions. Anisotropic interactions, however, contain valuable structural and dynamic information and can be reintroduced into the spectra by recoupling techniques *(20)*. Modern 2D pulse sequences allow us to exploit these parameters in a site-specific fashion, i.e., a structural or dynamical parameter can be obtained for each resolved peak in the spectrum.

In this chapter, methods for studying fast motions of rigid cartilage macromolecules are illustrated. The methodology is also suited for study of diseased cartilage. In the course of arthritis, the intact extracellular matrix of cartilage is degraded by enzymes. This molecular decomposition results in small peptides derived from the collagen moiety that are characterized by largely increased molecular mobility, which is probed by solid-state NMR spectroscopy *(17)*. Therefore, the molecular dynamics of articular cartilage molecules can be used as a parameter to differentiate healthy and arthritic cartilage.

2. Materials

Pig articular cartilage was obtained from local slaughter houses immediately after slaughter of healthy juvenile animals (about 1 yr old). The cartilage was separated from the joint and cut into small cubes with a typical dimension of about 1 mm using a surgical scalpel. For the measurements discussed here, approx 50 mg of the cartilage sample was placed in a 4-mm MAS rotor with a Teflon insert and sealed. It is possible to exchange part of the water in cartilage with deuterated water (D_2O) to lock the ^2H frequency for better field stability during the course of the experiment. Excess water should be removed (*see* **Note 1**) Cartilage can be stored at –78°C for several months.

3. Methods

The following description of solid-state NMR methods illustrates the acquisition of cross-polarization (CP) MAS spectra (*see* **Subheading 3.1.**), the measurement of ^1H–^1H widelines (*see* **Subheading 3.2.**), and the measurement of

^1H–^{13}C dipolar couplings by Lee-Goldburg (LG) CP (*see* **Subheading 3.3.**), as well as by DIPSHIFT (*see* **Subheading 3.4.**). Technical issues are provided in **Notes 2** and **3**. The information content of each of these spectra is discussed (*see* **Note 4**).

3.1. CP MAS Experiment

The CP experiment is the basic building block of almost all solid-state NMR experiments *(21)*. It involves one spin lock pulse on the ^1H and ^{13}C channel, respectively. If the Hartmann-Hahn condition ($\gamma_H\omega_{1,H} = \gamma_C\omega_{1,C}$) is fulfilled, polarization is transferred from the protons to the carbons, allowing one to observe the carbon signal with up to four times higher sensitivity. The signal is detected under high-power dipolar decoupling, yielding spectra dominated by the chemical shift anisotropy of all spins observed. In combination with MAS, high-resolution conditions are obtained for solid samples *(22)* yielding isotropic signals with the characteristic chemical shift dispersion of ^{13}C and a typical signal line width of approx 1 ppm. The CP MAS experiment is the basis for many 2D solid-state NMR experiments.

3.1.1. Pulse Sequence

The pulse sequence for the CP MAS experiment is shown in **Fig. 1A**. After a $\pi/2$ excitation pulse on protons, transverse ^1H magnetization is locked; ^{13}C magnetization is created if the spin lock fields match the Hartmann-Hahn condition. Subsequently, the signal is observed under high-power dipolar decoupling.

3.1.2. Experimental Parameters

The MAS rotation frequency should be chosen high enough to average out the chemical shift anisotropy but not too high because sample heating owing to friction of the rotor occurs (*see* **Note 5**). Typically, values between 5 and 10 kHz are reasonable for tissue samples at high magnetic field. The typical pulse length for the ^1H 90° excitation pulse should be on the order of 4 μs. The spin lock field on one channel should be set to approx 50 kHz; the corresponding spin lock field of the other channel is best determined experimentally for each sample since the Hartmann-Hahn condition turns out to be dependent on the MAS frequency, and shaped spin lock pulses may become necessary for efficient polarization transfer (*23*; *see* **Note 2**). Modern spectrometers allow for parameter optimization by sweeping through the power setting for the spin lock until maximum intensity is found. Typical contact times for maximal intensity of biological tissues are in the range of 0.5–1 ms. During acquisition, high power ^1H decoupling with a typical radiofrequency (RF) field strength of

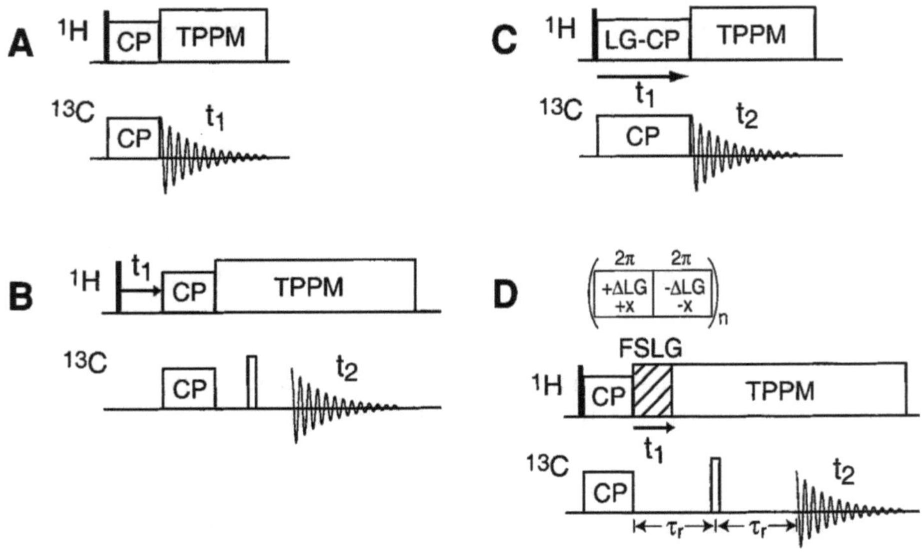

Fig. 1. Pulse sequences for the CP MAS experiment **(A)**, the WISE experiment **(B)**, the LG-CP experiment **(C)**, and the DIPSHIFT experiment **(D)**. Filled and open rectangles represent π/2 and π pulses, respectively. CP, cross-polarization, TPPM, two-pulse phase modulation decoupling, FSLG, frequency-switched Lee-Goldburg decoupling, τ_r: length of a rotor period.

60–80 kHz should be applied. Best results are obtained with the two-pulse phase modulation (TPPM) scheme *(24)*. Typical signal acquisition times should not exceed approx 25 ms to avoid RF heating (*see* **Note 5**), but since NMR lines of biological tissues are relatively broad, in most cases shorter acquisition times are sufficient. A relaxation delay of 3–5 s between successive scans should be allowed for protons to relax fully and to prevent sample heating.

3.1.3. Data Analysis and Information Content

A ^{13}C CP MAS spectrum of pig articular cartilage at 25°C is shown in **Fig. 2** (^{1}H Larmor frequency 750 MHz). The assignment of the collagen part of the spectrum is carried out according to **ref.** ***25***. Besides the dominating collagen resonances, there are signals of the rigid part of the glycosaminoglycans present in the spectra representing mostly hyaluronan. However, compared with the HR-MAS spectra shown in Chapter 14, the signals of the mobile carbohydrates are completely suppressed.

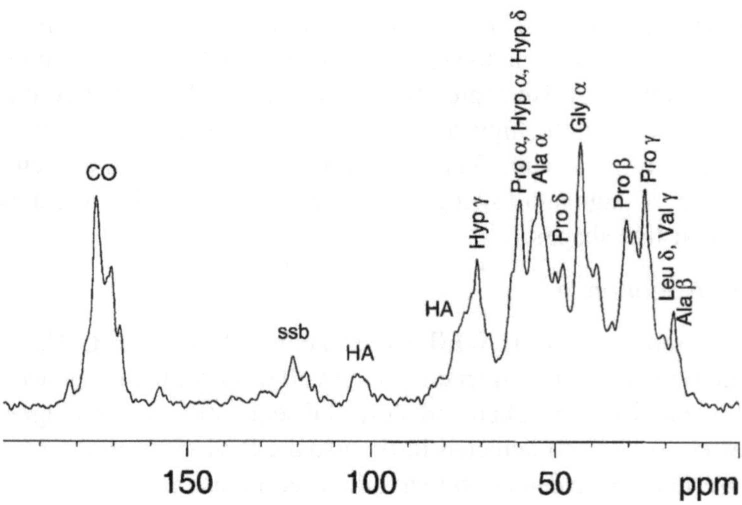

Fig. 2. A 188-MHz ^{13}C CP MAS spectrum of pig articular cartilage. Assignment of the collagen signals is given according to ref. ***25***. Besides the collagen signals, residual resonances of rigid carbohydrates (mostly hyaluronan) are detected (HA). ssb, spinning side band; Ala, alanine; Leu, leucine; Val, valine; Pro, proline; Gly, glycine; Hyp, hydroxyproline.

3.2. Wideline Separation (WISE) Experiment

Molecular motions scale down anisotropic interactions, for instance dipolar couplings between nuclear spins. The higher the mobility, the smaller the residual dipolar interaction, providing a measure of the motional amplitude typically expressed by an order parameter. It is desired to measure a dipolar coupling for each molecular site providing motional information for the entire molecule. However, the ^{1}H line shapes of rigid molecules represent a superposition of many dipolar spectra and cannot be analyzed quantitatively. A possible solution to that problem would be site-specific isotopic labeling, which is tedious, expensive, and particularly difficult for biological tissue samples. Alternatively, the idea separating anisotropic interactions in a 2D experiment evolved in the eighties, based on the ideas of Jeener, Ernst, Waugh and their coworkers ***(26)***. To date, a number of 2D pulse sequences have been available, in which the MAS spectrum is detected in the direct dimension and an anisotropic spectrum is measured in the indirect dimension for each resolved site. Thus, many motional parameters can be obtained site-specifically in a single experiment ideally without isotopic labeling.

The WISE experiment *(27)* represents a simple modification of the CP MAS technique, which allows one to separate isotropic and anisotropic interactions in a 2D experiment. Anisotropic ^1H–^1H dipolar couplings evolve during the first time domain, and the high-resolution ^{13}C MAS spectrum is detected during the second time domain. Thus, the dipolar spectrum can be detected for each resolved ^{13}C signal, allowing one to separate the overlapping anisotropic ^1H–^1H dipolar line shapes.

3.2.1. Pulse Sequence

The pulse sequence of the WISE experiment is shown in **Fig. 1B**. After the ^1H excitation pulse, proton magnetization evolves under the influence of dipolar coupling and isotropic chemical shift. Subsequently, proton magnetization is transferred to ^{13}C and detected in the usual CP MAS experiment. A Hahn echo is inserted before detection to avoid baseline distortions.

3.2.2. Experimental Parameters

Spectral parameters of the WISE experiment are identical to the CP MAS experiment except that only a short CP contact time on the order of 100 μs or less should be applied to prevent spin diffusion during CP. A short dwell time of the order of 10 μs in t_1 provides a sufficient spectrum width for the proton widelines in the indirect dimension. The MAS rotation frequency should be kept at an intermediate value (~5 kHz) that hardly affects the proton line shape, which is dominated by interactions that are about ten times stronger.

3.2.3. Data Analysis and Information Content

Figure 3 shows a 2D WISE spectrum of articular cartilage recorded at a ^1H Larmor frequency of 750 MHz. The 2D correlation spectrum is best analyzed by extracting ^1H–^1H dipolar spectra as slices at given isotropic ^{13}C signals, as indicated in the figure. The width of these proton lines is caused by the homonuclear dipolar interactions of the proton networks in the vicinity of the ^{13}C nucleus. Molecular motions average these dipolar interactions, which results in narrower ^1H widelines. Thus, qualitative mobility information can be obtained from this simple experiment: the narrower the lines, the more mobile the molecular site. Since the line shape of ^1H–^1H dipolar spectra is dominated by a superposition of several spin couplings of varying distance in the complicated proton network of organic molecules, there is no straightforward way to simulate ^1H widelines and to obtain quantitative information about the motion. For a qualitative discussion, the line width at half height of a signal in a biological tissue sample is best compared with that of a rigid powder (e.g., of a crystalline amino acid or peptide). Also, comparisons within the sample are

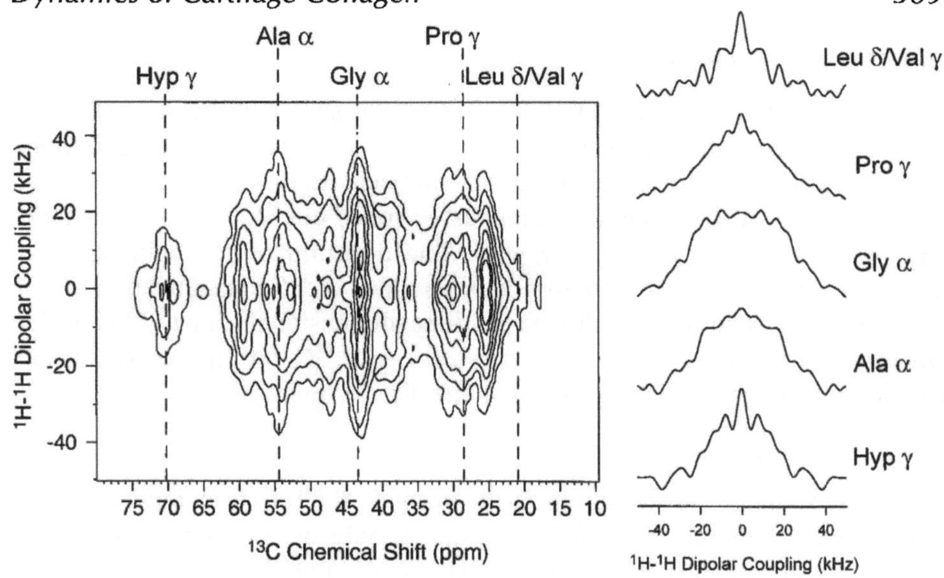

Fig. 3. 2D wideline separation spectrum of pig articular cartilage at a temperature of 25°C and a MAS frequency of 5 kHz (left). Slices taken for specific ^{13}C signals are shown on the right, 1D ^{1}H–^{1}H dipolar spectra. The width of the cartilage collagen ^{1}H–^{1}H widelines is 16, 32, 51, 41, and 37 kHz, from top to bottom, indicating differences in the mobility of the respective site.

instructive. For instance, in **Fig. 3** it can be seen that the collagen side chain signals (Leu δ/Val γ, Pro γ, Hyp γ) exhibit narrower proton widelines than the signals from the protein backbone (Ala α, Gly α).

3.3. Lee-Goldburg CP (LG-CP) Experiment

The disadvantages of analyzing proton widelines in a complicated structure can be overcome by measuring dipolar couplings of a well-defined geometry such as along the C–H bond. In first approximation, the dipolar coupling measured for a ^{13}C nucleus is only determined by the nearest covalently attached proton. Thus, the C–H dipolar coupling of any given molecular site can be determined quantitatively, which allows one to calculate an order parameter of that particular site. Two out of many experiments are discussed here that allow one to measure C-H dipolar couplings in a site-specific fashion, the LG-CP and the dipolar/chemical shift (DIPSHIFT) correlation experiment. In the LG-CP experiment *(28)*, dipolar powder spectra are measured in the indirect dimension for each resolved ^{13}C NMR signal. Thus, the dipolar coupling can be directly read off from the spectrum by measuring the frequency difference between the two characteristic maxima of the spectra.

3.3.1. Pulse Sequence

The pulse sequence of the LG-CP experiment is shown in **Fig. 1C**. After the proton excitation pulse, magnetization is locked along the effective field (tilted at an angle of 54.7° with respect to the external field) to fulfill the Lee-Goldburg condition *(29)*. A B_1 field is simultaneously applied on the ^{13}C channel matching the condition $\gamma_H\omega_{1,H,eff} = \gamma_C\omega_{1,C}$. The duration of the spin locks is incremented in t_1, leading to an oscillatory buildup of ^{13}C magnetization that is detected under proton decoupling in the direct dimension during t_2. 2D Fourier transformation yields a correlation spectrum with ^{13}C–^1H dipolar patterns in the indirect and isotropic ^{13}C signals in the direct dimension.

3.3.2. Experimental Parameters

For the setup of the ^1H spin lock, the normal ^1H CP field in the laboratory frame, which becomes the effective field, should be reduced according to $\omega_{1,H,lab} = \omega_{1,H,eff}\sin(54.7°)$. Also, the ^1H offset should be set to $\Omega = \omega_{1,H,eff}\cos(54.7°)$ but reset to the usual on-resonance value after LG-CP for dipolar decoupling. The contact time on the LG-CP spin locks is incremented in t_1 at a step width on the order of 10 μs to provide a sufficient spectrum width in the indirect dimension. The maximum of the t_1 evolution is determined by the end of the observed oscillation, which is typically achieved after a few ms. The experiment is designed for high MAS frequencies on the order of 10 kHz. All other parameters are identical to those of the CP experiment.

3.3.3. Data Analysis and Information Content

Figure 4 shows a 2D LG-CP spectrum of pig articular cartilage at a temperature of 25°C and a ^1H Larmor frequency of 750 MHz. Similar to the WISE spectrum, for each resolved ^{13}C NMR signal, a C-H dipolar spectrum can be extracted in the indirect dimension, as indicated in the figure. Since the LG-CP experiment is a γ-encoded pulse sequence, powder patterns are detected in the indirect dimension. The frequency splitting between the two maxima of the spectrum represents the dipolar coupling, scaled by 0.577. The ratio of the obtained motionally averaged dipolar coupling value ($\bar{\delta}$) and the rigid limit value (δ = 22.8 kHz for a C-H bond) defines the molecular order parameter of the C–H bond on the fast timescale according to

$$S_{CH} = \frac{\bar{\delta}}{\delta}. \qquad (1)$$

Unlike proton widelines, the C–H dipolar powder spectra of the LG-CP experiment can be simulated numerically. In the simplest case, the oscillation frequency of the CH dipolar interaction is given by

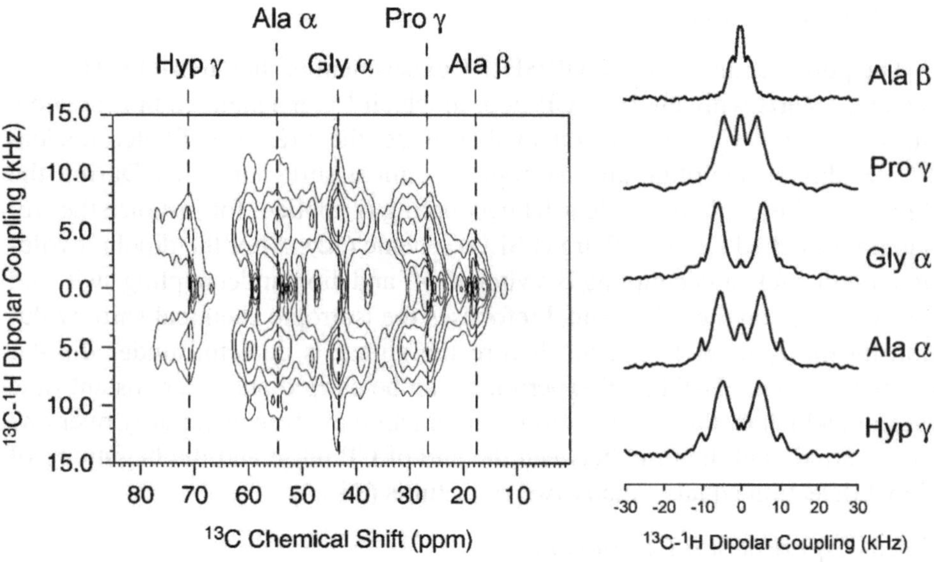

Fig. 4. LG-CP spectrum of pig articular cartilage at a temperature of 25°C and a MAS frequency of 10 kHz (**left**). Slices taken for specific ^{13}C signals are shown on the **right**, representing dipolar C-H powder spectra. The width of the experimentally observed splitting equals the dipolar interaction scaled by 0.577. From top to bottom, the dipolar couplings measured from the splittings of the spectra on the right side are 8.5, 18.0, 22.4, 21.0, and 20.5 kHz, respectively.

$$\omega_{CH} = -\frac{\sqrt{2}}{4}\bar{\delta}\sin\left(54.7^{\circ}\right)\sin\left(2\beta\right). \tag{2}$$

For powder averaging, the integration of β has to be executed from 0 to π. More elaborate theoretical treatments including distant protons ***(28)*** or nonuniaxially averaged dipolar interactions ***(30)*** can be found in the literature.

3.4. Dipolar-Chemical Shift Correlation (DIPSHIFT) Experiment

Like the LG-CP experiment, the DIPSHIFT pulse sequence ***(31)*** is designed to separate ^{13}C–^{1}H dipolar couplings according to the isotropic ^{13}C chemical shift. In the DIPSHIFT experiment, a MAS spectrum is measured in the indirect dimension that is modulated by the dipolar interaction manifested by the occurrence of spinning side bands. The motionally averaged dipolar coupling can be extracted from the MAS signal detected in the indirect dimension by analyzing either the time or the frequency domain. Numerical simulations are necessary to obtain the ^{13}C–^{1}H dipolar coupling value at the respective ^{13}C site.

3.4.1. Pulse Sequence

The pulse sequence of the DIPSHIFT experiment is shown in **Fig. 1D**. The sequence starts with a normal CP step, in which ^{13}C magnetization is created. Subsequently, ^{13}C magnetization evolves under the influence of heteronuclear ^{13}C-^{1}H dipolar coupling and isotropic chemical shift during t_1. During the dipolar evolution, homonuclear ^{1}H decoupling is applied, for instance the frequency-switched Lee-Goldburg (FSLG) scheme *(32)*. After the dipolar evolution, homonuclear decoupling is switched off and dipolar decoupling switched on. A π pulse on the ^{13}C channel refocuses the isotropic chemical shift evolution during t_1 in a Hahn echo before the signal is detected under dipolar decoupling. The DIPSHIFT experiment can be carried out in a constant time fashion, which means that the dipolar interaction evolves maximally over one rotor period, and the time between the end of CP pulse and the beginning of signal detection equals exactly two rotor turns *(33)*.

3.4.2. Experimental Parameters

The critical part of setting up a ^{13}C DIPSHIFT experiment is the homonuclear decoupling. As indicated in **Fig. 1D**, FSLG involves RF irradiation of 2π pulses on the proton channel switching between the +LG and the –LG condition, thereby executing a 180° phase shift. On modern spectrometers, FSLG can be implemented either by virtually switching the ^{1}H offset for each 2π pulse or by replacing the frequency change by an equivalent phase shift *(34)*. ^{1}H offset and field strength should be determined carefully, as described for the LG-CP experiment in **Subheading 3.3.** The ^{1}H RF field strength should be on the order of 60–100 kHz (*see* **Notes 2** and **5**). All other parameters are identical to the CP MAS experiment. The MAS frequency should be smaller than the dipolar coupling to be observed multiplied by the scaling factor for the homonuclear decoupling sequence (0.577 for FSLG). For rigid macromolecules in biological tissues, values between 2.5 and 8 kHz are recommended.

3.4.3. Data Analysis and Information Content

In DIPSHIFT spectra, dipolar coupling values are only obtained from numerical simulations of the time or frequency domain signal acquired in the indirect dimension. The time-dependent NMR frequency for a dipolar modulated MAS signal can be calculated according to *(35)*:

$$\omega_{CH}(t) = C_1 \cos(\omega_r t + \gamma) + C_2 \cos(2\omega_r t + 2\gamma) \tag{3}$$

where ω_r is the MAS angular frequency,

$$C_1 = -\bar{\delta}\frac{\sqrt{2}}{2}\sin(2\beta) \tag{4}$$

and

$$C_2 = -\bar{\delta}\frac{1}{2}\sin(\beta)^2 \tag{5}$$

The angles β and γ have to be integrated for powder averaging.

Equation 3 yields a periodic time domain signal that produces a MAS side band spectrum after Fourier transformation. Both time and frequency domain signals can be evaluated to obtain the dipolar coupling of the spectrum. In **Fig. 5**, examples are shown for a cartilage sample at 25°C and a ^{1}H Larmor frequency of 750 MHz. Since it is sufficient to measure the periodic MAS signal over one rotor period in a constant time DIPSHIFT experiment, time domain simulations according to **Eq. 3** can be compared with the experimentally determined MAS time domain signal, as shown in **Fig. 5A** and **D**. These DIPSHIFT spectra were only Fourier transformed in the direct dimension, which results in a pure time domain signal in the indirect dimension plotted in the figure. The best fit between measured and simulated signal determines the dipolar coupling. Alternatively, a 2D Fourier transformation of the DIPSHIFT spectrum provides an envelope of the MAS side band spectra, shown in **Fig. 5B** and **E**. Again, best agreement between measured and simulated signal allows one to determine the dipolar coupling of interest. Finally, the time domain signal can be reproduced over many rotor periods, which yields a true MAS side band spectrum after Fourier transformation, as shown in **Fig. 5C** and **F**. In our opinion, it is the best way to analyze these spectra in the time domain (**Fig. 5A** and **D**).

4. Notes

1. Excess water: natural cartilage contains up to approx 70 wt% water and high concentrations of monovalent ions. Since ^{1}H channels of MAS probes of high-field NMR spectrometers may have a relatively narrow bandwidth, this might result in difficulties in tuning the probe to the ^{1}H frequency. This problem can be overcome by allowing the freshly prepared cartilage to air-dry for several minutes to get rid of some of the excess water.
2. Spectrometer requirements: for the experiments introduced in this chapter, real solid-state NMR equipment is required (i.e., high-power probes and transmitters, fast digitizers, and hardware that allows for fast phase and frequency shifts within 1 μs). Typically, amplifiers with a power of 500–1000 W are required to create the desired RF field strengths. HR-MAS probes that have recently been introduced to investigate biological tissues are usually not designed to take the power required for solid-state NMR experiments. Since experiments have to be carried out at natural abundance ^{13}C, ^{1}H Larmor frequencies of 600 or 750 MHz are required to provide sufficient sensitivity for the 2D experiments.
3. MAS equipment: several MAS rotor diameters are available for modern spectrometers. Although larger rotors have the advantage of larger sample volumes,

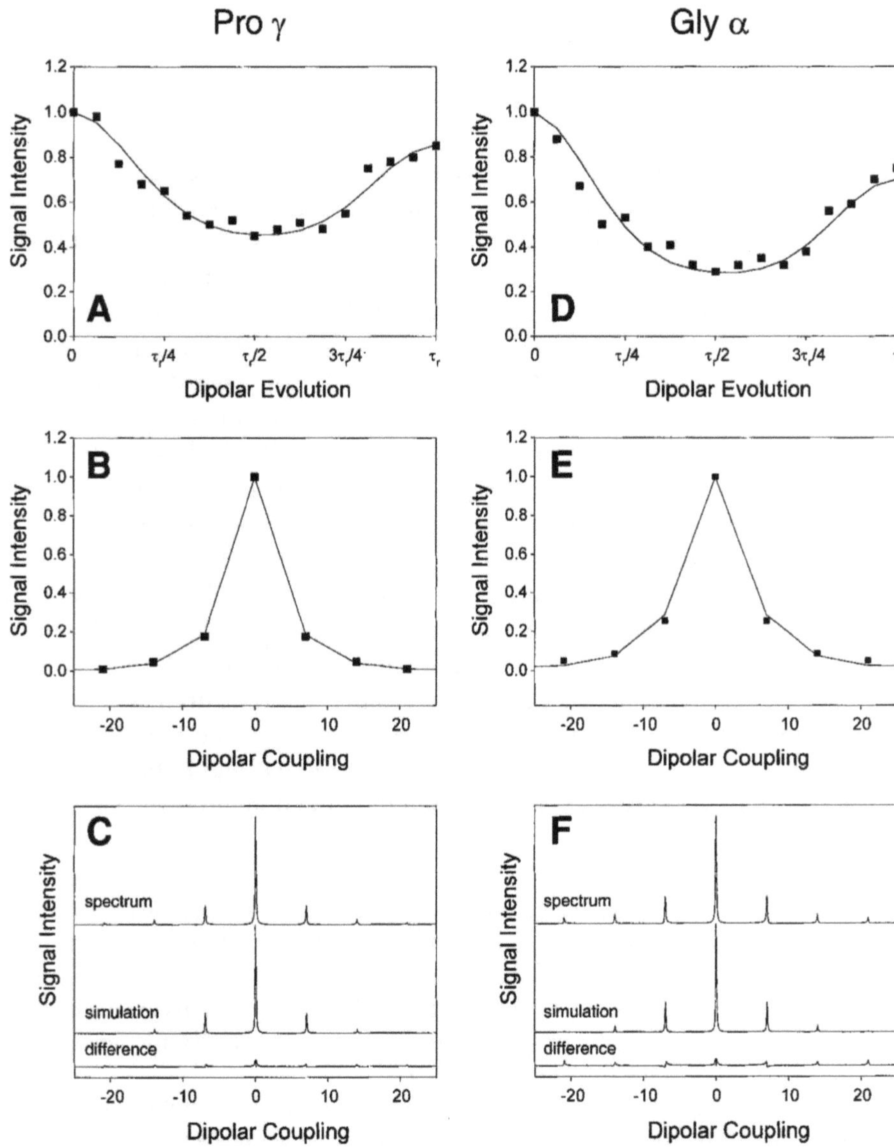

Fig. 5. Analysis of DIPSHIFT spectra of pig articular cartilage. The left column shows the time signal over one rotor period **(A)**, the Fourier transform of that signal **(B)**, and the Fourier transform of the time domain signal reproduced over many rotor periods **(C)** for the Pro γ signal. In the right column, the analogous spectra for the Gly α signal are depicted **(D–F)**. For (A), (B), (D), and (F), the points represent the experimentally measured signal intensities and the lines are the best fit numerical simulations. In (C) and (F), the spectra, best fit simulations, and difference between the two are given. The dipolar coupling that can be obtained from these spectra is 18.7 kHz for Pro Cγ and 22.3 kHz for Gly Cα.

maximum spinning speeds and RF performance of these probes are compromised. In our studies, 4-mm rotors were used that accommodate a maximum sample volume of approx 100 mg. Considering that cartilage contains on the order of 20 wt% collagen, this translates into about 20 mg of collagen for the measurement. Line shapes and RF performance can be improved by using rotor inserts (made of Teflon or Kel-F). The data presented in this chapter were acquired using 4-mm rotors with inserts providing a 50-μL sample volume, i.e., the total amount of collagen in the sample was on the order of 10 mg.

4. Which experiment to choose? Among the three experiments introduced to study the mobility of rigid cartilage collagen, the WISE experiment represents the simplest and most robust pulse sequence. However, the information content is also limited and only qualitative. The information content of LG-CP and DIPSHIFT is about comparable and quantitative. Since the LG-CP pulse sequence is γ-encoded, powder line shapes are measured, which allow one to distinguish between sites of higher and lower mobility by measuring a superposition of several dipolar splittings. However, the experiment is more time-consuming since more t_1 increments have to be acquired to record the magnetization buildup during the LG-CP experiment. For the DIPSHIFT experiment, only 8–16 t_1 increments have to be acquired for the full information content. Athough, other experiments are available to measure dipolar couplings under MAS ***(36–38)***, the experiments discussed in this chapter are simple modifications of the CP MAS experiments that can be conducted with relatively good sensitivity, which is necessary when working with biological tissues at natural abundance ^{13}C.
5. Sample overheating: at high proton Larmor frequency, absorption of the almost microwave energy of RF pulses and decoupling by the water molecules may result in sample overheating. Therefore, acquisition times should be kept to a minimum (typically about 10 ms is sufficient for the ^{13}C line widths observed for cartilage specimen), and a generous duty cycle of $\leq 1\%$ should be applied. As mentioned above, rotor inserts and smaller sample volumes also help to limit the RF heating.

Acknowledgments

The junior research group is funded by the Saxon State Ministry of Higher Education, Research, and Culture. The work was supported by the Deutsche Forschungsgemeinschaft (SFB294/G5) and by the Bundesministerium für Bildung und Forschung (BMB+F), Interdisciplinary Center for Clinical Research (IZKF) at the University Leipzig (01KS9504/1 Project A17).

References

1. Antzutkin, O. N., Balbach, J. J., Leapman, R. D., Rizzo, N. W., Reed, J., and Tycko, R. (2000) Multiple quantum solid-state NMR indicates a parallel, not antiparallel, organization of beta-sheets in Alzheimer's beta-amyloid fibrils. *Proc. Natl. Acad. Sci. USA* **97,** 13045–13050.
2. Ketchem, R. R., Hu, W., and Cross, T. A. (1993) High-resolution conformation of gramicidin A in a lipid bilayer by solid-state NMR. *Science* **261,** 1457–1460.

3. Lambotte, S., Jasperse, P., and Bechinger, B. (1998) Orientational distribution of α-helices in the colicin B and E1 channel domains: a one and two dimensional ^{15}N solid-state NMR investigation in uniaxially aligned phospholipid bilayers. *Biochemistry* **37,** 16–22.
4. Marassi, F. M., Ma, C., Gratkowski, H., et al. (1999) Correlation of the structural and functional domains in the membrane protein Vpu from HIV-1. *Proc. Natl. Acad. Sci. USA* **96,** 14336–14341.
5. Gr°bner, G., Burnett, I. J., Glaubitz, C., Choi, G., Mason, A. J., and Watts, A. (2000) Observations of light-induced structural changes of retinal within rhodopsin. *Nature* **405,** 810–813.
6. Tong, G., Pan, Y., Dong, H., Pryor, R., Wilson, G. E., and Schaefer, J. (1997) Structure and dynamics of pentaglycyl bridges in the cell walls of *Staphylococcus aureus* by ^{13}C-^{15}N REDOR NMR. *Biochemistry* **36,** 9859–9866.
7. van Beek, J. D., Beaulieu, L., Schafer, H., Demura, M., Asakura, T., and Meier, B. H. (2000) Solid-state NMR determination of the secondary structure of *Samia cynthia ricini* silk. *Nature* **405,** 1077–1079.
8. Petkova, A. T., Hatanaka, M., Jaroniec, C. P., et al. (2002) Tryptophan interactions in bacteriorhodopsin: a heteronuclear solid-state NMR study. *Biochemistry* **41,** 2429–2437.
9. Asakura, T., Yao, J., Yamane, T., Umemura, K., and Ulrich, A. S. (2002) Heterogeneous structure of silk fibers from *Bombyx mori* resolved by ^{13}C solid-state NMR spectroscopy. *J. Am. Chem. Soc.* **124,** 8794–8795.
10. Laws, D. D., Bitter, H. M., Liu, K., et al. (2001) Solid-state NMR studies of the secondary structure of a mutant prion protein fragment of 55 residues that induces neurodegeneration. *Proc. Natl. Acad. Sci. USA* **98,** 11686–11690.
11. Alia, Matysik, J., Soede-Huijbregts, C., Baldus, M., et al. (2001) Ultrahigh field MAS NMR dipolar correlation spectroscopy of the histidine residues in light-harvesting complex II from photosynthetic bacteria reveals partial internal charge transfer in the B850/His complex. *J. Am. Chem. Soc.* **123,** 4803–4809.
12. Isaac, B., Gallagher, G. J., Balazs, Y. S., and Thompson, L. K. (2002) Site-directed rotational resonance solid-state NMR distance measurements probe structure and mechanism in the transmembrane domain of the serine bacterial chemoreceptor. *Biochemistry* **41,** 3025–3036.
13. Smith, S. O., Smith, C., Shekar, S., Peersen, O., Ziliox, M., and Aimoto, S. (2002) Transmembrane interactions in the activation of the Neu receptor tyrosine kinase. *Biochemistry* **41,** 9321–9332.
14. Tuzi, S., Yamaguchi, S., Naito, A., Needleman, R., Lanyi, J. K., and Saito, H. (1996) Conformation and dynamics of [3-^{13}C]Ala-labeled bacteriorhodopsin and bacterioopsin, induced by interaction with retinal and its analogs, as studied by ^{13}C nuclear magnetic resonance. *Biochemistry* **35,** 7520–7527.
15. Yang, Z., Liivak, O., Seidel, A., LaVerde, G., Zax, D., and Jelinski, L. W. (2000) Supercontraction and backbone dynamics in spider silk: ^{13}C and ^{2}H NMR studies. *J. Am. Chem. Soc.* **122,** 9019–9025.

16. Huster, D., Xiao, L., and Hong, M. (2001) Solid-state NMR investigation of the dynamics of soluble and membrane-bound colicin Ia channel-forming domain. *Biochemistry* **40,** 7662–7674.
17. Schiller, J., Naji, L., Huster, D., Kaufmann, J., and Arnold, K. (2001) ^{1}H and ^{13}C HR-MAS NMR investigations on native and enzymatically-digested bovine cartilage. *MAGMA* **13,** 19–27.
18. Naji, L., Kaufmann, J., Huster, D., Schiller, J., and Arnold, K. (2000) ^{13}C NMR relaxation study on cartilage and cartilage components. The origin of ^{13}C NMR spectra of cartilage. *Carbohydr. Res.* **327,** 439–446.
19. Huster, D., Schiller, J., and Arnold, K. (2002) Comparison of collagen dynamics in articular cartilage and isolated fibrils by solid state NMR spectroscopy. *Magn. Res. Med.* **48,** 624–632.
20. Griffin, R. G. (1998) Dipolar recoupling in MAS spectra of biological solids. *Nat. Struct. Biol.* **5,** 508–512.
21. Pines, A., Gibby, M. G., and Waugh, J. S. (1973) Proton-enhanced NMR of dilute spins in solids. *J. Chem. Phys.* **59,** 569–590.
22. Stejskal, E. O. and Schaefer, J. (1976) Carbon-13 nuclear magnetic resonance of polymers spinning at the magic angle. *J. Am. Chem. Soc.* **98,** 1031–1032.
23. Hediger, S., Meier, B. H., Kurur, N. D., Bodenhausen, G., and Ernst, R. R. (1994) NMR cross polarization by adiabatic passage through the Hartmann-Hahn condition (APHH). *Chem. Phys. Lett.* **223,** 283–288.
24. Bennett, A. E., Rienstra, C. M., Auger, M., Lakshmi, K. V., and Griffin, R. G. (1995) Heteronuclear decoupling in rotating solids. *J. Chem. Phys.* **103,** 6951–6958.
25. Saito, H. and Yokoi, M. (1992) A ^{13}C NMR study on collagens in the solid state: hydration/dehydration-induced conformational change of collagen and detection of internal motions. *J. Biochem. (Tokyo)* **111,** 376–382.
26. Schmidt-Rohr, K. and Spiess, H. W. (1994) *Multidimensional Solid-Date NMR and Polymers.* Academic, San Diego, CA.
27. Schmidt-Rohr, K., Clauss, J., and Spiess, H. W. (1992) Correlation of structure, mobility, and morphological information in heterogeneous polymer materials by two-dimensional wideline-separation NMR spectroscopy. *Macromolecules* **25,** 3273–3277.
28. van Rossum, B.-J., de Groot, C. P., Ladizhansky, V., Vega, S., and de Groot, H. J. M. (2000) A method for measuring heteronuclear (^{1}H-^{13}C) distances in high speed MAS NMR. *J. Am. Chem. Soc.* **122,** 3465–3472.
29. Goldburg, W. I. and Lee, M. (1963) Nuclear magnetic resonance line narrowing by a rotating rf field. *Phys. Rev. Lett.* **11,** 255–258.
30. Hong, M., Yao, X., Jakes, K. S., and Huster, D. (2002) Investigation of molecular motions by magic-angle cross-polarization NMR spectroscopy. *J. Phys. Chem. B* **106,** 7355–7364.
31. Kolbert, A. C., de Groot, H. J. M., Levitt, M. H., et al. (1990) Two-dimensional dipolar–chemical shift NMR in rotating solids, in *Multinuclear Magnetic Reso-*

nance in Liquids and Solids—Chemical Applications (Granger, P. and Harris, R. K., eds.) Kluwer, Dordrecht, pp. 339–354.

32. Bielecki, A., Kolbert, A. C., and Levitt, M. H. (1989) Frequency-switched pulse sequences: homonuclear decoupling and dilute spin NMR in solids. *Chem. Phys. Lett.* **155,** 341–345.
33. Hong, M., Gross, J. D., and Griffin, R. G. (1997) Site-resolved determination of peptide torsion angle Φ from relative orientations of backbone N-H and C-H bonds by solid-state NMR. *J. Phys. Chem.* **101,** 5869–5874.
34. Vinogradov, E., Madhu, P. K., and Vega, S. (1999) High-resolution proton solid-state NMR spectroscopy by phase-modulated Lee-Goldburg experiment. *Chem. Phys. Lett.* **314,** 443–450.
35. Maricq, M. M. and Waugh, J. S. (1979) NMR in rotating solids. *J. Chem. Phys.* **70,** 3300–3316.
36. Bennett, A. E., Griffin, R. G., and Vega, S. (1994) *NMR Basic Principles and Progress*. Springer Verlag, Berlin, pp. 3–77.
37. Dusold, S. and Sebald, A. (2000) Dipolar recoupling under magic-angle spinning conditions. *Ann. Rep. NMR Spectrosc.* **41,** 185–264.
38. Brown, S. P. and Spiess, H. W. (2001) Advanced solid-state NMR methods for the elucidation of structure and dynamics of molecular, macromolecular, and supramolecular systems. *Chem. Rev.* **101,** 4125–4155.

17

Computerized Protocol for Anatomical and Functional Studies of Joints

Sandra Martelli and Stefano Zaffagnini

Summary

This chapter describes a new methodology for the acquisition and computer elaboration of joint anatomy and motion data and the study of their correlation. The method uses a commercial industrial *electrogoniometer*, custom tools, and software designed and developed by the authors for interactive display of the anatomical structures during joint motion, numerical interpolations of the articular geometries, and kinematic analysis of motion. The original data acquisition protocol and computer elaboration software are described in detail, and a final subheading describes briefly previous studies and future developments.

Key Words: Joint; anatomy; kinematics; electrogoniometer; biomechanics.

1. Introduction

Degenerative diseases such as osteoarthritis and rheumatoid arthritis produce both anatomical and functional deformations to human joints, which affect the patient's mobility and cause pain. We describe a method that allows the accurate analysis of joint biomechanics, quantifying its anatomical and kinematic features.

The acquisition of both anatomical and kinematic data is performed by an *electrogoniometer* (*for a definition of this and other technical terms in italics, see* **Subheading 5., Glossary**) known as a FaroArm. This equipment is commonly used in industry and was proposed for neurosurgery in the 1980s but has been recently used by the authors for computer-assisted knee surgery and kinematic animal studies ***(1,2)***. It consists of sensorized *linkages* with the structure of a 6-*degrees-of-freedom* arm, which can be used to record the position of the *end-effector* at the distal end of the "arm" either continuously or intermittently as required by the operator. The instrument is also capable of determining the

From: *Methods in Molecular Medicine, Vol. 101: Cartilage and Osteoarthritis, Volume 2: Structure and In Vivo Analysis*
Edited by: F. De Ceuninck, M. Sabatini, and P. Pastoureau © Humana Press Inc., Totowa, NJ

three-dimensional (3D) coordinates of a point in space with an accuracy guaranteed by the manufacturer of 0.3 mm/0.3°.

During the acquisition phase, the *electrogoniometer* either is used to *digitize* the articular surface by touching it with suitable *probes* or is attached to the mobile segment to *track* its motion with respect to the fixed one. The digitization of surfaces and the registration of motion can be repeated any number of times and used in any order. Switching from one to the other modality requires the so-called matching step, i.e., a double acquisition of reference points with the *digitizer probe* and of the reference *location* with the *electrogoniometer* attached to the mobile segment.

After acquisition, the software allows the simultaneous demonstration of the movement of one rigid segment relative to the other articular segment by conventional kinematic means as well as the relative shapes and positions of the contacting surfaces over a range of movement. These tasks can be carried out using 3D images and with movement occurring either continuously or in interrupted steps. Several observations can be quantified by computing geometrical fitting on sections, *least-square interpolation* of profiles, distances, range of motion and laxity, and decomposition of motion on the main axes and views.

Our method can deal with the relative motion of two articular surfaces of a joint similarly to other tracking systems such as Roentgen stereophotogrammetric analysis (RSA), light-emitting *diodes*, or *electrogoniometers* of various kinds ***(3–6)***. All these kinematic methods can be employed during gait analysis or normal activity since the motion of the bones can be sensed remotely, but they present the possible problem of kinematic *crosstalk* and of attaching stable markers to the skeleton by noninvasive means ***(7–10)***.

Our method can also be used to study the shapes of the surfaces as they move on each other to determine the nature of the relative movements, similarly to dynamic X-rays (in particular, computer tomography) or magnetic resonance ***(11–13)***. These methods, which depend on imaging of the surfaces, allow axes of rotation and translations to be located anatomically and are easy for clinicians to understand, but they can produce significant radiation on living tissues, and can track only static positions; also, the identification of displacement and rotation from anatomical features may be inaccurate.

The method we propose describes the shapes of the surfaces and their relative movements simultaneously and accurately with the use of remote kinematic markers; therefore it shares the potentialities of the aforementioned techniques while overcoming some of the cited limitations of previous methods ***(14)***.

Up to now the method has been applied in several cadaveric studies and laboratory tests because it requires the fixation of one articular segment. However, we are developing new tools to extend its use to computer-assisted interventions and eventually diagnostic examination, as the computerized analysis of joints shapes and motion provided by our protocol might be fundamental to understanding the severity of bone deformation and planning effective reconstructive treatments of joints.

2. Materials

2.1. Digital Equipment

The sensor used for recording motion and digitizing shapes is the FaroArm, model B06-01/02 (FARO Technologies, Lake Mary, FL; http://www.faro.com.). It is a commercial 6-degree-of-freedom passive *electrogoniometer* with an anthropomorphic structure (**Fig. 1A**) that can be easily moved by the user to record position and orientation of the end-effector. It can acquire data continuously at a 50 Hz rate (stream mode) or point by point at the user's request (point mode) with 0.3 mm/0.3° accuracy in a spherical workspace of diameter 1.8 m around its base. The FaroArm sensor is light (4 kg) and flexible, but it is mounted on a heavy, stable clamping base that is used to attach the sensor rigidly onto the experimental desktop and easily move it when necessary to fit the environmental obstacles.

The *electrogoniometer* is controlled by a standard PC, and the commercial software provided lets the user acquire locations, set the *resolution*, the *sampling rate* of motion, and the acquisition mode (stream or point), or choose end-effectors that have already undergone *calibration* and any user-defined coordinate system.

2.2. Probes and End-Effectors

The FaroArm *electrogoniometer* has to be equipped with suitable *probes* either to *digitize* surfaces or to track motion.

Anatomical acquisition is mostly carried out using the commercial point *probe* sold by the manufacturer, or custom ball probes with smaller tip diameters and therefore greater accuracy than the default one, and sometimes longer or bended point probes (**Fig. 1B**).

Motion tracking requires the FaroArm to be rigidly fixed to the mobile articular segment. We have designed and built an end-effector to secure the electrogoniomer on intracortical fiches, consisting of a modified short arm of the Orthofix (DMO, Bussolengo, Italy) external fixator (**Fig. 1C**).

2.3 Fixture and Consumables

The protocol needs one articular segment to be fixed to the experimental desk, which supports the FaroArm. Any standard clamping or immobilization

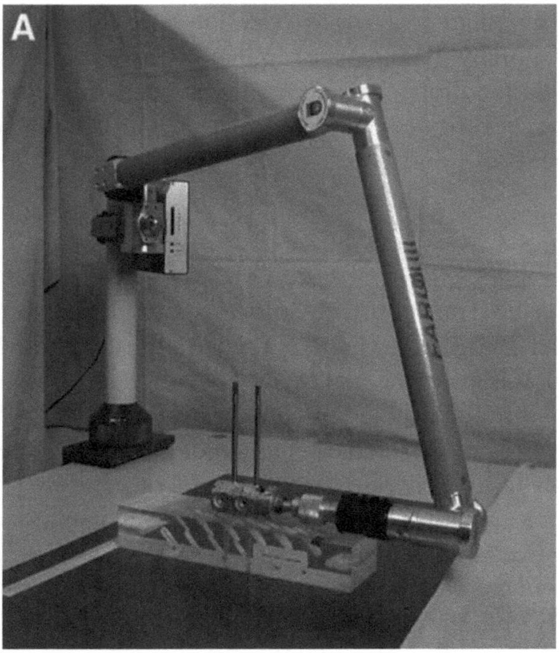

Fig. 1. FARO arm *electrogoniometer* (**A**) with probes for surface acquisition (**B**) and motion tracking (**C**) to be mounted at the last joint.

device can be used for this purpose. For short periods during the so-called matching phase, the mobile bone also has to be fixed with respect to the fixed bone, therefore an adequate clamping device or Kirschner threads should be available.

The protocol includes the identification of three reference landmarks on the two joint bones. Although the identification of anatomical landmarks is possible, we recommend using screw or mechanical markers.

Two or more external fixator pins are required to track the mobile bone. Standard anatomical equipment is necessary for dissection, as well as standard mechanical equipment such as a drill, hammer, and clamps.

2.4. Computer Software

Custom software has been developed by the authors to display and elaborate the acquired data. The original software was developed in MATLAB® code and is under the patent process. However, freeware versions of the programs are distributed at http://www.studyjoint.org. They run on a standard PC under Windows NT, 98 and successive, or XP operative system, and can be easily installed following on-line instructions.

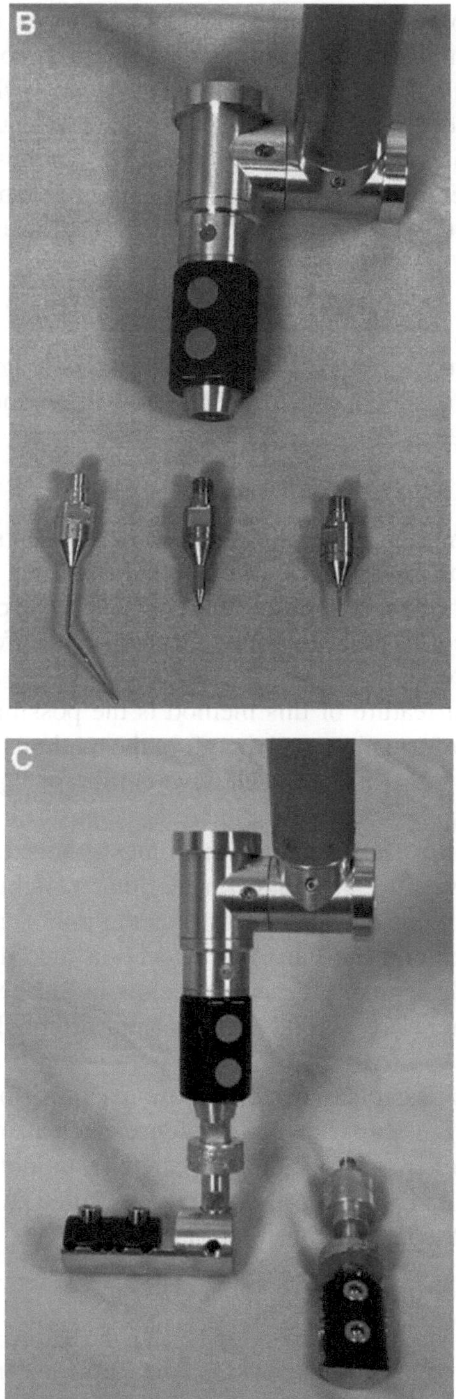
B
C

The software displays the acquired data (such as bones, ligaments' insertion areas, special anatomical points) during the recorded motion and allows the user to analyze bone geometry through *least-squares fitting* and dynamic observation of consecutive sections in an arbritary orientation (e.g., sagittal, frontal, coronal planes). Moreover, the physician can describe the ligament, tendon, or muscle elongation, analyze ligament fiber length and orientation during motion, or study rotations and translations of the articular segments in clinical frames.

3. Methods

The protocol requires both a physician and a computer scientist, and we recommend performing both experimental acquisition and off-line computer analysis of data together.

3.1. Design of the Experimental Protocol

Anatomical and motion acquisitions can be performed several times and in any order to study the joint under different conditions in a single experimental section. Therefore the first step of the study is indeed the careful design of the experimental protocol in order to obtain all the useful information as quickly as possible (*see* **Note 1**).

The most original feature of this method is the possibility to acquire anatomical-functional information, and therefore the method is particularly useful to track, for example, the effect of selective cutting of ligaments on the joint kinematics, or to display and analyze the relative position of the articular surfaces during kinematic tests, even with the joint still intact. In complex studies with several objectives, users should consider that switching from anatomical to functional acquisitions or vice versa needs the joint (or at least the mobile structure) to be fixed and the FaroArm's location recorded before and after fixation to the mobile segment (described below in **Subheading 3.5., Matching Procedure**). Therefore a good experimental protocol tends to minimize multiple switching.

In most cases it is possible to perform motion acquisition first and anatomical ones at the end of the experimental sequence, such as in the examples cited in refs. ***15–17***. However, any design and change from motion tracking to anatomical acquisition and vice versa, correctly executed, will ensure the same overall accuracy to the final reconstruction (*see* **Note 1**).

3.2. Experimental Setup (see *Fig. 2)*

1. Secure the fixed bone to the desktop and clamp the FaroArm around 50 cm from the joint. Switch on the computer and run the FaroArm control software.

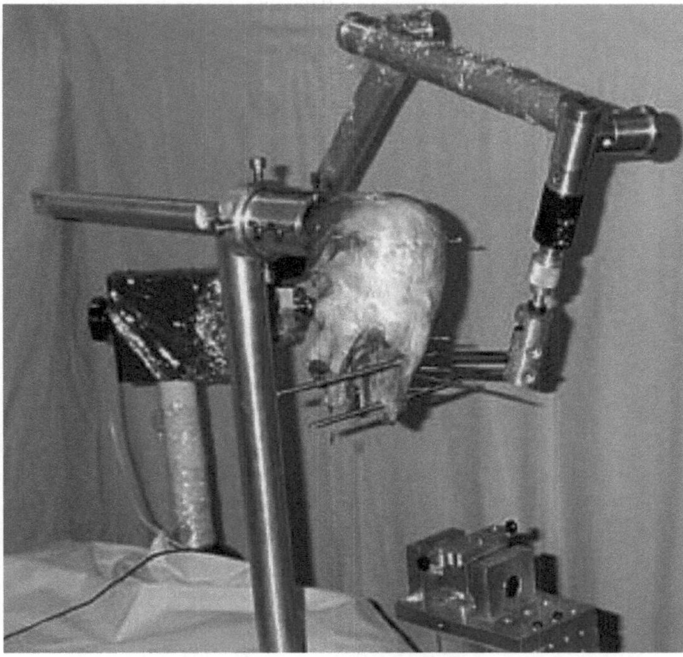

Fig. 2. Setup for knee study. The FaroArm is ready for trajectory acquisition.

2. Adjust the orientation and the position of the *electrogoniometer*, testing the planned motion and simulating the surface acquisition (*see* **Note 2**).
3. Set three landmarks (screws, needles, or wires) per bone onto the joint, in such a position that the planned motion can be performed, the markers are in the FaroArm workspace, and they are not aligned (*see* **Note 3**).
4. Fix two pins on the mobile bone for the tool used to attach the electrogoniometer and test the planned motion by attaching the FaroArm. If the electrogoniometer constrains the motion, change its position so that the passive movements can be correctly executed.
5. Use the point probe for the FaroArm, with 1-mm resolution in point mode. Define the reference frame for display and computations, by choosing the mediolateral direction as the *x*-axis and the anteroposterior direction as the *y*-axis in the Faro acquisition frame.

There are two different kinds of acquisition: surface points and trajectories. Each modality is performed using specific tools and the commercial FARO software; passing from one to the other requires the so-called matching procedure.

To carry out the designed experimental protocol, repeat the following steps as many times as necessary.

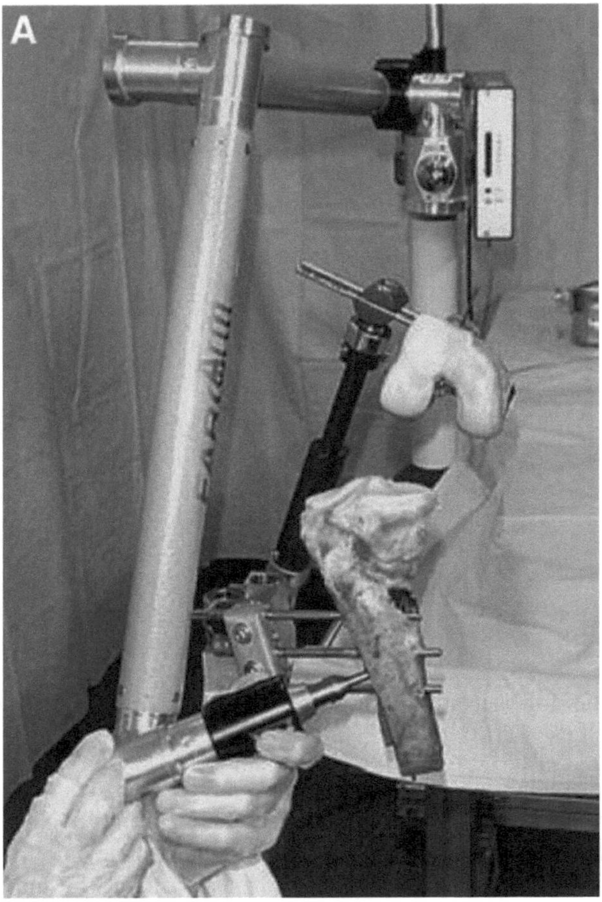

3.3. Acquisition of Surface Points (see Fig. 3)

1. Use a suitable point probe for the FaroArm (usually the standard point probe, but also bent probes for deep posterior areas especially accessed in arthroscopy or a small ball probe on very delicate soft tissues). Be careful to select the calibration file associated with the probe used and change it every time you change the probe.
2. Choose a suitable acquisition mode (or stream, i.e., continuous data collection, or point). Usually areas can be acquired in stream mode with low resolution (1 mm standard, 0.5 mm for very accurate acquisition, 1.5 mm for fast acquisitions of large areas); significant points or sharp edges are acquired in point mode (*see* **Note 4**).
3. Scan the surface to be acquired regularly, for example, by acquiring the boundary and a regular grid inside in stream mode. Keep the edge of the probe on the surface, e.g., keep the probe as perpendicular as possible to the acquired areas (*see* **Notes 5** and **6**).

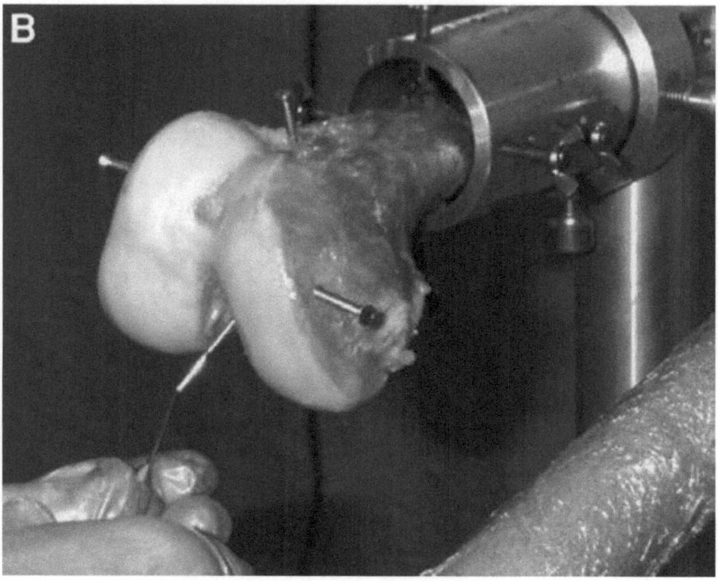

Fig. 3. Surface acquisition of tibia **(A)** and femur **(B)** during a knee study. Note that different probes can be used for the acquisition, and bones can be fixed in any convenient position.

3.4. Acquisition of Trajectories (see *Fig. 4*)

1. Use the custom fixture for pins, such as the Faro end-effector, and select the point probe calibration file (by convention).
2. Choose a suitable acquisition mode (stream, i.e., continuous data collection, or single point). Usually passive motion and diagnostic tests are acquired in stream mode with high resolution (5–10 mm for "big" joints); extreme positions used to compute range of motion or laxity are acquired in point mode (*see* **Note 7**).
3. The acquisition of motion can be either fast or slow, but you should perform each maneuver at an almost constant speed, whatever it is. You can acquire the same or different kinds of motion at different speeds, by adjusting the acquisition resolution of the *electrogoniometer* (*see* **Note 8**).

3.5. Matching Procedure

1. Fix the mobile bone to the experimental desktop (*see* **Fig. 5**, and **Note 9**).
2. Choose point mode on the FARO control software.

3.5.1. Matching Procedure for Switching From Trajectory to Surface Acquisition

1. Record the FaroArm position in a file (usually called *FAROREFn.mtr*; *n* = progressive index).

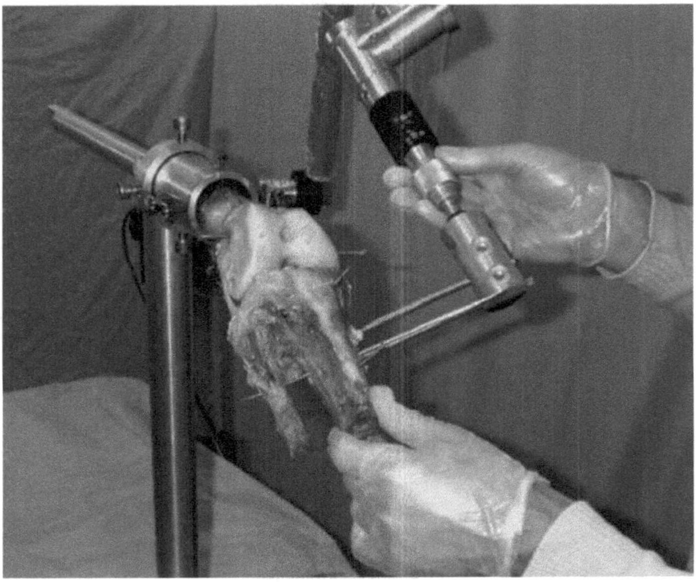

Fig. 4. Acquisition of the passive range of motion during a knee study.

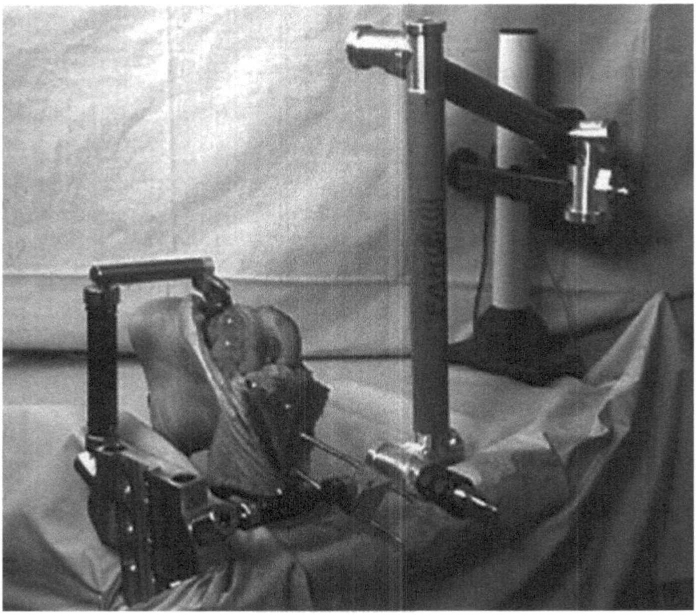

Fig. 5. Example of joint fixation for matching procedure. After fixation of the mobile segment (tibia) the FARO arm is equipped with a point probe for landmark (white screws) digitization.

2. Detach the FaroArm from the mobile bone and mount the point probe on the FaroArm.
3. Acquire the landmarks of the mobile bones in the established order and record them in a file (usually called *boneREFn.mtr*; *bone*= name of the bone, *n* = the index used for *FAROREF* file).
4. You can now move bones or start surface acquisition.

3.5.2 Matching Procedure for Switching From Surface to Trajectory Acquisition

1. Acquire the landmarks of the mobile bones in the established order and record them in a file (usually called *boneREFn.mtr*; *bone* = name of the bone, *n* = progressive index).
2. Remove the point probe and mount the Faro fixture for the mobile bone.
3. Attach the FaroArm to the mobile bone.
4. Record the FaroArm position in a file (usually called *FAROREFn.mtr*; *n* = the index used for *boneREF* file).
5. You can now move bones and start trajectory acquisition.

Note that some errors in the acquisition procedure can be recovered if detected before the end of the experiment (*see* **Notes 9–11**). Therefore, we recommend checking fixtures, setup, and acquisition accuracy regularly.

3.6. Computer Analysis of Data

All data acquired by the *electrogoniometer* (that is, articular surfaces or insertion areas on bones, trajectories, bone landmarks, and Faro reference positions) are processed to create single files describing each structure (i.e., fixed and mobile bone, separate insertion areas on fixed and mobile bone for ligaments, tendons, and muscles) and a separate file for each trajectory performed (*see* **Notes 12** and **13** for details and http://www.studyjoint.org for the format of input files).

In **Subheadings 3.6.1.–3.6.4.**, we describe the complete set of information that the user can obtain from our software package in a standard sequence. According to the specific goal of the procedure defined by the user, some steps can be omitted and others can be resorted.

3.6.1. Overview (see *Fig. 6*)

1. Observe each structure in the 3D windows looking at it in standard clinical views (frontal and lateral) or from arbitrary angles and distances, chosen interactively using mouse buttons (*see* **Notes 14** and **15**).
2. Observe the 3D anatomical structures during motions, looking at the successive positions of all or selected objects during the recorded trajectories, using *forward/backward buttons* in software interface (*see* http://www.studyjoint.org for movies and on-line demonstration and **Note 16** for mathematical background).

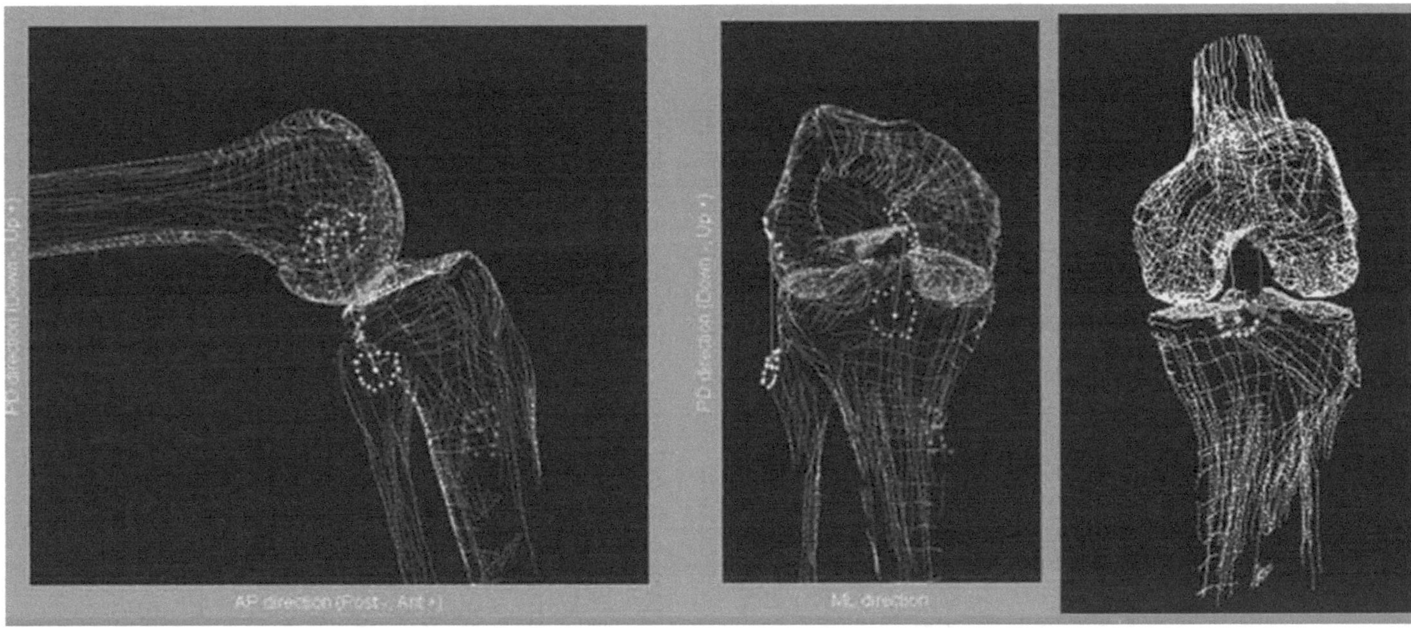

Fig. 6. Example of 3D reconstruction of a knee joint, displayed from different views.

3.6.2. Anatomical Analysis (see ***Fig. 7****)*

1. Examine successive sagittal sections (e.g., a section with 10-mm space distance and 2–3-mm thickness) in significant positions (e.g., in extension, flexion, or specific flexion or abduction angles), using *section tools* in the software interface.
2. Compute the best geometrical fitting for profiles of the fixed and mobile sections by test and trials (best = with minimal residual), using *fitting buttons* provided by the section interface (*see* **Note 17**).
3. Observe bone conformity.
4. Repeat section analysis for frontal and coronal sections, to obtain a complete 3D geometrical model of the joint.

*3.6.3. Soft Tissue Analysis (*see ***Fig. 8*** *and* ***Note 18****)*

1. Select one ligament or recorded soft tissue (defined by two insertion areas and fibers), using *ligaments list* in the software interface.
2. Compute fiber elongation and the distances between the centers of the insertion areas, using *ligaments tools* in software interface.
3. Compute fiber orientation with respect to sagittal, frontal, and coronal planes and with respect to the plane, fitting their insertion areas on the fixed and mobile bones, using *ligaments tools* in the software interface.
4. Repeat the analysis for each ligament or deformable structure in order to have a map of its function during joint motion.

*3.6.4. Kinematic Analysis (*see ***Note 19****)*

1. Display and observe the motion of special lines or points (e.g., transepicondylar line or center of rotations or geometrical fitting ***[13,18]***), using *display options* in the software interface.
2. Compute instantaneous Euler angles in the chosen anatomical frame to obtain plotting of flexion-extension angle and abduction-adduction and internal-external rotation, using *kinematic tools* in the software interface.
3. Compute instantaneous helical axes/angles (displayed at the user-defined origin), using *kinematic tools* in the software interface.

3.7. Examples and Future Development

This method can be used to analyze any diarthrodial joint. It has been used to study the anatomy and the passive motion of normal cadaveric knees, to study the role of cruciate ligaments in human joints, or for purely kinematic analysis of the knee motion ***(15–17,19)***.

At present the procedure has been tested on "big" joints (knee, shoulder, hip) but can easily be adapted to smaller ones (e.g., elbow, ankle) using smaller pins and clamping devices.

The authors are also developing a new version of the methodology using the main navigation system used for computer-assisted intervention, in order to

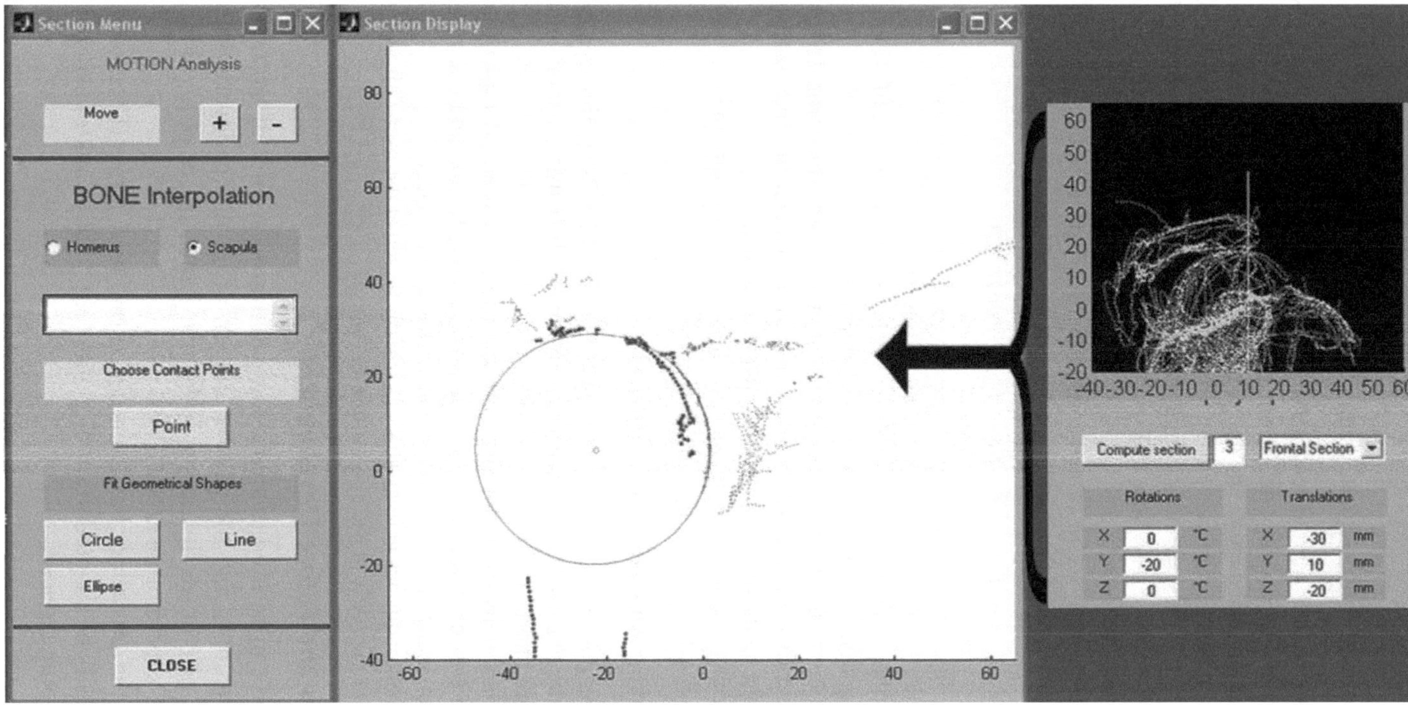

Fig. 7. Example of frontal section of the scapular (gray profile of acromion)-humeral (black profile) joint with the interpolation of the scapular cavity (circle).

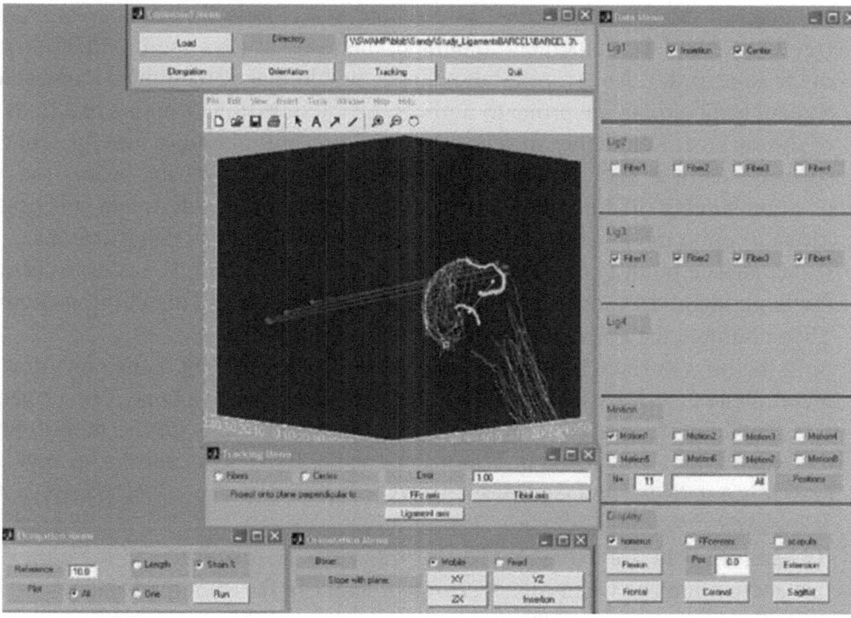

Fig. 8. Example of ligament tools to analyze the coracohumeral ligament and supraspinosus muscle fibers.

apply this method intraoperatively, in both navigated open surgery and arthroscopy.

Future development of new tools for commercial spatial linkages and optical digitizers is being investigated by the authors to reduce the method morbidity and allow diagnostic use and acquisition of active motion.

4. Notes

1. Under laboratory conditions, the method yields data with the following accuracy limits: the anatomical structures are reconstructed with 0.3-mm precision, the kinematic features are computed with 0.3- and 0.8°-precision, and all computations concerning the use of both geometrical and kinematic data are computed with less than 1 mm/1.5° accuracy. We have verified that a trained physician can acquire cadaveric data with 2-mm/degree uncertainty also on human joints, although the presence of soft tissues and ligaments can pose several difficulties ***(19)***.
2. The FaroArm must be distant enough from the joint to allow the use of the arm not completely extended and not near the vertical position. In addition, the choice of a position that allows the complete motion of the joint without constraint is critical for 6-degrees-of-freedom joints, such as the knee or hip. We therefore recommend using the FARO kinematic tools to fix it in the middle of the range of motion of its wrist; test the planned motion carefully.

3. Landmarks should be as spread as possible and closely form a regular triangle (*see* **Figs. 3** and **4**). Remember to number them and always acquire their position in the same order. An error in the sequence would make anatomical data useless.
4. Stream acquisitions are prone to outliers, i.e., acquisition of points and lines out of the surface. Remember to release the acquire-button before moving from the surface, scan the shot portion of the surface, stop, and set the probe in a new position staying off-line. Slow down the acquisition near edges and soft tissues. Move to point mode when the bone presents osteophytes or calcifications.
5. If the surface point is not reachable, move the joint (which is easier) to acquire the bone landmarks, or move the FaroArm to perform the matching procedure. Then continue the acquisition in the new configuration.
6. Split the huge surface file into smaller ones. Use significant names for files: we recommend *boneN* for bones (*N* consecutive indexes when a bone is described by several files), *lig_nameN_mb* for ligament insertion areas on the mobile bone, *lig_nameN_fix* for ligament insertion areas on the fixed bone, *muscle_nameN_mb*, *muscle_nameN_fix*, and significant shorts for motion, such as *PROMsurgeonA* or *IEwithACL*...
7. Be careful to choose the resolution for trajectory acquisition, and increase it for fast acquisitions or when the *electrogoniometer* is far from the joint center. For example, several-centimeter resolution can be suitable for sampling humerus flexion every 10°, when the Faro is fixed around half the human arm under examination.
8. If the motion of the joint is constrained by the FaroArm, move or reorient the base of the *electrogoniometer* to acquire the *FAROREFn* file as in the matching procedure, before and after the displacement. The experimental acquisition can continue normally.
9. If the FaroArm moves with respect to the fixed bone or mobile bone, the acquisition protocol is affected by a serious error. However, if you are able to reposition the *electrogoniometer* with respect to the joint, you can continue the acquisition with a few millimeters of additional error. Otherwise stop and start again.
10. If the mobile bone moves during the matching procedure, try to recover the position or restart the experiment.
11. If landmarks on the bones move, try to recover their position or restart the experiment.
12. Each rigid structure, such as the articulating surfaces, ligament attachment areas, or bundles, is a separate object for the elaboration software. The same anatomical structure is reconstructed as a single cloud of points (eventually filtering outliers) even if acquired in multiple positions, using an algorithm based on the single value decomposition ***(20,21)***, to compute the transformation between the different configurations of reference landmarks (referred to as SVDM).
13. The trajectories acquired by the FaroArm control software of the mobile segment (and relative anatomical structures) are transformed from three spatial coordinates plus three Euler angles into 4 × 4-rototranslation matrices in homogeneous coordinates.

14. If **step 5** of the experimental setup (**Subheading 3.2.**) is omitted, the reference frame for display and the definition of sagittal-frontal view must be adjusted by eye on the joint reconstruction interface.
15. The conventional coordinate system used for displaying the joint follows the clinical conventions on axes (*y*-axis in the anterior-posterior direction and *z* as the "vertical" proximal-distal axis; compare with ref. *8*) and normalizing nonorthogonal relationships. However, there is not a general agreement on the definition of the ideal coordinate system to describe either anatomy or kinematics, and often medical doctors have personal conventions and habits for joint examination. Therefore, the program allows the definition of an optional file containing the "adjustment" to the acquisition frame that meets the user's needs (for example, according to RSA conventions, a special alignment in the lateral view and in the frontal view, or setting the origin in a significant anatomical point). This information is stored as a rototranslation around the acquisition axes, called *frame* input file.
16. The positions of an anatomical structure during motion (S_i) is computed from motion and anatomical input data (S) according to the following formula:

$$\forall P \in S \quad P_i = M_i \times M_0^{-1} \times F_0 \times (P)$$
$$S_i = \{P_i\}_i$$

where: M_i is the *i*th location of the recorded motion;
M_0 is the location of the recorded trajectory used during the matching phase (usually the first, e.g., full extension during the passive range of motion);
F_0 is the SVDM transformation from the acquisition position of the examined anatomical structure into the matching position; and
S_i is the position of the mobile structure at the *i*th instant of the examined motion.
17. The circle and ellipse fitting needs an arc of > 50° to be reliable; smaller fittings show a trend, more than an accurate interpolation, and are sensitive to addition-subtraction of a few points. To verify the reliability of the fitting, try and change the point selection and look at the results on the same section and a few sections in the neighborhood. The result is within the method accuracy when the interpolation changes less than 1.5 mm/degee.
18. Up to four different ligaments or muscles can be defined together in the present version of the software. For each ligament, if insertion areas on fixed and mobile bones are present, the program computes the line between their centers; in addition, up to eight different fibers can be input for each ligament (recognized automatically by the software). All computations (distances and angles during the recorded motion) can be performed for one or more fibers, according to the user's specification
19. The availability of motion and anatomical data allows the computation of all the kinematic descriptions proposed in the literature, based on anatomical decompositions *(3,8,9)* or purely kinematic computations *(2,7)*. Although purely anatomical and kinematic elaborations are possible with our software, the most typical study consists of the computations described in **steps 3–10** of **Subheading 3.6.**

5. Glossary

Calibration An interactive procedure to determine the correct size and shape of FaroArm end-effectors, performed by using the sensor's software and setting the end-effector in particular positions.

Crosstalk Errors owing to the sum and the interaction of different causes that amplify each other.

Degree-of-freedom Any one of the number of ways in which a space configuration of a mechanical system may change.

Digitize To convert the position of a point in the space into three numbers describing the numerical value of its coordinates.

Digitizer probe An instrument used to digitize points and surfaces.

Diodes A semiconductor emitting infrared signals.

Electrogoniometer An instrument used for determining the position and the orientation of a point in the space, which consists of a series of electrical encoders to measure spatial and angular displacements.

End-effector A structure that is mounted at the end of the FaroArm to perform a specific task.

Least square interpolation A technique of fitting a curve close to some given points, which minimizes the sum of squares of the deviation of the given points from the curve.

Linkage A mechanism that converts motion into numbers by using some combinations of bar links, slide pivots, or rotating members.

Location Position and orientation of a tool in the space, expressed by six numbers.

Probe An instrument used to get numerical information about a specific event or structure.

Resolution The minimum distance that the sensor can measure reliably.

Sampling rate The rate at which the measurements of physical quantities are made.

Track (motion) To follow the movements of an object by monitoring its location at frequent intervals.

Acknowledgments

This work was partly funded by the Italian Ministry of Health Care. The authors gratefully acknowledge Carmelo Carcasio for the construction of the custom tools designed in this work and Mr. Giampaolo Bernagozzi and Maurizio Bonfiglioli for assistance in preparation of the manuscript.

References

1. Martelli, S., Marcacci, M., Nofrini, L., et al. (2002) Computer and robot assisted total knee replacement: analysis of a new surgical procedure. *Ann. Biomed. Eng.* **24,** 230–236.
2. Martelli, S., Zaffagnini, S., Falcioni, B., and Marcacci M. (2000) Intraoperative kinematic protocol for knee joint evaluation. *Comp. Methods Programs Biomed.* **62,** 77–86.
3. Chao, E. Y. S. (1980) Justification of triaxial goniometer for the measurement of joint rotation. *J. Biomech.* **13,** 989–1006.
4. Hefzy, M. S., Kelly, B. P., Cooke, T. D., al-Baddah, A. M., and Harrison, L. (1997) Knee kinematics in-vivo of kneeling in deep flexion examined by bi-planar radiographs. *Biomed. Sci. Instrum.* **33,** 453–458.
5. Huiskes, R., Kremers, J., de Lange, A., Woltring, H. J., Selvik, G., and van Rens, Th. J. G. (1985) Analytical stereophotogrammetric determination of three-dimensional knee-joint geometry. *J. Biomech.* **18,** 559–570.
6. Quinn, T. P. and Mote, C. D. (1990) A six degree-of-freedom acoustic transducer for rotation and translation measurements across the knee. *J. Biomech. Eng.* **112,** 371–378.
7. Blankevoort, L., Huiskes, L. R., and De Lange, A. (1990) Helical axes of passive knee joint motions. *J. Biomech.* **23,** 1219–1229.
8. Grood, E. S. and Suntay, W. J. (1983) A joint coordinate system for the clinical description of three-dimensional motions: application to the knee. *J. Biomech. Eng.* **105,** 136–144.
9. Pennock, G. R. and Clark, K. J. (1990) An anatomy-based coordinate system for the description of the kinematic displacements in the human knee. *J. Biomech.* **23,** 1209–1218.
10. Piazza, S. J. and Cavanagh, P. R. (2000) Measurement of the screw-home motion of the knee is sensitive to errors in axis alignment. *J. Biomech.* **33,** 1029–1034.
11. Ando, Y., Fukatsu, H., Ishigaki, T., Aoki, I., and Yamada, T. (1994) T. Analysis of knee movement with low-field MR equipment—a normal volunteer study. *Radiat. Med.* **12,** 153–160.
12. Niitsu, M., Akisada, M., Anno, I., and Miyakawa, S. (1990) Moving knee joint: technique for kinematic MR Imaging. *Radiology* **174,** 569–570.
13. Pinskerova, V., Iwaki, H., and Freeman, M. A. R. (2001) The shape and relative movements of the femur and tibia in the unloaded cadaveric knee: a study using MRI as an anatomical tool, in *Surgery of the Knee*, vol. 1, 3rd ed., (Insall, J.N. and Scott, W.N. eds.), WB Saunders, Philadelphia, pp. 255–283.
14. Hirokawa, S. (1993) Biomechanics of the knee joint: a critical review. *Crit. Rev. Biomed. Eng.* **21,** 79–135.
15. Martelli, S. and Pinskerova, V. (2002) The shapes of the tibial and femoral articular surfaces in relation to tibiofemoral movement. *J. Bone Joint Surg. Br.* **84,** 607–613.
16. Martelli, S. and Visani, A. (2002) Computer investigation into the anatomical location of the axes of rotation in the knee. *J. Mech. Med. Biol.* **2,** 433–447.

17. Martelli, S., Zaffagnini, S., Falcioni, B., and Motta M. (2002) Comparison of three kinematic analyses of the knee: determinatation of intrinsic features and applicability to intraoperative procedures. *Comput. Methods Biomech. Biomed. Engin.* **5,** 175–184.
18. Hollister, A. M., Jatana, S., Singh, A. K., Sullivan, W. W., and Lupichuck, A. G. (1993) The axes of rotation of the knee. *Clin. Orthop.* **290,** 259–268.
19. Martelli, S. (2003) New method for simultaneous anatomical and functional studies of articular joints and its application to the human knee. *Comput. Methods Programs Biomed.* **70,** 223–240.
20. Arun, S. K. and Clostein, S. D. (1987) Least-square fitting of two 3-D point sets. *IEEE Trans PAMI* **9,** 698–700.
21. Hanson, R. J. and Norris, M. J. (1981) Analysis of measurements based on the singular value decomposition. *SIAM J. Sci. Stat. Comput.* **2,** 363–373.

Index

MIX
Papier aus verantwortungsvollen Quellen
Paper from responsible sources
FSC® C105338

If you have any concerns about our products,
you can contact us on
ProductSafety@springernature.com

In case Publisher is established outside the EU,
the EU authorized representative is:
Springer Nature Customer Service Center GmbH
Europaplatz 3, 69115 Heidelberg, Germany

Printed by Libri Plureos GmbH
in Hamburg, Germany